AF443269

WISECARE

Studies in Health Technology and Informatics

Editors

Jens Pihlkjaer Christensen, European Commission, Luxembourg; Arie Hasman, EFMI and
University of Maastricht; Ilias Iakovidis, European Commission, Brussels; Zoi Kolitsi, University of Patras;
Olivier Le Dour, European Commission DG Research, Brussels; Antonio Pedotti, Politecnico di Milan;
Otto Rienhoff, Georg-August-Universität Göttingen; Francis H. Roger France, Centre for Medical Informatics,
UCL, Brussels; Niels Rossing, National University Hospital, Copenhagen;
Faina Shtern, National Institutes of Health, Bethesda, MD

Volume 73

Previously published in this series

ISSN: 0926-9630

WISECARE

Workflow Information Systems for European Nursing Care

Edited by

Walter Sermeus

*Faculteit Geneeskunde, Katholieke Universiteit Leuven,
Leuven, Belgium*

Nora Kearney

*Nursing and Midwifery School, University of Glasgow,
Glasgow, UK*

Juha Kinnunen

*Department for Health Policy and Management, University of Kuopio,
Kuopio, Finland*

Lieve Goossens

*Faculteit Geneeskunde, Katholieke Universiteit Leuven,
Leuven, Belgium*

and

Morven Miller

*Nursing and Midwifery School, University of Glasgow,
Glasgow, UK*

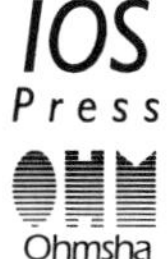

IOS
Press

Ohmsha

Amsterdam • Berlin • Oxford • Tokyo • Washington, DC

ISBN 1 58603 048 5 (IOS Press)
ISBN 4 274 90399 0 C3047 (Ohmsha)
Library of Congress Catalog Card Number: 00-107166

Publisher
IOS Press
Nieuwe Hemweg 6B
1013 BG Amsterdam
The Netherlands
fax: +31 20 620 3419
e-mail: order@iospress.nl

Distributor in the UK and Ireland
IOS Press/Lavis Marketing
73 Lime Walk
Headington
Oxford OX3 7AD
England
fax: +44 1865 75 0079

Distributor in the USA and Canada
IOS Press, Inc.
5795-G Burke Centre Parkway
Burke, VA 22015
USA
fax: +1 703 323 3668
e-mail: iosbooks@iospress.com

Distributor in Germany
IOS Press
Spandauer Strasse 2
D-10178 Berlin
Germany
fax: +49 30 242 3113

Distributor in Japan
Ohmsha, Ltd.
3-1 Kanda Nishiki-cho
Chiyoda-ku, Tokyo 101
Japan
fax: +81 3 3233 2426

LEGAL NOTICE
The publisher is not responsible for the use which might be made of the following information.

PRINTED IN THE NETHERLANDS

v

Preface

Christine HANCOCK, General Secretary, Royal College of Nursing (UK)
President, Standing Committee of Nurses of the European Union (PCN)

Nurses are natural collaborators. As a profession we work in teams and develop skills of communication and adaptability. Every day we meet people from different backgrounds and disciplines. We are good listeners and negotiators. These are the nursing strengths, which the WISECARE project harnessed in an initiative with implications for cancer nursing practice, and also, more widely, for how nursing and other types of research are undertaken in Europe.

Willingness to collaborate is born out of nurses' recognition that sharing good practice, experience and research is an imperative for achieving high quality patient care. Nurses are, first and foremost; interested in what will benefit the people for whom they are responsible. They want to base their practice on the best evidence available. The great appeal of this project is the involvement of clinically based nurses from the start. The nurses who provided the hands-on care were also responsible for collecting the data. The research was generated and owned by the same practitioners who then went on to implement the findings. This approach transcends the barriers, which continue to exist between research and practice. The level of patient involvement is also to be commended, with patients experiencing improvements to their own care derived from a research project in which they were participating.

This sense of intimacy and immediacy linking nurse, patient, research and outcomes was greatly assisted in this project by the use of new technology. By using a mini-electronic patient record to monitor a patient's symptoms, nurses could collect data by a patient's side, share 'instant feedback' to evaluate the impact of aspects of nursing care and access the experience of colleagues and patients involved in the project in other countries.

The use of new technology also leads to speedier and more convenient communication, which is of particular value for international research projects. As nurses are discovering across the world, the use of e-mail offers enormous potential for the creation of nursing networks. Those involved in the WISECARE project found the flexibility of e-mail provided a supportive link to allow problems to be shared and solutions found.

The potential of new technology and nurses' appetite for collaboration and evidence-based practice bode well for the future of nursing research in Europe. The approach adopted by WISECARE is eminently transferable to other fields and disciplines. Joining forces with colleagues in different countries makes sense financially; a consideration particularly pertinent for nursing research with its chronic underfunding. Collaboration is also efficient, with different partners bringing complementary expertise and resources to a project, creating synergy and avoiding duplication.

For nursing, pan-European projects are set to become increasingly important, clinically, professionally and politically. A project like WISECARE, which encourages European nurses to compare their practice with other clinical sites, could eventually lead to the creation of benchmarks, international guidelines and protocols. The European Oncology Nursing Society (EONS), the organisation which pioneered WISECARE, is also active on professional issues, working with the Standing Committee of Nurses of the European Union (PCN) to create a framework for specialist nurse education across Europe. The political dimension of collaborative working is most powerful when it addresses the challenge all nurses face in defining and conveying the value of nursing care. This issue takes on a greater significance in an expanding Europe where interpretations of what we mean by nursing are becoming more and more varied.

I congratulate all the partners involved in WISECARE on a project with tangible benefits for patients and which contributes to our shared desire to make the nursing voice heard in Europe, loud and clear. Collaboration is not a straightforward option; much hard work lies behind the successful completion of this project and the securing of the European Commission funding which made it possible in the first place. I believe WISECARE will inspire many more nurses, both as individuals and groups, to look for opportunities to work and network with colleagues across Europe.

Acknowledgements

It is our pleasure to acknowledge everyone who has been involved in the process of WISECARE.

We thank the European Commission for funding the WISECARE project in the 4th Telematics for Health Care Programme We want to thank Mr. J. Lacombe and Mrs. M. Fitzgerald, EU-project officers for their support. We are indebted to EONS for their unique contribution to the project from the start. The development of a unique oncology nursing network connected through internet will be of great value for the future.

Thanks to the management and board of participating hospitals for their support of this project. Thanks also go to all the nurses from both the Validation and Demonstration Sites who participated in the project. We want to thank all the patients who gave their time and effort complete the questionnaires.

Special recognition goes to the peer reviewers Prof. H. Hansen, Prof. E. Halloran and Prof. J. Sansoni, for their comments and suggestions which have contributed to the success of the WISECARE project.

Contents

Part I

Introduction

WISECARE: an Overview

Walter Sermeus, Lieve Goossens, Kris Vanhaecht

1 Setting the WISECARE Scene

Throughout Europe, costs for nursing services take up 40-60% of the health care budget, but the impact that nursing has on the quality of care for Europe's citizens is not evaluated. Given the changes in health care financing that are taking place across Europe it is imperative that hospitals focus their cost-containment efforts in this area. Furthermore, it is essential that the relationship between costs of nursing and outcomes of care be established. One could argue that the vast amounts of data generated by nursing staff should be used constructively for the development and evaluation and improvement of nursing protocols and guidelines. However, the vast majority of data stored in patient records are only used for individual and operational communication between individual caregivers, hospitals and community care [1].

It is within this European situation that the Workflow Information Systems for European Nursing Care (WISECARE) Project has been conceived. WISECARE turns actual clinical care information into data which can be used for the development and evaluation of protocols and guidelines. Through dissemination and sharing of information, the WISECARE project aims to provide international guidelines and protocols and the facility to compare actual practice with benchmarks. While the focus of the project is nursing care, concentrating on oncological care has allowed a wide range of clinical settings and nursing care to be incorporated.

Using clinical problems as the vehicle for the project, WISECARE aims to quantify and make visible factors vital to patient care and nursing practice. These include the diversity of patient populations, the variability of patient care across Europe, patient outcomes and nursing resources. Using this information and pooling the experiences of cancer nurses across Europe will lead to the development of a knowledge base of best practice and facilitate a move away from individual knowledge to knowledge sharing and ultimately improved patient care [1] [2].

State-of-the-art information technology (IT) systems allow these nurses to communicate and compare their current practices and patient outcomes in a way that has not hitherto been accessed by clinically based nurses on a pan-European basis. Communicating in this way has the potential to markedly alter the way that knowledge is transferred and nursing practice is developed. Traditional education strategies and transfer of knowledge will be superseded by inductive experience-based knowledge development, driven by clinical practice and patient requirements. Additionally WISECARE aims to meet the needs of nursing management in Europe, addressing issues such as nursing workload and nurse staffing to ensure better quality care.

The project is designed in workpackages according to the EU-proposal framework. Overall co-ordinator of the project is the Centre of Health Services Research & Nursing, Katholieke Universiteit Leuven, Belgium. The Centre is doing research in health care management since 1962. Since 1985, they are involved in a national endeavour to develop, test, implement and exploit minimum data sets, including a nursing minimum data set for Belgian general hospitals. The daily co-ordination of project (WP1) is subcontracted to Arthur Andersen. The European co-ordination of the health care practice is based in Brussels. They had long tradition in performance measurement, process alignment, change management and management information systems.

The co-ordination of the usergroup (WP2) has been done by European Oncology Nursing Society (EONS). The Society was established in 1984 and aims to promote and develop cancer nursing throughout Europe through the advancement of education of nurses engaged in caring for individuals with cancer and their families. For reaching that goal, they co-operate very closely with the University of Edinburgh and the University of Glasgow, UK.

The data collection tools and datawarehouse (WP3) are developed and maintained by the Department of Nursing and Community Health at Glasgow Caledonian University (GCU), Scotland. The Management Executive of National Health Service in Scotland (NHSiS) is supporting this effort.

The data analysis (WP4) is done by the Centre of Health Services Research & Nursing, Katholieke Universiteit Leuven (KUL), Belgium. The practical modelling of the feedback tools is subcontracted to An Teallach (AT), Scotland, a small to medium-sized Enterprise (SME) which is specialised to describe and animate business processes for health care management.

Technology assessment (WP5) was undertaken by HISCOM, the Netherlands. HISCOM, formerly BAZIS supports health care institutions in implementing Hospital Information Systems (HIS). HISCOM developed one of the first operational integrated nursing information system called VISION. In the WISECARE project, it is supported in this quality review process by the Department of Health Policy and Management, University of Kuopio (Finland). This department performs research on the quality of health services, outcome measures, innovation, productivity, efficiency and effectiveness of health care organisations and evaluation research.

The final workpackage (WP6) concentrates on networking through developing and maintaining the WISECARE webserver (http://WISECARE.dn.uoa.gr). The work has been undertaken by the Laboratory of Health Informatics of the University of Athens (Greece), which is widely recognised in the field of Health Care Informatics.

Research must be brought closer to the practice of nursing and so consequently nearer to the practitioners in nursing [2]. In an attempt to achieve this and to ensure that the nurses involved in WISECARE have a sense of ownership of the research, clinically based nurses in five European cancer centres, Scotland, Finland, Sweden, Belgium and The Netherlands are involved in validation efforts. In September 1997, five settings across Europe agreed to participate as Validation Sites to the project:

- Academic Hospital Groningen, the Netherlands
- Beatson Oncology Centre, Scotland, UK
- Helsinki University Central Hospital, Finland
- Huddinge University Hospital, Sweden
- University Hospitals Leuven, Belgium

These sites had the advantage of participating in the identification of clinical focus and priorities and in specifying data collection and feedback.

In September 1999, another six settings across Europe agreed to participate as Demonstration Sites. These were:

- Aalborg Hospital, Aalborg, Denmark
- Institut Gustave-Roussy, Paris, France

- Institut Jules Bordet, Brussels, Belgium
- Royal Marsden NHS Trust, London, UK
- Red Cross Hospital, Athens, Greece
- University Medical Centre, Ljubljana, Slovenia.

2   Design of the Project

2.1 Objectives

The original objectives, as formulated in the WISECARE proposal [3] were:
- To create a workflow information model to systematically exploit clinical nursing data, stored in electronic patient records, for clinical and resource management. The diversity of the patient population, the variability of care, patient outcomes and nursing resources will be quantified using existing patient classification and coding systems. This information will be made visible using state-of-the-art data presentation techniques. Relations and links between the data will be analysed in a multivariate way, using state-of-the art statistical and analysing tools.
- To establish a network of oncological care centres by using network software (WWW, Workplace servers) in which the clinical practice information will be shared. This will lead to state-of-the art knowledge dissemination and sharing through the network partners.
- The impact of the availability of information on the diversity of the patient population, the variability of care, patient outcomes and nursing resources that have been used and the links between these components, will be evaluated.
- The WISECARE project seeks to provide a workflow model to monitor nursing activities in relation to the clinical care process, measure the outcomes and the costs of services to patients. The WISECARE project wanted to use the existing clinical nursing care data for evaluation and development of guidelines and protocols. The WISECARE project aimed to disseminate and share the state-of-the-art international guidelines and protocols and to provide tools in comparing the actual practice with the benchmarks. The WISECARE project focuses on oncological care as a domain of demonstration, as oncological care covers by its nature a variety of nursing care in a diversity of clinical settings.

Based on these objectives, the focus was to create tools to support the complete 'WISECARE Data Cycle': data collection (Figure 1), processing for the data warehouse, feedback and communication of the developing knowledge base for the user defined patient groups. The WISETOOL helps to collect clinical data across the Validation Sites. Within the WiseTool local feedback is generated. At the same time, the data are transferred to the WiseHoos data warehouse, as input for further analysis and generating global feedback. See also Chapter 3 (Impact of WISECARE on Clinical Behaviour of Oncology Nurses).

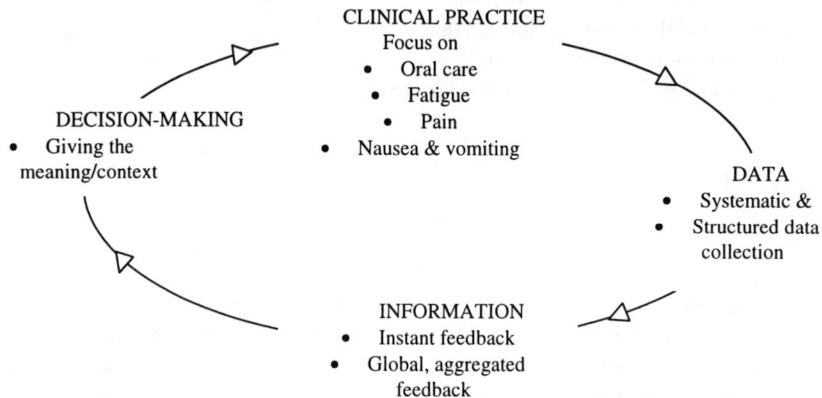

Figure 1   The Workflow Framework of the WISECARE Project

2.2 Observations

Six patient groups (lung cancer, osteosarcoma, Non-Hodgkin's lymphoma, breast cancer, acute lymphoblastic leukaemia and acute myeloid leukaemia) were included in the project. Every patient admitted for chemotherapy or surgery is eligible. In total, 282 patients were included in the sample. For these patients, a total of 590 treatment episodes were recorded.

2.3 Data and Sampling Design

Three types of data were recorded during the project. All three have a different set of variables and require a different sampling design. The first type of data was related to clinical management. The second type of data was related to resource management. The third type of data was related to technology assessment.

2.3.1 Data for Clinical Management

In the WISECARE-project, the choice was to use instruments and measures that are imbedded in clinical oncological practice. Because of a lack of clinical relevancy and specificity, no general classification schemes for nursing care (e.g. NANDA, NIC, NOC, ICNP) were chosen.

Building on the work of Donabedian, four broad categories to measure patient outcomes are identified and thus determine what data is relevant for quality improvement: clinical end points, functional status, general well being and satisfaction with care. Based on these broad categories, the user group determined 4 priority domains in which nursing care could have impact: oral care, fatigue, pain and nausea and vomiting [3].

Standardised clinical scales have been used for data collection: the Oral Assessment Guide (OAG) for assessing mouth problems, Piper Fatigue Scale (PFS) for assessing fatigue problems and EORTC-QLQ-C30 (Quality of Life scale) for assessing quality of life.

Four periods can be identified in data collection. The first period of data collection takes from April 1998 until December 1998. Five Validation Sites (7 nursing units) started to collect data. On the date of admission for the first chemotherapy administration, the patient filled in 2 questionnaires: Piper Fatigue Scale (PFS) and the EORTC Quality of Life Questionnaire (EORTC-QLQ-C30). The nurse performed an oral assessment using the Oral Assessment Guide (OAG). This oral assessment was repeated daily during hospital stay. The Piper Fatigue Scale and the EORTC-QLQ-C30 was filled in every week on the same day as the day of admission. When the patient was discharged, they were asked to fill the PFS and EORTC-QLQ-C30 every week. At the final treatment, they were asked to fill in both questionnaires after 1, 2 and 3 months after discharge. In December 1998, after the first feedback, the variables, the instruments as well as the sampling design were adjusted. Based on the experiences of the Validation Sites with the data collection procedure and the first feedback, the PFS-measurement was stopped. Based on the same experiences and feedback, filling in the complete EORTC-QLQ-C30 didn't seem to be meaningful. Many aspects of quality of life don't change so frequently as foreseen in the data collection design, leading to a high non-response. Moreover, it became very clear that data were not comparable because of organisational confounds. Some nursing units were run as a one-day clinic. Some were run as a clinical unit in which patients stay for many days. It is quite obvious that the collecting data at the day of discharge had a complete other meaning for unit A than for unit B.

The second period of data collection takes from January 1, 1999 until April 15, 1999. In December 1998, the data collection design was discussed in the consortium meeting. A change in data collection was announced, but was not made very concretely. This data collection period is more fuzzy and probably less reliable.

The third period of data collection takes from April 16, 1999 until September 30, 1999. The complete EORTC-QLQ-C30 is replaced by focusing on 3 most relevant subscales (7 questions): pain, nausea and vomiting and fatigue. No change was made in oral assessment, done by patients rather than nursing staff. The concept of clinical time was introduced. Clinical time is the time between the clinical event and the day of recording. A clinical event is defined as an event which has a significant impact on the course of disease, treatment or functional status e.g. administrating chemotherapy or surgery. Clinical time became an extra variable in the data collection. The data collection design was organised according to the clinical time. For ten days after the clinical event (chemotherapy, surgery), all data (OAG, 3 subscales of EORTC-QLQ-C30) are recorded, regardless of length of stay in the hospital. It had the consequence that the nurse had to teach the patient how to evaluate the four symptoms at home. This had consequences for the design of the data collection form which had to be patient-friendly. It had an impact on the data input in that this had to be done when the patient returned to the hospital for the next treatment. The data collection took place in the 5 Validation Sites.

The fourth period of data collection took from October 1 until December 31, 1999. The same data collection design as in period 3 was used. The data collection was extended to include the new Demonstration Sites involving 11 Clinical Sites (15 nursing units) in 10 countries.

2.3.2 *Data for Nursing Resource Management*

For resource management, data on patients as well as on nursing staff are recorded. The data collection is cross-sectional, meaning that on a given day, data on all nurses and patients (also patients that are not included as WISECARE patients) are recorded. The major aim is to calculate a "nursing-hours-per-patient-day" measure as a variable to assess resource use in the various Clinical Sites and nursing units. Data collected:
- Personnel data: the number of nurses, the number of hours they actually worked, their qualification level

- Patient data: the number of patients in the nursing unit at the particular day, the hours stayed in the nursing ward, the Moffitt score for indicating the nursing intensity class.

Data collection started in July 1999. In each week a random day was assigned by the project team in which resource data should be collected.

2.3.3   Data for Technology Assessment

To evaluate the effect of the WISECARE-approach on nursing care delivery, a questionnaire has been developed. The questionnaire, called WiseCompass, has 59 questions concerning the impact of the WISECARE project on clinical oncological nursing practice, on patient outcomes, use of different project products and general management of the hospital/department/ward. The instrument was built using the EFQM model of quality assessment and was previously tested and developed by Rank Xerox.

Questionnaires were given to the Validation Sites to evaluate the impact of WISECARE. This was done in March 1999, before the first WISECARE feedback was generated. The second data collection was done in May 1999 and a third one in September 1999. Each Validation Site was asked for 5 responses in each data collection. Out of these five, three nurses should be wise-nurses, which means that they were actively participating in the WISECARE project in data collection or utilisation of the feedback. Two of them should be non-wise nurses, i.e. nurses who had not been directly involved in the project but were working on one of the nursing units. Altogether 66 questionnaires were returned. [4]

3   Evaluation

3.1   Impact on Clinical Management

During 18 months, more than 13000 patient assessments have made for 280 patients and 590 treatment cycles. The local feedback graphs are used to discuss symptom control with patients, nurses and physicians. Two global feedback reports were generated, a first report in December 1998, a second one in September 1999.

Figure 2 shows the main results. It reveals a decrease in the average fatigue score of 44% in the beginning of the project (04/98-12/98) to 33% in period 3 (04/98–09/99), a decrease in the average nausea & vomiting score from 11,8% to 5,6%, a decrease in the average pain score from 23% to 19% and a decrease in oral problems (OAG) from 22,3% to 18,5%.

3.2   Impact on Clinical Behaviour of Oncology Nurses

Nearly one third of the nurses (28 %, n = 32) indicated that WISECARE had improved the nursing assessment in their units. The experienced improvement in nursing assessment due to the WISECARE project related modestly positively (Kendall's tau_b correlation coefficient varying from .54 to .60, p = .01, n = 32) to the use of WISECARE products (i.e. the WiseTool, WiseWeb and WiseMailingList). About one fifth of the nurses (19 %, n = 32) stated that the use of WiseWeb had had a positive impact on the nursing assessment in their units; all of them were WiseNurses. Altogether 16 % of the respondents (n = 32) evaluated that the WISECARE-patients' needs were assessed better than those of the other patients.

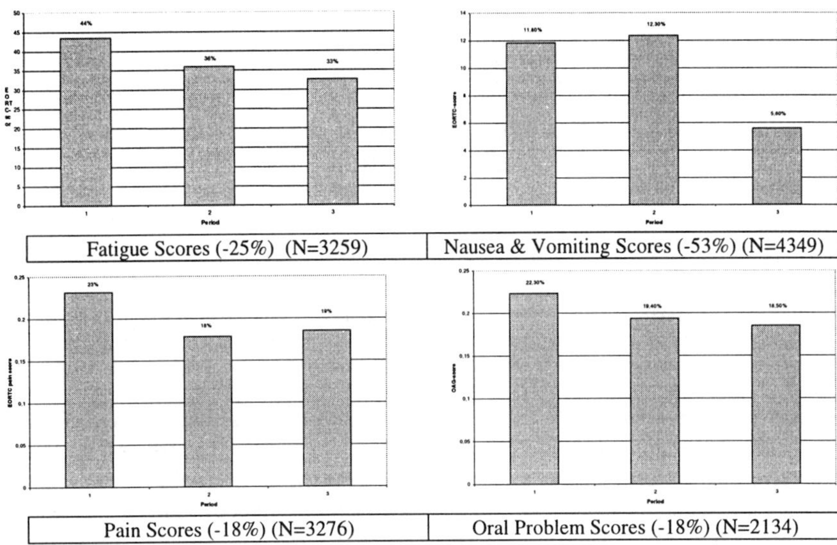

| Fatigue Scores (-25%) (N=3259) | Nausea & Vomiting Scores (-53%) (N=4349) |
| Pain Scores (-18%) (N=3276) | Oral Problem Scores (-18%) (N=2134) |

Figure 2   Evolution in Symptom Management from Beginning of Project Period 1 (04/98-12/98) to period 3 (04/98–09/99) for all Validation Sites (N=total number of patient assessments)

About one fifth of the nurses (19 %, n = 64) indicated that the WISECARE project had improved the planning of nursing care, i.e. the setting of nursing objectives for the care and deciding the interventions. There was a statistically significant difference in this matter between the WiseNurses and non-WiseNurses (Pearson chi-square value 8.150, df = 1, asymp. sig. (2-sided) .004; n = 64).

Table 1   Correlations between the experienced improvement in planning the nursing care and the WiseFeedback, team building and use of research results (n = 64)

	Planning nursing care
WiseFeedback	.732**
Team building (e.g. multi-professional teams, QI-teams)	.729**
Use of research results	.651**
Kendall's tau$_b$, ** p = .01 (2-tailed)	

As can be seen in Table 1 the experienced improvement in planning the nursing care due to the WISECARE project related positively to the WiseFeedback, team building initiatives and the increased use of research. These correlations were statistically significant (p = .01).

The WISECARE project has enhanced the use of research results as criteria for clinical judgement among one third of the respondents either a bit (25 %) or a lot (6 %). The difference between WiseNurses and Non-WiseNurses is significant (Pearson chi-square value 7.342, df = 1, p < .01, n = 64).

Nearly half of the nurses (42 %, n = 64) indicated that the WISECARE project had encouraged discussions about the best nursing practices in their units. There was a statistically significant difference in this matter between the WiseNurses and non-WiseNurses (Figure 3). Two thirds of the WiseNurses (66 %, n = 64) considered that the project had promoted discussions about the best nursing practices. WiseNurses from all Sites reported this positive impact.

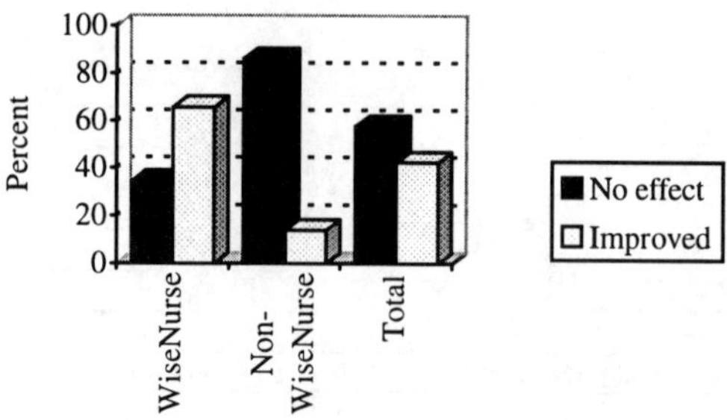

Figure 3   Difference between the WiseNurses and non-WiseNurses evaluating the experienced impact of the WISECARE project on encouraging discussions about the best nursing practices (Pearson chi-square value 17.530, df = 1, asymp. sig. (2-sided) .000; n = 64)

One quarter of the respondents (25 %, n = 64) indicated also that the WISECARE project had a positive impact on patient education. This improvement in patient education showed positive correlation with the improvement in written nursing procedures and the impact of the information concerning nursing interventions included in the WiseTool (Kendall's tau_b correlation coefficient varying from .66 to .69, p = .01, n = 64).

During the verification and validation phases of the project the different Validation Sites shared their written nursing procedures related to oral care, alleviation of fatigue, nausea and vomiting, and pain, which initiated a comparison between the Sites. A quarter of the respondents (27 %, n = 64) stated that they had improved their written nursing procedures during the project. Nearly half of the WiseNurses (49 %, n = 35) indicated that they had slightly altered the nursing interventions in their units due to the information obtained from the WiseTool. The same applied to the experienced development in nursing interventions due to the information nurses had obtained through the WiseWeb.

To the question whether the information obtained from the WiseFeedback had altered the nursing interventions, one fifth of the nurses (21 %, n = 64) answered positively.

About one fifth of the nurses (22 %, n = 64) stated that they changed their way of evaluating patient's progress during the WISECARE project so that it was now done better (11 %). There was no statistically significant difference between the WiseNurses and non-WiseNurses in this matter (Pearson chi-square value 1.012, df = 1, asym. sig. (2-sided) .31; n = 64).

Oral health as an indicator and its measurement tool had been part of the project since the beginning of the data collection in summer 1998. According to the respondents (42 %, n = 64) the project has been most successful during the verification and validation phases in promoting the patients' *oral health*. More than half of the WiseNurses (57 %, n= 35) and nearly a quarter of the non-WiseNurses (24 %, n = 29) were of this opinion. The difference between the two groups was statistically significant (Pearson chi-square value 7.083, df = 1, asym. sig. (2-sided) .008; n = 64).

The experienced impact on patients' oral health correlated positively with the experienced additional value of the WISECARE project on nursing practice (Kendall's tau_b correlation coefficient .66, p = .01, n = 64) and the use of structured language (Kendall's tau_b correlation coefficient .64, p = .01, n = 64).

Eleven percent of the nurses (11 %, n = 64) indicated that the project had had a positive impact on patients' fatigue and pain alleviation during the verification and validation period. Just three percent (3 %, n = 64) of the respondents indicated that about nausea and vomiting.

One fourth of the nurses (n = 64) indicated that they had been able to use the instant (WiseTool) and global feedback (WiseFeedback) as an evidence base in their work. There was a statistically significant difference in this matter between the WiseNurses and non-WiseNurses. See also .Chapter 3, Impact of WISECARE on Clinical Behaviour of Oncology Nurses.

4　Results and Achievements

Evaluating the impact of the WISECARE project on nursing care, it is clear that the opportunity to discuss and compare nursing interventions and consequently patient outcomes using the latest IT facilities on a pan-European basis has been an entirely novel concept for nurses. First the availability of computers and nurses' skills in their use was less than had been anticipated during the planning phase of the project. It took some time to supply each Validation Site with a computer, not to mention the Internet connection. In some Sites training was arranged for the nurses using electronic mail, World Wide Web and browsers, and the WiseTool. Secondly, the use and comparison of aggregated information and peer reviewing has meant a major change in professional culture. WISECARE has required a new way of thinking and developing nursing in the spirit of evidence-based nursing with a close connection to everyday nursing reality. Use of research findings or utilisation of feedback, which is received from outside one's own organisation, is not common in nursing care.

The added value of the WISECARE project is not in the software but in the knowledge network. Davenport & Prusack [4]. define knowledge as "a fluid mix of framed experience, values, contextual information and expert insight that provides a framework for evaluating and incorporating new experiences and information". The definition makes clear that knowledge is not neat or simple. It exists within people. If information has to become knowledge, humans must do virtually all the work.

The transformation happens through such C-words as:

- Comparison: how does information about this situation compare to other situations that we have known? Benchmarking activities can support this transformation process.
- Consequences: what implications does the information have for decisions and actions? The focus on outcomes and a systematic evaluation and review of effects and outcomes is supportive
- Context: how does this bit of knowledge relate to others?
- Conversation: what do other people think? Networking is the way to tackle this issue. Knowledge is widely generated within the project.

4.1　Standardised Scales for Measuring Clinical Outcomes

A first element in generating knowledge is done by providing standardised scales for measuring clinical outcomes that are useful for guiding clinical practice. They are useful to guide the communication among nurses, from nurse to doctor, from nurse to patient and vice versa. As for all scales, psychometric criteria such as reliability, validity, sensitivity are involved. Because of their use in daily practice, the scales should be not too time-consuming and be usable by nurses as well as by patients or their relatives. Within the WISECARE-project, following tools are selected and evaluated:

- The Oral Assessment Guide (OAG) [5], which is a concise, clinically useful tool comprising of 8 questions, developed through clinical expertise and literature review, to record and communicate oral cavity status and determine changes expected with stomatotoxic treatments. A clinical guide with photographic material was provided by

Glaxo Welcome as learning material for teaching patients or their relatives how to evaluate the mouth status in a valid and reliable way.

- The Piper Fatigue Scale (PFS) [6] which is composed of 22 numerically-scaled items (0-10) which measure 4 dimensions of subjective fatigue, behavioural/severity, affective/meaning, sensory and cognitive/mood. Both subscales and total fatigue scores can be calculated. The Piper Fatigue Scale was not retained in the third period of the project. Although very useful in a research environment, it was evaluated as too time-consuming for patients in a real life clinical environment.

- The European Organisation for Research and Treatment of Cancer Quality of Life Questionnaire (EORTC QLQ-C30) [7] which is a modular approach for evaluating quality of life. It incorporates 9 multi-item scales: 5 functional scales (physical, role, cognitive, emotional and social), 3 symptom scales (fatigue, pain, nausea and vomiting) and a global health and quality of life scale. Several single-item symptom measures are also included. From period 3 of the project, only the 3 symptom scales were retained for further evaluation.

The added value of WISECARE in using standardised scales:

- Although many scales are evaluated on their psychometric properties in literature, most of these evaluations are done in controlled research environments. The added value of WISECARE is on the evaluation of these standardised scales in real life environments.

- Most of the standardised scales are aggregated in a simple Likert-type way of adding up all item scores. The added value of WISECARE is in the more sensitive aggregation of the different item scores to improve the psychometric properties of the scale (e.g. sensitivity, validity, and reliability). In WISECARE, the Oral Assessment Guide has been processed as an example.

4.2 Risk Assessment Scales

A second element in generating knowledge has been developed in the evaluation of the toxicity level of chemotherapy according to some specific side effects as pain, fatigue, nausea and vomiting and mucositis. For measuring this level of toxicity, the Leuven Chemotherapy Risk Assessment Scale (LCRAS) has been developed. The scale shows the risk that 36 chemotherapy products can have on 47 side effects. It was developed in 1994 by an interdisciplinary group of Belgian nurses, pharmacists and doctors, in close co-operation with Glaxo Wellcome and the Flemish Oncology and Radiotherapy Society. It was part of the Nurses Cytostatic Compendium, Practical Guide For Nurses [8]. For 36 chemotherapy products, it provides information about the product, incompatibilities, skin contamination, eye contamination, spilling, extravasation, excretion and frequent side effects. The compendium was used as input for adjusting risk in WISECARE. The four risk levels were recoded in a score from 1 to 4 (from no/unknown risk to high risk). The risk on the WISECARE fatigue indicator was derived from two side effects mentioned in the compendium: fatigue and bone marrow depression. In WISECARE, the different treatment profiles are evaluated on their effect on fatigue, pain, nausea & vomiting, mouth problems. See also Chapter 2, Risk Assessment. The added value of WISECARE is:

- Sensitivity and specificity in evaluating the LCRAS in predicting the impact of the chemotherapy product on fatigue pain nausea & vomiting, mouth problems.

- Providing a standardised patient monitoring design per indicator. In the project, the data collection design has been standardised for 10 days after a clinical event. From the results, it becomes obvious that for some indicators, this period is much too long (e.g. nausea and vomiting). For other indicators such as fatigue and mucositis, it is much too short. Not only, recommendations can be made on the length of patient monitoring for side effects but also on the optimal frequency of data collection e.g. daily, every other day. This standard way of patient monitoring and data recording will enhance the comparability of data among different Clinical Sites and will enhance the knowledge on the course of side effects of chemotherapy. These data can be used to evaluate treatments on their impact on the course of chemotherapy.

- Providing benchmarking scores on fatigue pain, nausea & vomiting, mouth problems according to risk category of chemotherapy product and per day after chemotherapy. Although, the scores are adjusted by the LCRAS (on toxicity level of chemotherapy) and clinical time (days after chemotherapy), there is still a high variability between centres. The scores can be used to evaluate their clinical performance in the management of side effects of chemotherapy. See also Chapter 3: Global Feedback on Clinical Management.

Besides the LCRAS, the nurses' team in the University Hospital Groningen has developed a Groningen Breast Cancer Risk Assessment Scale (GBRAS). A Delphi-echnique has been used to assign risk scores to the various surgical procedures.

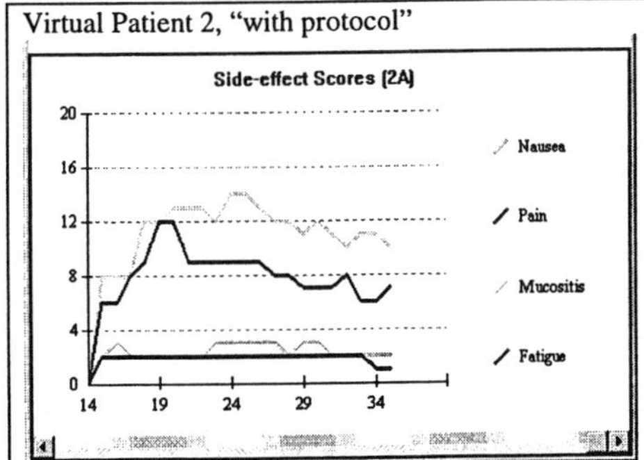

The chart shows the side effect profile from the day of the patient's first chemotherapy (day 14 of the simulation).
The virtual patient exhibits low levels of nausea (3) and pain (2). Over the next 20 days, these remain at about the same levels, with pain finally decreasing to level 1.
The patient's mucositis score rises to 12 within 5 days of chemotherapy, peaking at 14 and then gradually falling, but only to 9 or 10.
The patient also experience high levels of fatigue, rising to 12, and remaining at 6 or higher

Figure 4   : "With-protocol" Model for Virtual Patient 2

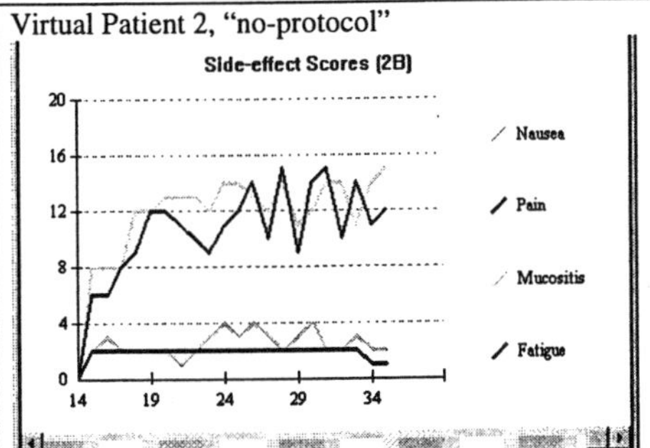

These are the simulated charts for the same virtual patient with a "no-protocol" model.
Again side effects of mucositis and fatigue dominate.
There appears to be an interesting oscillatory effect on fatigue. This arises from the nature of the simulation using a daily event interval, and thus showing a daily average.

Figure 5   : "No-protocol" Model for the same Virtual Patient 2

4.3 Development of Patient Models

A third element in generating knowledge is in enhancing the level of understanding of the relations between problems, interventions and outcomes, by developing patient models. The developed model is coded in a simulation language EpiScript. The language executes according to a discrete event mechanism. In this study, it was set to be day by day. Based upon WISEdata, the model generates virtual patients that will undergo chemotherapy. As an example, the side effect profiles of a virtual patient who has their first chemotherapy on day 14 of the simulation. Figure 4 simulates "with-protocol" model whereas Figure 5 simulates the "no-protocol" model.

See also Chapter 3, Modelling and Simulation of patients undergoing Chemotherapy.

4.4 Feedback

A fourth element in generating knowledge is feedback. Two types of feedback are generated. The first type of feedback is instant feedback, in which the feedback loop is very short. The recorded data are plotted in a graph (Figure 6). The 'instant feedback' facilitates the demonstration of the impact of nursing interventions on individual patient outcomes, going some way to prove the tangible difference that nursing interventions confer to patient outcomes. It allows nursing staff to:

- identify when a symptom is becoming problematic for patients
- implement nursing interventions accordingly
- Systematically evaluate their impact.

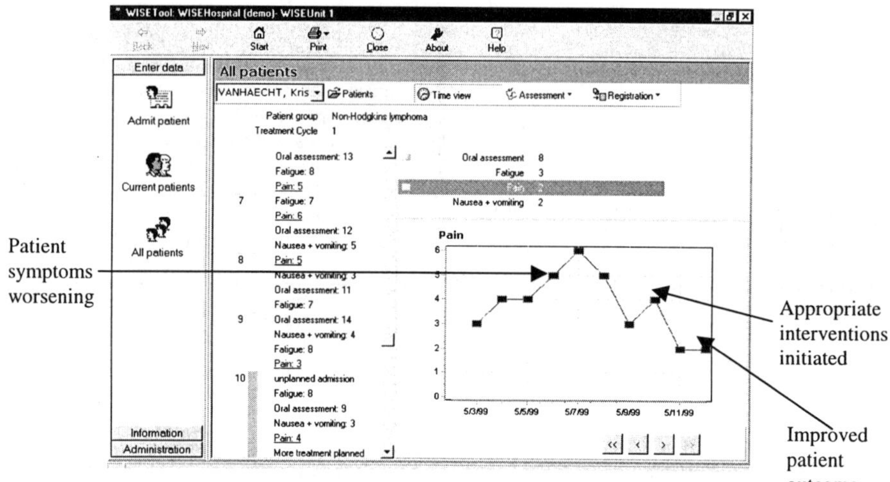

Figure 6   : Instant Feedback Graph

Exercising this level of control over their nursing empowers nurses to prove the value of their care. In addition, the use of these tools as a classification system has improved the communication between nurses and patients. Comments from patients have illustrated that their participation in the project has allowed them to be important contributors in their care, as opposed to passive recipients. They perceive that their feelings and experiences have been increasingly considered in the treatment plan. Completing the standard questionnaires would appear to have given patients a vehicle and a common language that allows them to express feelings or concerns that they may otherwise have found difficult to raise with members of the health care team, emphasising the importance of enhanced communication.

The second level of feedback is 'global' feedback, which requires a much larger feedback loop. Data are sent regularly (with an agreed periodicity: e.g. every 6 weeks, every 2 months) to the datawarehouse in which the data from all Clinical Sites are stored.

Before transfer, the data are anonymous and encrypted. These data are processed for the global feedback (Figure 7). Before producing feedback, data have be cleaned and organised. Developing and selecting the right indicators, the right reports in the right presentation format for the first time can take quite some time, even when all data are ready in the right format and content. International experiences reveal that, when there is agreement on the indicators and the standard way of reporting, it takes about six weeks to have the data analysed and to produce the global feedback report [9].

Global feedback reports are on paper using a graphic interface. They are made available on the Website. Their main goal is to position every Clinical Site in their achievements to manage side effects of chemotherapy (fatigue, nausea & vomiting, pain, mucositis) in relation to all other Clinical Sites in the network. If the other Sites were to remain anonymous, they would serve as benchmarks for the Clinical Site. However when they are not anonymous (as chosen by the WISECARE partners and Validation Sites), the feedback becomes much more powerful. Clinical Sites can make contact with each other to understand their positioning and to learn from other Sites how to improve their performance.

Next to the global feedback on clinical management, the WISECARE project provides feedback on nursing resource use: qualification level, staffing levels. The purpose is similar as for the clinical management feedback: positioning and understanding.

The information (clinical and resource use) can be used in team meetings to discuss team performance in relation to resource utilisation.

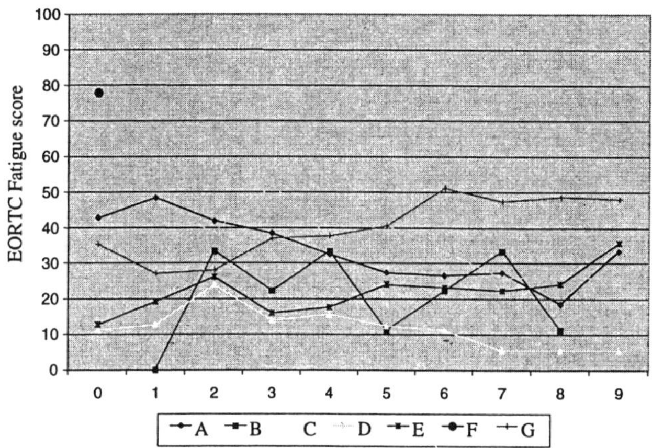

Figure 7   Example of Clinical Management Global Feedback. On the Y-axis: the EORTC-fatigue-score (0-100 X). On the X-axis: clinical time (days after clinical event). Each line is representing each of the Clinical Sites.

The more advanced level of feedback is in integrating instant and global feedback. This can be done by completing the instant feedback score with a reference score (according to the clinical time and risk score for that particular patient). See also Chapter 3, Global Feedback on Clinical Management. From the global feedback, reference scores can be regularly uploaded into the instant feedback module.

The added value of WISECARE is:

- The design of instant feedback graphs for various clinical indicators
- The design of clinical and nursing resource indicators and standardised reports for the management in oncological care settings

- The availability of reference scores (average, median, range,....) which can uploaded in instant feedback module on clinical management.

4.5 Networking

A fifth element in generating knowledge is networking. There is a large agreement in management literature that three types of assets of an organisation can be identified [13]: the financial capital (the numbers, plain resources), the human capital (the knowledge, skills, experiences, attitudes of all people: what you know) and the social capital (the accessible networks with specific resources: who you know). Burt [10] shows that real value of a network is not in the number of contacts, but in the quality of the contacts. Well-structured networks obtain much higher results than non-structured networks. Benefit-rich networks have (1) contacts established in the places where useful bits of information are likely to air, (2) provide a reliable flow of information to and from those places. Networks are most effective when there is a good balance between cohesion and diversity.

It is this kind of network that has been built in WISECARE. The Clinical Sites were carefully selected to be part of the network. Most of them were recommended by the European Oncology Nursing Society. All Sites have a high level of clinical expertise and legitimacy. There is a mix of oncological, haematological and even surgical wards. They were all required to have computer and Internet access on the nursing ward.

The networking in the project was very diverse in nature:
- sharing information on clinical management and nursing resource management by contributing to the global feedback,
- exchanging clinical guidelines and protocols,
- asking/ giving advice using e-mail, electronic discussion platforms for general of very specific patient problems,
- taking on the telephone,
- half-yearly project meetings with representatives from the various Clinical Sites.

All five elements of knowledge generation (standardised scales, categorising patients according to their risk, modelling for understanding relations between problems, interventions and outcomes, instant and global feedback, networking) are incorporated in the software tools that have been developed within the project: the WiseTool, WiseWeb and WiseCompass.

4.6 Supporting Tools

4.6.1 WiseTool

The WiseTool has to support all specific activity of clinical networking, from local data collection, to aggregation in the data warehouse, analysis, and finally feedback of new information. At each Site a tool was required which would support data collection and management, and would provide feedback on clinical effectiveness from the project. Users spoke multiple languages, were not generally experienced in the use of IT and had poor systems support. Therefore the tool had to be: very easy to use by nurses at the Sites; require minimal training; easy to install and maintain by non-IT professionals; secure and confidential; and support local customisation. The agreed requirement was for a stand-alone PC-based software tool with minimal duplication with existing local systems. Further, there should only be one integrated tool for data collection and local feedback. The WISETool was developed to meet these requirements.

The WISETool was developed for Windows 32bit operating systems (Windows 95/98/NT) using the Borland Delphi development environment. Delphi offered: support for stand-alone, client-server, or web-enabled applications; good control of user interface; rapid application development; flexible database links; support for Microsoft distributed computing technology (DCOM, COM, Activex, OLE, DDE...), and CORBA and very good third party support. A proprietary relational database was used which supported stand-alone, client-server and network operation. This was low cost, with no licence fees, and proved to be robust, fast enough in use, and simple to administer. It required exporting of data to allow use of 'open' tools.

The WISETool architecture involved three layers: user interface, application modules, and server modules. The WISETool used one main window for most operations. The interface was similar to the familiar Microsoft Outlook style, with a *button bar* for common operations and *pages* holding *function icons* in related groupings. This produced a simple, clean design, without complex multiple forms. Various application modules run on the WiseTool.

Examples of application modules are:

- Patient record module
- Data editors, combined into larger data entry forms.
- Information pages for providing access to protocols, local information (RTF format)
- Web pages, which can be linked into the WISETool, with hyperlinks and graphics.
- Data export is done through a custom module

Server modules can be shared by application modules and provide common services across the whole application. For example, a data access module centralises all data access to a small set of generic functions, simplifying testing and maintenance of the system. It also allowed replacement of the database system as the WISETool moved from prototype to a production version. A knowledge base server offers simple services including links to protocols (in HTML) and risk factors for treatments. Another server module manages links to other applications, with the first prototype link being to the HISCOM MIRADOR system by Windows Dynamic Data Exchange, leading in the final edge to a "WiseStation".

The terminology and dialogue services were combined and delivered through one *terminology server* module. This server used model files that were separate from the WISETool application to allow for flexibility in development and maintenance. One model file defined the concept space and semantic links within it. A separate lexicon file held the term labels for these concepts, with a set for each language required. Languages could be changed dynamically while the WISETool was running. Project team members at each Validation Site were able to translate terms using a simple spreadsheet, which was then compiled into a lexicon file. The actual WiseTool can be used in 8 different European languages: English, Dutch, Swedish, Finnish, French, Greek, Slovenian and Danish. Within the model file were the links required to group concepts to meet dialogue requirements.

Figure 8 shows the main patient record view. To the left is the *time line*, which shows a list of data items in an agenda format. Admissions, clinical events (for example, chemotherapy) and assessments are shown. Above this are some data items that change very slowly, such as *patient group*. Below are *indicator headings*, which show the current values of assessments for each indicator. The *feedback* graph shows the scores for selected indicators. Clicking on points on the graph selects that assessment on the *time line*, which can be double-clicked to open that assessment record for review. So, on seeing a high score, a user can quickly look at the assessment to see what was the cause. Clicking on the *protocols* button opens a window with protocols for the currently selected heading.

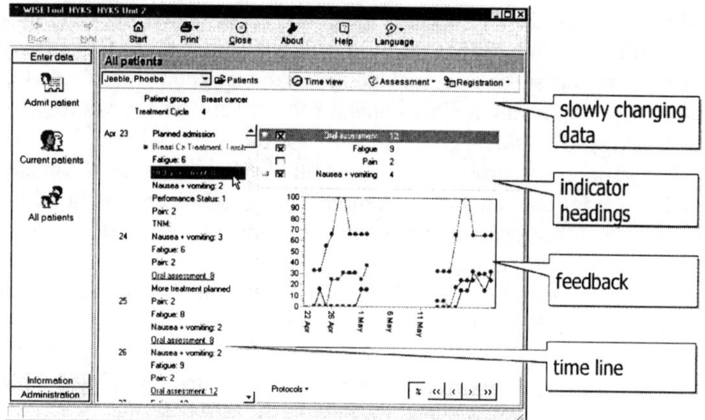

Figure 8   Patient Record View

See also Chapter 2, WiseTool.

4.6.2   *WiseWeb*

The WiseWeb is the communication module within the WISECARE project. The WiseWeb is organised in the WiseWeb and the WiseNet. The WiseWeb is a common Webserver (http://wisecare.dn.uoa.gr) for communicating the project to external visitors. Some interesting functions are provided: e.g. The WISECARE DISCUSSION FORUM. It is developed using the PERL Programming Language and it is, as the name implies, a Web-based bulletin board.

The WiseNet is a BSCW-server (Basic Support for Cooperative Work). The BSCW enables collaboration over the Web (Figure 9). BSCW is a 'shared workspace' system which supports document uploads, event notification, group management and much more. To access a workspace you only need a standard Web browser. The BSCW system supports collaboration by providing shared workspaces over the Internet. A shared workspace allows storage and retrieval of documents and sharing information within a group. This functionality is integrated with an event mechanism to provide each user with an awareness of the activities of others within the workspace. It comprises numerous features, e.g., support for threaded discussions, version management of documents, group management, search features and many more. The system is designed primarily to support self-organising groups.

The BSCW supports asynchronous and synchronous co-operation with your partners over the Internet, in your Intranet or in a network with your business partners (Extranet).

The essential *advantages*:

- With a BSCW workspace, workgroups can share documents — independent of the specific computer systems that the members use.

- You need not install any software before using BSCW. You only need a standard Web browser.

- You access BSCW workspaces, browse folders and download documents to your local system just like "normal" Web pages.

- BSCW keeps you informed of all relevant events in a shared workspace.

- You can upload documents to a shared workspace using any standard Web browser [11].

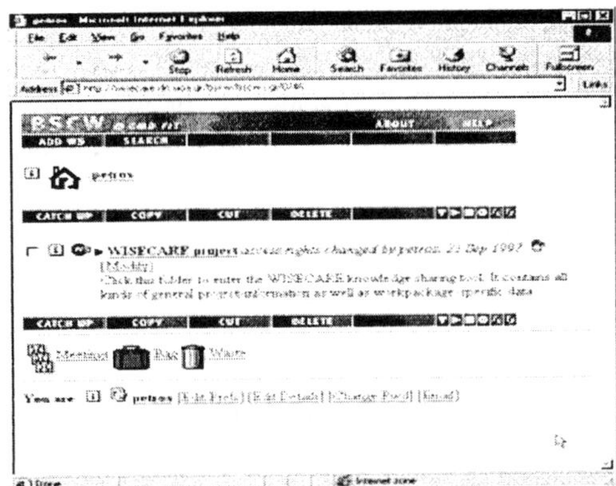

Figure 9   The BSCW Server

4.6.3   *WiseCompass*

WiseCompass is the adaptation of ComPass for use in the WISECARE environment. ComPass is based on the European Foundation of Quality Management (*EFQM*). The objective of ComPass is to provide Quality Assessors with a software tool according to a pre-defined Management Model, Business Framework, Functional Checklists or a Quality Model. The level of the assessment exceeds ISO 9000 and 14000 standards and can be enhanced with any other standard, like HACCP. WiseCompass is used in the project to assess the impact of WISECARE on clinical behaviour of oncological nurses. WiseCompass, as a means for systematic evaluation of the change in the organisation, is seen as an integrative part of whole WISECARE commitment to focus on outcome and quality.

5   Conclusions and Future Plans

A major commitment at the start of WISECARE was the intention to hand over the ownership of the outcomes of WISECARE to EONS that has played a vital role in the development and support of the project over the last three years. EONS would be responsible for the dissemination of the project throughout the European cancer nursing community. In order to achieve this, the Society has considered the most appropriate method for dissemination and proposes the development of a WISECARE Steering Committee to oversee future developments of the project.

Ten WISECARE-products have been identified. Eight of them will be internally exploited within the new WISECARE consortium: The Leuven Chemotherapy Risk Assessment Scale (LCRAS), the standardised clinical scales for measuring fatigue, nausea and vomiting, pain, oral problems and nursing intensity, the patient models, the instant and global feedback, the WiseTool-HIS links, the WiseWeb, the WiseHoos and the WiseCompass. Two products can be externally exploited. For the WiseTool a license will be taken, in order to incorporate it in any Hospital Information System. Special rights are reserved for EONS and the partners in the project. For the WISECARE network, a trademark on name and logo will be taken. Moving into the world of evidence-based clinical practice, the whole WISECARE-project has to breathe a spirit of trust: trust in the reliability and validity of the scales, the design frames, the analysis, the guidelines, the links, the partners in the network, the feedback. A WISECARE Trademark should help to support a high level of trust. Protecting the WISECARE name and logo by a Trademark allows assigning the label very selectively to highly reliable and valid standardised scales, guidelines. It can be used to help software vendors to build in the WiseTool functionality in the electronic patient record as 'WISECARE compatible', meaning that the required functionality is incorporated to load reference scores into instant feedback modules, to generate global feedback reports etc.

Is there a market for WISECARE? The WISECARE project has been designed as a general application system within health care. Although the demonstration domain is oncological care, it has limited impact on the software, which has a very flexible and open design. The highest impact is on the WISECARE knowledge server which is very oncology specific given the standardised scales, data collection design and risk appraisal tools. The first aim to launch the project in a production environment will be in oncological care. In a second phase, the project knowledge could be expanded to other health care domains.

Extrapolation of some national (Belgium) and international figures [12] to the EU (375 million inhabitants) results for oncological care in 3,8 million admissions/year; 33,3 million inpatient days (a bed capacity of 90000 beds) and 6,3 million chemotherapy administrations/year. Combined with the serious quality of life -problems, patients are facing during treatment (70% of oncology patients in hospitals perceive fatigue problems, 2 out of 3 has some oral problems, 50% experience pain and 25% has nausea & vomiting problems), there is a need to manage nursing care more properly.

Potential stakeholders are patients and their representatives: social insurance companies and governments; professionals represented by health care organisations and professional associations, pharmaceutical companies, ICT-companies.

The benefit of the WISECARE-project for *oncological patients* is obvious. Oncological care is not only life threatening but has a very high impact on the quality of life of patients under treatment. The WISECARE approach proves a reduction of the negative impact on the quality of life of patients. The benefit is not only due to better procedures and better monitoring, but also by an active involvement of patients in the care process. It is of utmost importance that patients or their family members are taught how to handle these problems effectively. Professional care is only appropriate when patients or family members are not able to provide it. Nurses should put every effort into improving the self-care abilities of the patient and the family rather than ritualistically taking over that care. The WISECARE-service should be expanded freely to patients in an easily accessible way.

The feedback from Validation and Demonstration Sites shows clearly that the network is seen as very valuable to *health care professionals,* mainly nurses. Nine out of eleven Clinical Sites want to continue WISECARE networking after finishing the project. There is an agreement among partners and Clinical Sites to continue at least for 6 months, without further development, with limited maintenance support and only one global feedback report in April 2000. Even based on these limited conditions, more than 100 new patients have been entered in the WiseHoos database. Based on this success, the European Oncology nurses Association maintained their commitment in the project, supporting the development and maintenance of the WISECARE network.

Pharmaceutical companies are highly interested in the WISECARE project, because it provides information regarding effectiveness of therapeutic drugs instead of information about efficacy as usually is obtained from the randomised clinical trials. A second interest is the changing role of pharmaceutical companies from pure sellers (a marketing focus) to become partners in care delivery. They can fulfil an well-appreciated role behind the scenes in providing up-to-date information toxicity levels, leaflets, teaching packages, clinical management software. Several interest groups of pharmaceutical companies have been identified.

There is high interest in WISECARE from the wide range of *ICT-companies:* specifically from those in the field of developing hospital or health care information systems. The high potentiality of the electronic patient record is in the exploitation. It is always taught that the use of this data for further exploitation purposes will be driven by its simple availability. From WISECARE it becomes increasingly obvious that the structure and content of the EPR will not determine its exploitation. It is the need for exploitation that will determine the structure and content. For developers of EPR-software it is important that they are involved in a project such as WISECARE as soon as possible. HISCOM is one of the major partners in WISECARE. A link between the WiseTool and Mirador has been built. HISCOM intend to invest in WISECARE in the future. A second group of ICT-companies interested in WISECARE are the EPR-exploitation companies. All kind of applications are offered by these firms: Resource Enterprise Systems, executive information systems, management information systems, data mining, scheduling and planning systems. A third group of ICT-companies interested in WISECARE is the group of the networking companies. Networking across Europe, setting up knowledge centres and creating virtual organisations by providing a highly performant network environment is the main goal.

The further development of the WISECARE consortium, requires three basic roles: network co-ordination, knowledge development (guidelines, indicators, scales, feedback) and IT-development. Given some fixed costs in setting up the WISECARE Knowledge Centre (knowledge development and IT), an average cost of 10000 Euro/year is estimated when at least 50 Clinical Sites subscribe in the Network. Extending the network to 500 Clinical Sites, subscription rates can be reduced to less than 2500 Euro/year. Because there is little tradition in European hospitals to spend money on this kind of information, the cost-benefit analysis shows that this kind of activity still needs to be subsidised.

References

[1]　Sermeus W, Hoy D, Jodrell N, Hyslop A, Gypen T, Kinnunen J, Mantas J, Delesie L, Tansley J and Hofdijk J. The WISECARE project and the impact of information technology on nursing knowledge in Nursing Informatics: the impact of nursing knowledge on health care informatics. IOS press, 176-184, 1997.

[2]　Kearney N, Campbell S & Sermeus W. Practising for the future: utilising information technology in cancer nursing practice European Journal of Oncology Nursing, 1998 Vol 2 No 3 pp169-175.

[3]　Sermeus W, Hoy D, Jodrell N, Hyslop A, Gypen T, Kinnunen J, Mantas J, Delesie L, Tansley J and Hofdijk J. WISECARE: Workflow Information Systems for European Nursing CARE, Technical Annex Report HC 4113 Health Care Sector, EU-DGXIII, Telematics, Fourth Framework, 1996.

[4]　Davenport T & Prusack L Working kowledge: how organizations manage what they know, Harvard Business School Press, Boston, 1998.

[5]　Eilers J, Bergen AM, Petersen MC. Development, testing and application of the oral assessment guide, *Oncology Nursing Forum* 1988 15:325-330.

[6]　Piper BF, Lindsey AM, Dodd MJ, Ferketich S, Paul SM, Weller S. The development of an instrument to measure the subjective dimension of fatigue. In management of Pain, Nausea and Fatigue Funk SG Torniquist EM Champagne MT Copp LA Wiese RA (Eds) Springer Publishing Company: New York, 1993.

[7]　Aaronson N, Ahnedzai S, Bergman B, Bullinger M, Cull A, Duez N, Fiiberti A, Fletcher H, Fleischman S, de Haes J, Kaasa S, Klee M, Osoba D, Razari D, Rofe P, Schraube S, Sneeuw K, Sullivan M, Takdea F. The European Organisation for the Research and Treatment of Cancer QLQ-C30: a quality of life instrument for use in clinical trials in oncology. Journal of the National Cancer Institute, 1993 **85**(5): 365-376.

[8]　Dhaenekint C. et al. Nurses Cytostatic Compendium, Practical Guide for nurses, Glaxo Wellcome, 1994.

[9]   Kazandjian VA & Lied T.R. Healthcare Performance Measurement: Systems Design and Evaluation.
      ASQ Quality Press, Milwaukee, Wisconsin, 1999.
[10] Burt R.S. The social structure of competition in Networks and Organisations: Structure, Form an
      Action. Harvard Business School, 1992: 57-91.
[11] Dounavis P, Karistinou E & Mantas J.   WISECARE www-server.   Deliverable 6.1, WISECARE
      project, 1998.
[12] OECD. The reform of health care systems: a review of 17 OECD countries. *Health Policy Studies*,
      1994, **5**.

Information Needs of Oncology Nurses

Nora Kearney

1   Nursing Interventions and Patient Outcomes

The nursing profession requires outcome measurements to demonstrate both the value of care delivered by nurses, and the qualified nurses providing that care. Outcome measures offer the opportunity for defining the unique contribution of nurses and to assert the value of this contribution. In measuring outcomes of nursing it is necessary to consider a number of issues. There is a difficulty in defining what are the distinctly nursing ventures in differentiating nursing practice for the improvement of patient care [2]. During an illness, patients are exposed to interventions from numerous other health care professionals and relatives acting in a caring role. The problem for nursing is to determine whether nursing alone is responsible for a particular patient outcome - whether there needs to be mono or multi-disciplinary evaluation [3]. There are some authors who believe that it is possible to measure outcomes specifically related to nursing intervention [4, 5] although examples of how to achieve this are not presented in their work. Kitson [6] has probably done most in an attempt to define in a generic way the articulation of nursing outcomes with her Therapeutic Nursing Function Indicator with which nursing may find evidence to support its claims.

Patient outcomes are influenced by other external factors beyond the sphere of nursing and the input of other health care professionals, such as restorative processes unique to the individual and environmental and social influences. The aim of outcome research should be to ascertain which nursing interventions, under which circumstances, and with which patients, result in optimal patient outcomes. Evidence is beginning to emerge about the effectiveness of nurse-led interventions from a range of health settings; for example, the treatment of leg ulcers [7] and other types of wound care, urinary incontinence [8], and catheter care, stoma care [9], diabetes care [10], breast cancer and counselling [11], management of acute pain [12] and management of dyspnoea in patients with lung cancer [13]. Nurse-led services are also key components in the treatment of asthma, hypertension, and in cardiac rehabilitation programmes. There are however, limitations in the body of nursing knowledge, which make scientific measurement of nursing interventions difficult. French [14] claims that nurses operate in an 'information vacuum' and lack the means to determine the effectiveness of nursing activity, while desiring feedback for the identification of best nursing practice [14]. Kirkevold [15] calls for 'integrative research' to further develop the science of nursing. Integrative research asserts that related knowledge from separate studies can be integrated to give comprehensive understanding, and therefore cumulative knowledge development. She comments that studies in nursing do not tend to build on prior work - researchers devise different study-specific tools, with various methodological approaches and theoretical inconsistencies, so weakening the science of nursing [15]. This view is echoed by French [14] who contends that whilst a range of measurement tools is exciting it is not progressive. Collating nursing intervention studies on to a database would be incredibly complex because of inconsistencies of language (keywords) and classification terms [14]. Kirkevold [15] believes that integrative research allows general appraisal of contexts and findings, rather than becoming bogged down in critique of methodologies. In this way, the appropriateness and relevance of studies can be assessed and their clinical implications discussed. Many authors are in disagreement with this notion of a 'broad brush' approach, fearing that generic conclusions and broad application of results is not helpful, asserting that measuring the complexities of nursing care requires methods to be sensitive, specific and scientifically robust in terms of reliability and validity, to be of value to the progression of the body of knowledge [16, 17]. The product of a nursing service is not nursing care, but outcomes of that care i.e. the expected results of a nursing intervention [2]. As the literature reveals, measuring patient outcomes is a multifactorial and complicated endeavour.

In her review of British outcome studies between 1990 and 1994, French [14] discovered a host of outcome variables, which she categorised as physical status, psychosocial status, functional status, well-being, health behaviour and knowledge, service utilisation, and satisfaction. Of the 228 studies she reviewed, no fewer than 119 formal measurement tools were identified. Bond and Thomas [3], list the fifteen outcome categories classified by Marek [18] from a review of the literature: physiological, psychosocial, functional, behavioural, knowledge, symptom control, home maintenance, well-being, goal attainment, patient satisfaction, safety, nursing diagnosis resolution, frequency of service, cost, and re-hospitalisation. Clearly, what constitutes an outcome is entirely arbitrary. Thomas and Bond [17] assert that a vital component of patient outcomes must be patient satisfaction with nursing care, as sometimes nurses make patients feel better when they do not always get better [17]. It is lamented however that the literature fails to reveal any sensitive, valid or reliable quantitative measures of patient satisfaction with nursing based on patients' views. Poor questionnaires censor patients' opinions and subsequently nurses are in danger of thinking they are performing better than they really are [17].

Hegyvary [4] states that the desirability of a particular outcome will vary depending on the values, preferences and expectations of patients. It is a subjective variable founded in individual human experience and therefore difficult to quantify [4]. Other factors to consider in outcome measurement should be the quality of the practitioner [characteristics, level of expertise), and the care element of practice delivery [4].

2   Evidence-based Nursing

To improve knowledge and patient outcomes, WISECARE sought to utilise evidenced-based practice. As Mulhall [19] concurs: "Research-based practice must be embedded in the culture of practitioners" [19]

From a medical perspective, evidence-based practice has been widely used to inform management of disease and to assess the outcome of treatments. It is defined as: "The conscientious, explicit and judicious use of current best evidence in making decisions about the care of individual patients integrating individual clinical expertise and external clinical evidence from systematic research" [20].

Evidence-based practice has been criticised as being conducted from so-called ivory towers with little meaningful contribution from clinical settings. Sackett et al [20] refute this claim citing evidence-based practice studies by clinical teams on the shop floor. They describe it as utilising the bottom-up approach by necessity, integrating external evidence, individual clinical expertise and patient choice. They assert quite categorically that external clinical evidence can only inform, never replace, clinical expertise. It is this expertise which decides how clinical evidence applies, if at all, to an individual patient's predicament, and then how best to apply it [20]. There has also been concern voiced that this approach to practice will serve the needs of the managers and purchasers charged with ensuring that costs are contained. The contrary situation may in fact arise as evidence-based medicine guides a physician to utilise the most efficacious interventions to maximise quality and quantity of life for patients; clearly this may lead to the incurring of greater costs to the financiers [20]. A particularly pertinent issue when applying evidence-based practice in nursing, is consideration of the quality of evidence on which practice is to be based. Sackett et al [20] acknowledge that randomised controlled trials are the 'gold standard', but where these do not exist, drawing on less scientifically produced knowledge to formulate external evidence is acceptable.

Evidence-based practice will assist nurses in naming their skills and defining outcomes, which isolate nursing interventions. Patient outcomes are the end result of treatments [2], whether they are medical or nursing, and linking nursing interventions to patient outcomes is critical [21]. Evidence-based nursing can demonstrate the cause and effect of nursing on patient outcomes of a particular intervention i.e. the implementation of nursing interventions in response to nursing assessment supported by evidence-based knowledge.

3   Identifying Priorities of Care

The WISECARE project seeks to harmonise cancer-nursing care across Europe, and priorities of care have to be determined as a starting point. Ownership of research is integral to relevance and acceptability in practice [16]. Fitch and Thompson [21] claim that a bottom-up approach in setting a research agenda will reflect concerns in clinical practice and be in keeping with the strengths and research interest of the staff. Nurses are aware of knowledge gaps and are best placed to identify priorities [21,22]. Consistent with these views from the literature, nurses in the relevant clinical areas were asked to identify common topical issues and specific areas of care on which WISECARE would focus.

However, it is beyond the scope of the WISECARE project to address, in any meaningful way, the problems encountered by all patients with cancer, which require nursing intervention. In an attempt to optimise the opportunity WISECARE affords cancer nurses, specific areas of care were identified by the clinically based nurses in the project. Following discussion and assessment of the needs of these nurses' patient population, it was decided that fatigue and oral care were two significant nursing issues within the clinical area. Additionally the whole concept of satisfaction with care was considered integral to the study. The users described satisfaction of care as the satisfaction derived by nurses by delivering care in their own area and the satisfaction patients experience as a result of receiving this care. However, patient satisfaction with care is extremely difficult to measure and given the added complexity of cultural differences, it is unlikely that this area will be addressed in the WISECARE project. What may be more relevant would be an assessment of patients' quality of life in the clinical area and this issue required further exploration. Indeed, the availability of the EORTC QLQ-C30 quality of life questionnaire, which has been validated throughout Europe, affords the means of collecting meaningful data in this important area of patient care. It was believed that evaluating patients' quality of life would measure the impact of treatment on this. Measuring quality of life in this way provides a patient-centred method of measuring 'success' in all patient groups, including those receiving palliative treatment. Quality of life measurement has an intuitive appeal for cancer nurses: identifying what makes patients' lives worthwhile and the caring aspect of nursing. Consequently the three patient issues of quality of life, oral care and fatigue were identified as the specific issues on which the project would focus.

However, the clinical reality of data collection was somewhat different than anticipated. The broad nature of the concept of quality of life made it problematic to link patients' outcome with specific nursing interventions. Not only was the quality of life QLQ-C30 questionnaire cumbersome and difficult for patients to complete, the assessment for fatigue issues the Piper Fatigue Scale was also reported by patients to be unwieldy. A drive for a change to the data collection also came from the data managers who believed that a large amount of data was being collected, from which only a small amount was being used in the project. Consequently, a change to data collection was negotiated. Further discussion with nursing staff revealed that their clinical priorities were oral care, fatigue, pain and nausea and vomiting and the resultant change was based on this.

For the majority of the project, data collection has occurred for each patient for 10 consecutive days for each treatment cycle. Patients complete 7 questions (derived from QLQ–C30) relating to their perceptions of pain, fatigue and nausea and vomiting over the previous 24-hour period. The patient is also educated to complete the Oral Assessment Guide daily between days 1-10. This duration of time is likely to capture the patients' nadir, when most side effects of treatment would be expected, nursing interventions initiated and patient outcomes evaluated

4   Nursing Data

Hegyvary [4] suggests there should be three core elements when collecting nursing data in a systematic way to create a minimum data set; nursing care (nursing diagnosis, interventions, outcomes, and intensity of care), patient demography, and service elements. Nursing Minimum Data Set (NMDS) is defined as:
"Systematic registration of the smallest number possible of unequivocally coded data, with respect to or for the purpose of nursing practice, making information available to the largest group possible of users according to a broad range of information requirements" [23]
Belgium is the only country so far that uses information from nursing activity data to inform decisions about financing and resource management. This data collection, or NMDS, has been compulsory in Belgium since 1988, and consists of patient demographics, medical diagnosis, dates of admission and discharge, 23 nursing activities, hours and numbers of nurses, and activities of daily living. The Belgian NMDS is a comprehensive, valid and reliable instrument, which the WISECARE project may utilise. Data was collected from each of the five sites to determine baseline information and the priority areas of nursing care. Information from the sites is detailed in Table 1.

Table 1   Clinical Sites Data

Clinical Site	Postbasic education	Average length of stay/patients	Nursing outcome measures	Number of wards
A	yes	9 days	no	2
B	yes	10 days	no	1
C	no	7 days	no	3
D	yes	18 days	no	1
E	yes	2 days	yes	2

It is evident from the information presented in table 1 that there are differences in relation to the Clinical Sites in a number of areas. In all but one of the countries nurses have access to specialist education in cancer nursing but only one of the countries currently employs nursing outcome measures in clinical practice. The average length of stay also varies considerably therefore further discussion is required to determine more specifically which patient group(s) will be considered in this project.

4.1 Fatigue

The major priority, which is common to all sites, is cancer, or cancer treatment related fatigue. Fatigue is experienced by more than 90% of patients with cancer [24] and is the most frequently reported symptom of cancer and cancer treatment [25]. Yet despite this there is no common definition of fatigue identifiable in the literature. This fact is compounded when one considers fatigue from a European context adding the variable of culture to the problem.

From the nurses involved in the WISECARE project fatigue has been identified as one of the most significant problems for the patients in their care and is a problem, which is not always dealt with adequately, either in terms of assessment or effective intervention strategies.

4.1.1 Incidence

Fatigue is associated with both cancer treatment and the disease process. Most nursing research has concentrated on fatigue associated with chemotherapy [26,27,28,29,30], radiotherapy, [31,32,33,34] and biological therapies [35,36, 37]. With the exception of Cimprich [38] limited research has been conducted into the fatigue associated with cancer surgery.

4.1.2 Aetiology

There are many factors thought to be responsible for cancer related fatigue but as yet there remains no definitive scientific rationale to explain this phenomenon. Rather what is presented throughout the literature is a description of the concept of fatigue rather than clearly defined scientific knowledge. There is a limited amount of knowledge developing and this incorporates both physical and psychological factors but little is understood regarding correlations between the different factors and indeed if correlations do exist.

The range of factors associated with cancer related fatigue include; sleep disturbances, various biochemical alterations associated with disease or treatment, nutritional status, psycho social factors, environmental factors, level of activity and numerous inherent factors [38,39,41].

4.1.3 Understanding

The knowledge base to date in relation to fatigue has been hampered by a number of issues which have been raised by numerous authors. These include the lack of a clear theoretical framework [25,26], methodological issues associated with recent research [26,42,25], and the validity and reliability of assessment tools [26,43].

However despite these obvious limitations there is a need to explore further the problem of fatigue, given the negative impact it has on the lives of individuals with cancer and their families and the unknown amount of nursing resource utilised in addressing this problem.

4.1.4   Knowledge Development

Developing new knowledge about fatigue and its management will add to the limited body of knowledge that currently exists.

By utilising the experience of the nurses in each of the Clinical Sites information regarding the prevalence of fatigue will be ascertained in relation to specific patient groups. This approach is contrary to most previous research, which has utilised small sample sizes and heterogeneous patient populations [30,26,42]. Involving a more homogeneous patient population in WISECARE should produce more reliable data for sub sections of the cancer population facilitating the development of more specific nursing interventions. What is anticipated in the first stage is an exploration of the prevalence of fatigue in the patient populations to be included in the project and the way in which this patient problem is currently assessed and addressed by the nurses involved in the WISECARE project.

Utilising this baseline data it should be possible to demonstrate the following:

- Current state of knowledge of clinical nurses in relation to management of fatigue
- Utilisation of research findings in practice both at the start of the project and development over time
- Nursing resource being utilised to manage this problem
- Changes in nursing practice

4.1.5   Assessment

There are a number of assessment tools to measure the incidence of fatigue available which could be utilised and/or adapted for the project. The most reliable is likely to be the Piper Fatigue Scale. Although developed for use with American patients it has been utilised reliably in a number of European countries.

However, as previously mentioned, patients found using the Piper Fatigue Scale cumbersome and time consuming. Despite the benefits of reliability and validity of using such a scale, patient compliance was an essential component of the project. Consequently, the collection of information regarding patient's fatigue was modified based on the fatigue related questions of the EORTC QLQ-C30, with a resultant improvement in compliance.

4.2   Oral Care

The lack of a systematic approach to oral care for patients receiving chemotherapy was also identified as an important nursing issue for the nurses involved in the project. Maintaining good oral health is necessary to prevent infection, for eating, and communicating either through speech or non-verbal expression such as smiling [44,45,46,47,48]. There is a prevalence of oral complications in oncology, and mouth care for these patients is particularly significant.

Mouth care is a basic nursing activity, essential for effective prevention or minimising of side effects from cancer therapies and for symptom management in good palliative care [47,49,46]. It has been found, however, that this area of care engenders negative attitudes in nurses who find it unrewarding and unpleasant, making it a low priority and often delegating the role to unqualified care assistants [44,50]. Mouth care has become a ritualistic and banal activity, a topic of conflicting advice and subjective conclusions from sporadic research [51,52]. In the management of cancer, oral dysfunction is a potential hazard for the majority of patients and is therefore a major oncology nursing concern. Mouth problems arise where there is primary oropharangeal malignancy, as sequelae of cancer treatments, and as a consequence of general debilitation from advancing disease. They impact on patients' quality of life, are significant dose-limiting factors potentially affecting prognosis, and can result in prolonged hospital admission for treatment of infections and nutritional support.

Accurate assessment of the mouth and knowledge of treatment procedures is vital for effective individualised care. As Sweeney et al [53] report in a survey of mouth care provision by nurses for cancer patients in Scotland, there is a demonstration of positive interest in this area. The acknowledgement of patchy knowledge with a need for more training leads to improve standards of oral hygiene for the terminally ill both in the hospice and the community [53].

4.2.1   Cancer Therapies

Oral complications during cancer therapies result from one of two mechanisms: direct effect of a treatment on the oral mucosa (direct stomatotoxicity), or an indirect result of cytotoxic agents' myelosuppressive effects (indirect stomatotoxicity). Radiation damage will occur 7-14 days after commencement of treatment [54], and chemotherapy-induced effects will be seen as quickly as 3 days following initiation of treatment [55]. Within the layers of the epithelial cells of the oral mucosa lie indigenous pathogens which, in health, present no threat to the host, but in immuno-compromised patients cause opportunistic infection which can spread through the blood and lymphatic systems with potentially life threatening effect [56]. Age and tumour type are also significant.

Patients with haematological malignancies develop oral complications more frequently than patients with solid tumours probably because their underlying malignancies render them immunosuppressed prior to treatment. Young patients (< 20 years of age) are at greater risk of oral problems attributable to the decreased rate of cell renewal in older people [55,56].

4.2.2   Chemotherapy

Direct stomatitis results from a cytotoxic drug's non-specific effects on cells undergoing mitosis. Chemotherapy decreases the renewal rate of the basal epithelium resulting in mucosal atrophy, localised or diffuse ulceration of the mucosa and inflammation [56]. Cytotoxic agents primarily associated with stomatitis (inflammation of the oral cavity) are anti-tumour antibiotics, anti-metabolites and plant alkaloids.   Biological response modifiers also cause oral complications. The secondary effect of reduced nutritional intake and subsequent protein deprivation increase the severity of oral mucositis (inflammation of the mucous membrane). Indirect stomatotoxicities, due to disease-related or bone marrow suppressive treatment, are infection and haemorrhage which correlate to the intensity and duration of mucositis [56]. Minimising the sequelae of inevitable oral side effects is an oncology nursing challenge and an integral part of oncology nursing practice [45]. Strict oral hygiene is essential for these patients, which if not adhered to, can have serious consequences - sepsis, cachexia, suspension of treatment [56]. Mouth care protocols for chemotherapy patients remain largely subjective and unit driven, with varying levels of consultation of multi-disciplinary personnel including dental health practitioners and dieticians.

4.2.3   Understanding

Mouth care, as with other symptom management has suffered from what Hogan [57] describes "we-have-always-done-it-this-way" syndrome. Over the past thirty years there has been an attempt to investigate and evaluate the efficacy of a multitude of cleansing agents and implements, and oral hygiene protocols producing confusion and sometimes contradictory findings [51]. Comparisons between studies are difficult due to different assessment tools being used, small sample sizes, and heterogeneity of patients and treatment regimes.

In the Clinical Sites identified as part of the WISECARE project there is no consistency in the delivery of oral care. However by utilising the experience of the nurses involved in the project we should be able to determine what patterns of care are common to all sites in relation to oral care.

Utilising this baseline data it should be possible to demonstrate the following:

- Current state of knowledge of clinical nurses in relation to management of fatigue
- Utilisation of research findings in practice both at the start of the project and development over time
- Nursing resource being utilised to manage this problem
- Changes in nursing practice

4.2.4 Assessment

The Oral Assessment Guide (OAG) devised by Eilers et al. [58] is the only tool designed to be used by nurses to assess the oral cavity in patients receiving chemotherapy. It has tested nurse-nurse inter-rater reliability and content validity although in an American setting. This would seem the most appropriate tool to be utilised in this project but initial pilot work to determine cultural reliability would be required.

Nursing staff did not experience any problems with the use of the OAG, however, following the adjustments to data collection, it was decided that the OAG should be completed daily for the 10 day duration of clinical indicator data collection. Although a member of the nursing staff usually completes the OAG, it was felt that, following education, there was no reason why patients could not routinely evaluate their own oral status using the OAG. Patient compliance has been good and assessment in this way proved successful.

4.3 Nausea and Vomiting

In the oncology setting, nausea and vomiting are most often associated with chemotherapy administration however, considering the chronic and occasionally critical condition of patient with cancer, the potential aetiologies for such symptoms are many and varied [59]. Chemical, structural, metabolic and physiological factors may all be responsible in causing the sensation of nausea or the emetic event.

Persistent vomiting can result in dehydration, electrolyte imbalance and metabolic alkalosis to name but a few [60]. Symptoms such as delayed and anticipatory nausea and vomiting have the potential to negatively impact on quality of life, causing anxiety, depression, restricted social life, job loss and even suicide [60]. Patients receiving chemotherapy have ranked 'being sick' as their most distressing symptom and 'feeling sick' as second [27] and the burden of this distressing symptoms can result in patients refusing further treatment [61]. This failure to receive the benefits of the prescribed treatment has the potential to lead to unnecessary and premature patient deaths. Consequently, the nurses involved in the project identified developing better methods of managing these side effects as critical for improving patients' quality of life and disease outcomes.

4.3.1 Incidence

Although pharmacological developments have improved many patients' experience of nausea and vomiting, the myth that the vast majority of patients can now obtain complete control of emesis with currently available anti-emetics can be challenged [62]. Forty to fifty percent of patients receiving chemotherapy experience emesis at some point in their treatment [62]. The unacceptable nature of this fact drove the nurses involved in the project to attempt to further improve their assessment and management of nausea and vomiting, and ensure rational decision making regarding patient management.

4.3.2 Aetiology

Although nausea and vomiting are distinct entities, the terms used to describe them are used interchangeably and simultaneously, leading to confusion and inadequate clinical practice. Nausea is medically defined as a highly subjective conscious recognition of the need to vomit [63] accompanied by symptoms of increased salivation, swallowing and tachycardia. Vomiting is easily objectively measured and has been defined as the oral expulsion of the stomach contents occurring as a result of a positive change in intrathoracic pressure [46]. The focus for treatment induced emesis has been chemotherapy, leaving radiation induced emesis less well studied. Factors such as site, dose, size of treatment field and concomitant administration of chemotherapy all influence the severity and incidence of radiation induced emesis [63]. In addition to radiation therapy, patients can experience nausea and vomiting as a result of 4 main reasons: chemical visceral, central nervous system and vestibular.

4.3.3 Understanding

The cornerstone of the management of nausea and vomiting remains in-depth, individual patient assessment [63] and, regardless of the care setting, it could be argued that nurses are in the best position to consider the symptoms of nausea and vomiting within the context of the individual patient. Due to ease of measurement, nausea and vomiting data tends to focus primarily on vomiting [64]. However, this narrow focus does not facilitate the comprehensive assessment of antiemetic therapies and patients' experiences. Rhodes [65] advocated the importance of considering nausea, vomiting and retching as well as the patients' reported distress accompanying these symptoms. Indeed, it could be suggested that only through the use of standardised, simple, accurate and reproducible assessment of nausea and vomiting and an understanding of the symptom experience that correct information will be gathered to ensure appropriate patient management. However, although people may seem to experience similar symptoms, the cause of the symptoms as well as the individual's response to the symptoms can vary enormously. Despite the knowledge already available, the nurses involved in the project were of the opinion that the care delivered could be improved and so the problems of nausea and vomiting have been included in the project.

4.3.4 Knowledge Development

Developing new knowledge about patients experience of nausea and vomiting in relation to specific cancer treatments will add to the knowledge base that already exists for nurses planning care for patients receiving treatment for cancer.
Utilising this baseline data it should be possible to demonstrate the following:

- Current state of knowledge of clinical nurses in relation to the management of nausea and vomiting
- Utilisation of research findings in practice throughout the project
- Nursing resources being utilised to manage this problem
- Changes in nursing

4.3.5 Assessment

A number of assessment measures exist for evaluating nausea and vomiting. For the purpose of the project however, and considering that no sites currently utilise any of these, nausea and vomiting was evaluated using 2 questions based on those of the EORTC QLQ-C30. One question concerns nausea and the other vomiting and both are concerned with the patient's experience during the previous 24 hours.

4.4 Pain

Patients with cancer may experience pain caused by cancer progression or treatment as well as pain caused by complications such as pathological fractures and infections [66]. Cancer associated pain is a complex phenomenon comprising of physiological, sensory, affective, cognitive, behavioural and sociocultural dimensions [67]. The psychological effects of cancer pain can lead to loss of hope, fear of worsening or progressive disease, rejection of treatment programmes, loss of enjoyment of family and societal roles, disruption of productive work and in some patients, thoughts of suicide [67].

4.4.1 Incidence

The prevalence of cancer related pain is great. It is estimated that 50-70% of patients with early stage cancer and 60-90% of those with advanced or terminal cancer experience pain [68].

4.4.2 Aetiology

Pain in cancer may be due to *the tumour itself, related to the cancer e.g. muscle spasm, constipation, related to the cancer treatment e.g. post-operative scar pain, caused by a concurrent disorder e.g. spondylosis [69].*

However, many patients with advanced cancer can have multiple pains related to several of these categories. An accurate diagnosis of the cause of pain is essential as this has significant implications for the treatment and patient outcome.

4.4.3 Understanding

Although the pharmacology of pain management is now better understood than ever before giving nurses a wide variety of analgesic medications with which to address patients' cancer pain, non-pharmacological methods of pain relief are also highly recommended [70]. However, despite the means and the knowledge to manage most pain with relative ease, many patients continue to endure unnecessary suffering [71]. Patients and families hold numerous misconceptions regarding pain management and unwarranted fears about drug addiction, drug tolerance and respiratory depression and these often result in the undertreatment of patients' pain [72].

4.4.4   Knowledge Development

A variety of pain theories exist, such as the Gate Control Theory of Pain [73]. However, the subjective nature of pain can complicate its assessment and management. Conflicting evidence characterises the most appropriate assessment and no single tool has been identified as appropriate for universal use. Individualised care should be the guiding principle for effective pain management. Optimistically, varying combinations of pharmacological and non-pharmacological treatment, appropriately applied, can control pain in most patients [72]. Given the conflicting nature of advice regarding assessment and management, sharing of information and the resultant harmonisation of the nursing care delivered to patients experiencing pain should lead to the improvement in patient outcomes.

4.4.5   Assessment

A plethora of assessment tools exist to evaluate patients' pain. All the Clinical Sites involved in the project use no standardised tool. As a consequence, patients' pain experiences were evaluated using 2 questions based on the EORTC QLQ-C30 that ask the patient to evaluate their pain experiences of the previous 24 hours.

5   Utilising information technology

Participants in the project will be able to compare and measure their performances against the best practices of other institutions via state of the art information technology systems. Information technology is impacting the way we live both personally and professionally. WISECARE has the potential to alter markedly the way we transfer knowledge and develop nursing practice. It will move away from the direct transfer of knowledge and traditional educational strategies currently employed in nurse education.

References

[1]   McVie JG. Current areas of treatment, *Semin.Oncol* **23** (suppl 1) (1996): 1-3.
[2]   Moritz P. Innovative nursing practice models and patient outcomes, *Nursing Outlook* **39** (1991): 111-114.
[3]   Bond S. and Thomas L. Issues in measuring outcomes of nursing, *Journal of Advanced Nursing* **16** (1991): 1492-1502.
[4]   Hegyvary S. Patient care outcomes related to the management of symptoms. In: Fitzpatrick and Stevenson (eds), Annual Review of Nursing Research Vol II Springer, New York, 1993.
[5]   Higgins M., McCaughan D., Griffiths M & Carr-hill. Assessing the outcomes of nursing care, *Journal of Advanced Nursing* **17** (1992): 561-568.
[6]   Kitson A. A framework for quality. A patient centred approach to quality assurance in health care. Scuttari Press, London, 1993.
[7]   Cullum N. & Rowbottom B. Leg ulcers, *Nursing Management* (1995).
[8]   O'Brien J., Austin M., Sethi P., O'Boyle P. Urinary incontinence: prevalence, need for treatment and effectiveness of interventions by nurses, *British Medical Journal* **303** (1991): 1308-1311.
[9]   Wade B. Colostomy patients' psychological adjustment, *Journal of Advanced Nursing* **15** (1991): 1297-1304.
[10] Mallows C. et al. An evaluation of nurse specialists diabetic clinics, *Practical Diabetes* **7** (1990): 21-23.
[11] Wilkinson S. Factors which influence how nurses communicate with cancer patients, *Journal of Advanced Nursing* **16** (1991): 677-688.

[12] Mackintosh, S. and Bowles S. Evaluation of a nurse-led acute pain service; Can clinical nurses specialists make a difference? *Journal of Advanced Nursing* **25** (1997): 30-37.

[13] Corner J. Beyond survival rates and side effects; cancer nursing as therapy, *Cancer Nursing* **20** (1997): 3-11.

[14] French B. British studies which measure patient outcomes 1990-1994, *Journal of Advanced Nursing* **26** (1997): 320-328.

[15] Kirkevold M. Integrative nursing research-an important strategy to further the development of nursing science and practice, *Journal of Advanced Nursing* **25** (1997): 977-984.

[16] Redfern, S. and Norman I. Measuring the quality of nursing: a consideration of different approaches *Journal of Advanced Nursing* **15** (1990): 1260-1271.

[17] Thomas S. and Bond S. Measuring patients' satisfaction with nursing: 1990-1994, *Journal of Advanced Nursing* **23** (1996): 747-756.

[18] Marek K.D. Outcome measurement in nursing, *Journal of Nursing Quality Assurance* **4** (1989): 1-9.

[19] Mulhall M. Nursing research: our world or theirs, *Journal of Advanced Nursing* **25** (1997): 969-976.

[20] Sackett D.L., Rosenberg W.M., Gray J.A., Richardson W.S., Evidence based medicine: what it is and what it isn't, *British Medical Journal* **312** (1996): 71-72

[21] Fitch M. and Thompson L. Fostering the growth of research-based oncology nursing practice, *Oncology Nursing Forum* **4** (1996): 631-637.

[22] Fitch M. Creating a research agenda with relevance to cancer nursing practice, *Cancer Nursing* **19** (1996): 335-342.

[23] Sermeus W. Variabiliteit van verpleegkunding verzorging in algemane ziekenhuizen. Doctoraal proefschrift School Maatschappelijke Gezondheidszorg, KU Leuven (1992).

[24] Richarson A. and Ream E. The experience of fatigue and other symptoms in patients receiving chemotherapy, *European Journal of Cancer Care* **5** (Suppl 2) (1996): 24-30.

[25] Winningham M. et al, Fatigue and the cancer experience: the state of the knowledge, *Oncology Nursing Forum* **21** (1994): 23-36.

[26] Richardson A. Fatigue in cancer patients: a review of the literature, *European Journal of Cancer Care* **4** (1995): 20-32.

[27] Coates Abraham A.S. & Kaye SB. On the receiving end - patient perception of the side effects of cancer chemotherapy, *European Journal of Cancer and Clinical Oncology* **19** (1983): 203-208.

[28] Nerenz D. et al, Factors contributing to emotional distress during cancer chemotherapy, *Cancer* **50** (1982): 1020-1027.

[29] Rhodes V.A., Watson V.M., Hanson B.M. Patients' descriptions of the influence of tiredness and weakness on self care abilities, *Cancer Nursing* **11** (1988): 186-194.

[30] Tierney A., Taylor J., Closs J. A study to inform nursing support of patients coping with chemotherapy for breast cancer, Department of Nursing Studies, University of Edinburgh (1989).

[31] Fobair P. et al, Psychosocial problems among survivors of Hodgkins disease, *Journal of Clinical Oncology* **4** (1986): 805-814.

[32] Nail P. Coping with intracavitary radiation treatment for gynaecologic cancer, *Cancer Practice* **1** (1993): 218-224.

[33] Oberst M.T., Hughes S.H., Chang A.S., McCubbin M.A. Self-care burden, stress appraisal and mood among persons receiving radiotherapy, *Cancer Nursing* **14** (1991): 71-78.

[34] King K.B., Nail L.M., Kraemer K., Strohl R.A., Johnson J.E. Patients' descriptions of the experience of receiving radiation therapy, *Oncology Nursing Forum* **12** (1985): 55-61.

[35] Quesada J., Talpaz M., Rios M. Clinical toxicity of interferons in cancer patients: a review, *Journal of Clinical Oncology* **4** (1986): 234-243.

[36] Piper B.F., Rleger P.T., Brophy L., Haeuber D., Hood L.E., Lyver A., Sharp E. Recent advances in the management of biotherapy-related fatigue, *Oncology Nursing Forum* **16**(Supp) (1989): 27-34.

[37] Skalla K., Lacasse C. Patient education for fatigue, *Oncology Nursing Forum* **19** (1992): 1537-1541.

[38] B. Cimprich, Development of an intervention to restore attention in cancer patients, *Cancer Nursing* **16** (1993): 83-92.

[39] Nail L. and King K. Fatigue...a side effect of cancer treatments, Seminars in Oncology **3** (1987): 257-262.

[40] Winningham M. et al, Response of cancer patients on chemotherapy to a supervised exercise programme, Medicine and Science In Sports and Exercise **17** (1985): 292.

[41] Piper B. Alterations in energy: the sensation of fatigue. In: Baird et al (eds), Cancer Nursing, WB Saunders, Philadelphia 1991.

[42] Irvine D., Vincent L., Graydon J.E., Bubela N., Thompson L. The prevalence and correlates of fatigue in patients receiving treatment with chemotherapy and radiotherapy, *Cancer Nursing* **17** (1994): 367-378.

[43] Varrichio V. Selecting a tool for measuring fatigue, *Oncology Nursing Forum* **12** (1985): 122-127.

[44] Boyle S. Assessing mouth care, *Nursing Times* **88** (1992): 44-46.

[45] Daeffler R. Oral hygiene measures for patients with cancer III, *Cancer Nursing* (1981): 29-35.

[46] Dodd M.J., Larson P.J., Dibble S.L., Miaskowski C., Greenspan D., MacPhail C., Hauck W.W., Paul S.M., Ignoffo R., Shiba G. Randomised clinical trial of Chlorhexidine versus placebo for prevention of oral mucositis in patients receiving chemotherapy, *Oncology Nursing Forum* **23** (1996): 921-927.

[47] Krishnasamy M. Oral problems in advanced cancer, European Journal of Cancer Care **4** (1995): 173-177.

[48] Turner G. Oral care for patients who are terminally ill, *Nursing Standard* **8** (1994): 49-56.

[49] Sweeney M.P., Bagg J. Oral care for hospice patients with advanced cancer, *Dental Update* December (1995): 424-427.

[50] Wallace K.G., Koeppel K., Senko A., Stawiazk K., Thomas C., Kozar K. Effect of attitudes and subjective norms on intention to provide oral care to patients receiving antineoplastic chemotherapy, *Cancer Nursing* **20** (1997): 34-41.

[51] Daeffler R. Oral hygiene measures for patients with cancer I, *CancerNursing* (1980): 347-356.

[52] Moore J. Assessment of nurse-administered oral hygiene, *Nursing Times* **91** (1995): 40-41.

[53] Sweeney M.P., Bagg J., Doig P., McGill M., Milligan S., Malarkey C. Provision of mouthcare by nursing staff for cancer patients in Scotland: current status and the role of training, NTResearch **1** (1996): 389-395.

[54] Little J. Head and Neck cancer: oral care during radiotherapy, *Nursing Standard* **10** (1996): 39-42.

[55] Graham K.M., Pecorara D.A., Ventura M., Meyer C.C. Reducing the incidence of stomatitis using a quality assessment and improvement approach, *Cancer Nursing* **16** (1993): 117-122.

[56] Madeya M. Oral complications from cancer therapy: part 2-Nursing implications for assessment and treatment, *Oncology Nursing Forum* **23** (1996): 808-819.

[57] Hogan C. Cancer nursing: the art of symptom management, *Oncology Nursing Forum* **24** (1997): 1335-1341.

[58] Eilers J., Bergen A.M., Petersen M.C. Development, testing and application of the oral assessment guide, *Oncology Nursing Forum* **15** (1988): 325-330.

[59] Fessele K.S. Managing the multiple causes of nausea and vomiting in the patient with cancer, *Oncology Nursing Forum* **23** (1997): 409-415.

[60] Joss R.A., Brand B.C., Buser K.S., Cerney T. The symptomatic control of cytostatic drug-induced emesis. A recent history and review, *European Journal of Cancer* **26** (1990): S2-S8.

[61] Laszlo J. Nausea and vomiting as a major complication of cancer chemotherapy, *Drugs* **25** Suppl 1 (1983): 1-7.

[62] Martin M. Myths and realities of antiemetic treatment, *British Journal of Cancer* **66** Suppl 19 (1992): S46-S51.

[63] Hogan C.M., Grant M. Physiologic mechanisms of nausea and vomiting in patients with cancer, *Oncology Nursing Forum* **24** Suppl (1997): 8-12.

[64] Troesch L.M., Blust C., Rodehaver G., Delaney E.A., Yanes B. The influence of guided imagery on chemotherapy-related nausea and vomiting, *Oncology Nursing Forum* **20** (1993): 1179-1185.

[65] Rhodes V.A. Nausea, vomiting and retching, *Nursing Clinics of North America* **25** (1990): 885-900.

[66] McMillan S.C. Pain and pain relief experienced by hospice patients with cancer, *Cancer Nursing* **19** (1996): 298-307.

[67] Zimmerman L., Story K.T., Gaston-Johansson F., Roules J.R. Psychological variables and cancer pain, *Cancer Nursing* **19** (1996): 44-53;

[68] Ho R.S.C. Pain in the cancer patient, *CA: A Journal for Clinicians* **44** (1996): 259-261.

[69] World Health Organisation, Cancer pain relief and palliative care. Report of a WHO Expert Committee. WHO Technical Support Series 804 WHO, Geneva, Switzerland (1990).

[70] Wallace K.G. Analysis of recent literature concerning relaxation and imagery intervention for cancer pain, *Cancer Nursing* **20** (1997): 79-87.

[71] Hanks G.W. Problem areas in pain and symptom management for cancer patients: case study and analysis, *Journal of Pain and Symptom Management* **9** (1995): 116-170.

[72] Miaskowski C. The deleterious effects of unrelieved cancer pain on patient outcomes. In: C. Miaskowski (ed), Helping patients manage cancer pain: challenges and opportunities. Discovery International, Deerfield (1997).

The WISECARE Environment

Derek Hoy

1 Introduction

As a starting point, the following is a statement of the 'challenge' the WISECARE tools attempt to solve: *Design and develop a computer-assisted system for supporting the delivery of efficient and effective nursing care, for use by clinical nurses and nurse managers at the point of care.* We can break this down into four key components: [1]

- The form of solution is a *'computer-assisted system'*, using existing information systems where possible, and adding facilities where these do not exist.
- The supported activity is *'supporting the delivery of efficient and effective nursing care'*, by recording patient characteristics (assessment data), clinical judgements (identified problems, evaluation of outcomes), and nursing actions, with the active support of feedback tools linked to appropriate knowledge bases.
- The users are *'clinical nurses and nurse managers'*, within the domain of oncology nursing, in the selected units of the Validation Sites.
- The level of support must be *'at the point of care'*, meaning the tools must be accessible and usable in the work area of the users.

1.1 Users

For the first phase of the project, WISECARE users were clinical nurses within oncology units in the five Validation Sites. Relevant characteristics were:

- registered nurse practitioners,
- nurse managers,
- different working languages (Dutch, English, Finnish and Swedish) and
- varying previous experience with computers.

1.2 Supported Activities

The main activities are: the recording of patient characteristics; recording judgements of need or outcome; and decision-making regarding the plan of care.
Table 1 illustrates the levels of patient data:

- atomic assessment data (descriptions, facts etc) and
- 'judgements' (diagnoses, problem statements, evaluation of outcomes etc).

Table 1 Levels of Patient Data

Patient characteristics		Care activity
Judgements	'Mucositis' 'Mouth better'	Nursing interventions 'encourage oral fluids'
Assessment data	'Sore gums' 'Chemotherapy...'	...

To do this the system must allow the nurse to start or edit a specific patient record, record assessment data, descriptions of problem, outcomes, and interventions. This must be done in a secure way, maintaining confidentiality and data integrity.

The system must offer access to appropriate knowledge bases to speed up or guide the nurse user in doing what they want, for example protocols or research-based reviews.

1.3 Level of Support

The tools must be accessible and usable in the clinical areas where the users work. Access will depend on the positioning, number of terminals, and level of use of workstations. Usability will be a feature of the tools and the attention to user requirements and fitness for tasks.

1.4 Form of Solution

The Validation Sites had varying level of computer-based systems, and for most of the project there was no Validation Site with a clinical system for routine use by nurses.

Yet it is clear that WISECARE aims to use data in clinical systems. To that extent, the project is complementary to the ongoing development of clinical systems, and stimulating the use of clinical data. It could be argued that the Validation Sites represent a fair sample of clinical practice across Europe, as it is still a minority of Sites that have clinical systems for nursing use. Reviews of nursing systems in the UK for example have indicated serious problems in those that have been used.

WISECARE aims to 'learn from the best, and improve the rest'. The WISECARE tools must:

- provide support from shared knowledge bases;
- help with the maintenance of the nursing record;
- support the aggregation of data across Sites and systems;
- provide analysis of this data;
- feed the results into a knowledge base; and
- present this in a meaningful way (with other relevant data) to users.

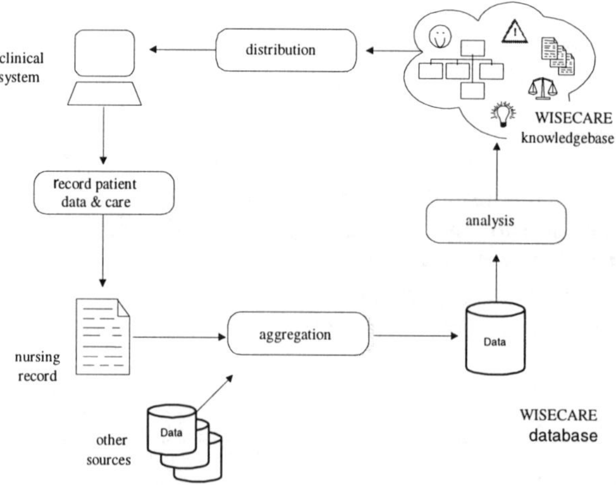

Figure 1   The WISECARE Data Cycle

1.5 The WISECARE Cycle

This cycle of data collection, analysis and feedback can be summarised in Figure 1. The left side of the cycle takes place at the Validation Sites, while the right side is done by the WISECARE consortium.

2 Summary of Validation Site Survey

A questionnaire survey was carried out, with follow-up communication via phone, email, and one Site visit. Table 2 to Table 7 show the results.

Table 2 Nursing Data related to Individual Patients

data	record system	coding scheme
nursing assessment	all Sites using paper	One Site had local scheme. Others free text
problem or nursing diagnosis	One Site not recording. Others using paper	None
goal or expected outcome	One Site not recording. Others using paper	None
interventions	One Site use Activity Module. Others using paper	One Site used local scheme and National NMDS. Others free text
evaluations	One Site not recording. Others using paper.	None

Table 3 Other Scales/Measures used

Norton pressure sore risk assessment.   Pain scales (varying).   Glasgow Coma Scale.   Discomfort Scale.   **** None used consistently across Sites. ****

Table 4 Other Data related to Individual Patients

data	record system	coding scheme
medical diagnosis	All recorded in computer-based systems	ICD9 or ICD10
medical procedure	All recorded in computer-based systems	varies: Belgian scheme, OPCS (UK), NCSP (FI)
DRG (Diagnosis Related Grouping)	All recorded in computer-based systems	to be confirmed
medication	All use paper records	
admission date	All recorded in computer-based systems	
discharge date	All recorded in computer-based systems	
age	All recorded in computer-based systems	
sex	All recorded in computer-based systems	

Table 5 Management Data

data	record system	coding scheme
Nursing workload or patient dependency	All different. 3 computer-based.	Local, or 1 San Joaquin
Nursing staffing levels	1 paper-based, 3 computer-based.	

Table 6 Do Nurses involved in WISECARE have access to...

standalone computers	-
locally-networked computers	all had access to networked computers, using MS Windows, 3.11 or 95.
computers connected to the internet	3 Sites had access available.

Table 7 Computer-Based Systems

Systems and suppliers	Various. None held clinical nursing data. Some used by nurses for ordering tests and retrieving laboratory results. All others were part of Hospital Information System/Patient Administration Systems and held patient demographic/episode data and case-mix data that was mainly medical.
Access to nursing staff (is it used by RNs, in all areas in the test Site, number of terminals)	All had ward-based terminals.
Database used (proprietary, Oracle, Sybase...)	Sybase, M/SQL, Oracle.
Are there tools for taking data/reports from the system?	All had reporting tools, though support required from IT staff except for standard reports.
Plans for further development in next 2 years	2 Sites had plans to implement nursing systems within the next 2 years, but only 1 Site was near achieving this by the end of the project.

3   The Role of Clinical Vocabularies and Classifications

3.1 Vocabularies and WISECARE

There are two quite different requirements in the WISECARE cycle.
- recording specific clinical characteristics, patient care, and data describing the nursing resource; and
- analysis of aggregated data, and linking of knowledge bases.

The first requirement needs a detailed, flexible vocabulary with terms that are natural to the clinical user. The second requires a more controlled vocabulary, with definitions and some hierarchical structure to support analysis at varying levels of detail. See next Chapter on Classification Systems.

3.2 Validation Site Findings

The Validation Sites were still recording most clinical nursing data using free text in paper records. Where data was more formalised, it was still using local coding schemes or single-purpose scales or other measures, for example pain assessments.

4   System Architectures

It is increasingly accepted that any non-trivial information system is best considered on a modular basis, separating out the levels. A simple three-tier architecture served as a logical model for our planning (see Figure 2).

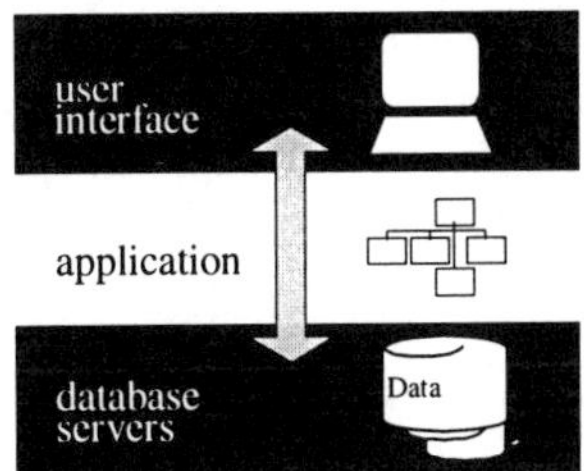

Figure 2   A simple Three-tier Architecture

4.1 Validation Site Findings

As mentioned earlier, nursing records at the Validation Sites were paper-based. Other relevant data, for example patient demographics, medical diagnosis, were mainly held in computer databases and managed by other systems. This data was accessible through reporting tools.

5   Options for WISECARE

Given the absence of suitable clinical systems for WISECARE nurses, some development of tools was necessary. There were some severe constraints on the possible choices. Firstly, using an available commercial system was not possible because:
- some Sites already had contracts with existing (different) suppliers;
- there were not resources within the project to cover costs of procurement and
- there were not resources at all the Validation Sites to support implementation and support of a 'large' system.

Other important constraints were:
- no internet access at some Sites, which ruled out a distributed system; and
- very poor information services support at some Sites, which meant that a solution must be very simple to install and maintain.

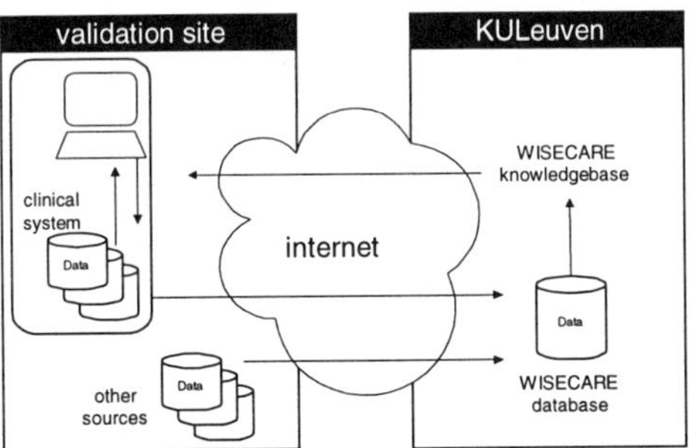

Figure 3   The Internet as Communication Medium

For these reasons, it was decided to develop a specific set of tools for WISECARE, designed on a modular basis, with separate interface and application logic. Relational database management systems are standard now, and the Validation Sites all held some relevant data on them. WISECARE could use RDBMS, and draw in this other data via extraction tools, or by direct query of data (with appropriate control to ensure data protection). For the external links between each Validation Site and the WISECARE centre responsible for processing and change control of the knowledge base material, the internet could be used as a carrier medium, again given appropriate controls to ensure data protection (see Figure 3).

References

[1]   Newman MN, Lamming MG. Interactive System Design. Harlow: Addison-Wesley, 1995.

Part II

Planning and Design

WISECARE
W. Sermeus et al. (Eds.)
IOS Press, 2000

Classification Systems and their Applicability to the Needs of Oncology Nurses

Nora Kearney, Morven Miller

1   Introduction

The development of nursing science has resulted in the emergence of knowledge that attempts to define the unique contributions made by nurses to the promotion of health across the life span [1]. Although it is crucial that the nursing contribution to clinical effectiveness is identified, to date this agenda has been virtually medically dominated [2]. It could be suggested that nursing's unique contribution to contemporary health care could be identified through organising nursing concepts in a way that would facilitate their utilisation and understanding. The lack of a system or language that makes explicit what nurses 'do' has resulted in nursing's invisibility within health care systems with its value and importance being unrecognised and unrewarded [3]. However, recognised or not, clinical judgements, decisions and classifications are a part of professional nursing practice. Within this context, classification systems may provide an element of organisation, linking patient problems, nursing interventions and patient outcomes.

The work to classify nursing began in earnest in the early 1970s with the development of Gebbie and Lavin's [4] nursing diagnoses and this work has evolved through various endeavours into a number of nursing classification systems. These include the North American Nursing Diagnosis Association (NANDA) [5], the International Classification of Nursing Project (ICNP) [3], The Omaha Classification System (OCS) [6], the Nursing Intervention Classification System (NIC) [7] and the Home Healthcare Classification (HHC) [8].

Through review of pertinent literature and reflection on experience gained during the WISECARE project, this report will explain the rationale behind the recent drive towards classification systems, define the various types of systems that exist and explain the development and advantages of the classification system utilised within the WISECARE project. To conclude, it will offer suggestions regarding the applicability of classification systems to the needs of oncology nurses.

2   Why have Classification Systems been developed?

The development of classification systems has previously been described as abstract theorising that has little to do with the real practice of nursing [9]. However, that practising nurses often fail to recognise both the complexities and intellectual underpinnings of their practice [10] encourages the movement towards developing a universal language that describes clinical judgements made by nurses. Clark and Lang [3] have identified four worldwide developments that further highlight the need for a systematic orientation to care:

- The increased use of IT in health care to sort and classify information makes the use of classification systems possible.
- Increasing emphasis on cost constraints within health care calls for the use of sound, reliable information to be used for local, national and international comparisons.
- Increased use of medical classification systems such as International Classification of Disease and Diagnosis Related Groups to organise health care is leading to decisions based on disease-orientated medical classifications.
- Nursing's goal to control its own work and practices.

3   What are Classification Systems?

Classification systems, like information technology, are best not thought of as a tool, but as a 'tool for making tools'. They can be used to build useful tools, for example, to help nurses in different clinical settings improve practice through comparing data. While their specific purposes can vary, they generally aim to describe nursing practice, what nurses do (nursing interventions) in relation to specific patient conditions (nursing diagnoses) with which effect (nursing outcomes). As such, they aim to support the understanding that informed practice is good practice. However, it is paradoxical that the simplest classification system for people, natural language, is the most complex model for technology to process. This paradox is at the heart of current classification systems, in that to develop tools that are simpler and more transparent in use, the necessary systems are becoming increasingly sophisticated and complex.

That classification systems provide standard descriptions and a universal language to describe nursing practice is indisputable. Behind this work is the belief that data can flow from clinical records to meet demands for aggregated or summarised data for a variety of other purposes such as local or area audit and strategic planning. While the simplicity of this vision makes the use of classification systems attractive for the nursing profession, myriad complexities lurk behind the idea of a 'common language'. Ingener [11] provided a categorisation of health care vocabularies that may be useful when evaluating classification systems.

Natural language is the most common representation of informal communication used in, for example, clinical conversations and hand written care plans. While natural language is a very powerful representation and requires no change in the way we think about information, it is not only difficult to analyse but also not well suited for purposes other than describing day-to-day nursing care. This leads us to consider the use of lists within classification systems. However, in constructing a list it becomes obvious that the number of terms actually needed to describe nursing care is unmanageable. A cascading dialogue could be used to enhance their effectiveness, for example, select a problem, generate a list of possible goals, select a goal, generate a list of possible actions etc, however no mechanism exists for grouping terms, causing problems with organising, accessing, retrieving and analysing information. Taxonomic vocabularies are systems in which concepts are related using hierarchical relations, for example, 'is a' or 'is part of'. Examples of these are NANDA [5] and INCP [3]. These vocabularies provide a structure for retrieving and using data from automated systems and have been said to formalise and expand nursing knowledge about nursing practice, facilitate determining the cost of nursing, assist in appropriate targeting of resources and make explicit the role of nurses in health care. However, although the extensive number of concepts required to describe nursing care in any detail is unmanageable, restricting the scope of the vocabulary and using only general concepts may create unacceptable ambiguity. Additionally, vocabularies may be unnatural to use.

The problems of these three vocabularies in classification systems have led to increasing interest in alternative representations, using a combination of terms to connect concepts with links to express relationships between them. Combining concepts to provide large numbers of possible expressions may be more clinically meaningful.

Combinational vocabularies are the result of breaking down complex concepts into their component parts, making a list of them and then combining them according to a predefined template. However, despite their increased expressiveness, there is the problem of combinational explosion and the potential of creating nonsensical concepts. Furthermore, cross-referencing between concepts is difficult and the large number of potential synonyms makes the analytical ability of the representation questionable. Compositional vocabularies have attempted to overcome the difficulties associated with these less structured representations. These have been developed as a terminological language that provides a means of capturing the knowledge underpinning clinical terminology.

Considering the various vocabularies available for use in classification systems went some way to evaluating their meaningfulness for clinical practice, and devising an appropriate system for use within the project. This knowledge was complemented with an evaluation of classification systems in clinical practice.

4　The use of classification systems in clinical practice

While one cannot dispute the importance of worldwide communication between nurses, the fact that within the UK alone, nurses use very different language to describe similar patient problems, highlights the need to develop a common language in relation to nursing's own culture [12]. Without a universal language, nursing remains invisible within the health care system [3]. Nursing must systematically demonstrate that it alone brings particular skills that make a tangible difference to the outcomes of patient care [2], articulating its professional value and credibility. The use of classification systems may provide nursing with an identifiable structure, through which, patient problems, nursing interventions and subsequent patient outcomes can be linked to justify nursing's existence. Through focusing on what they do in the health care system rather than what they assist others to do, nurses may at last be able to establish themselves as health care providers in their own right [13]. Such a universal language will additionally lead to a clearer definition of the difference between professional and non-registered health care workers [14].

However, it is important to recognise that the vast majority of work regarding classification systems has been concentrated in the United States of America and although literature is available within Europe, it primarily targets an audience that is culturally, managerially and professionally different to both the UK and Europe [12]. Having said this, nursing diagnoses and classification systems have reached some European countries such as Sweden, Belgium and France [15,16,17]. Nevertheless, major transcultural issues should be considered before nurses agree to adopt classification systems wholeheartedly. These issues are not merely confined to diagnoses nurses make, but also to the language nurses use to make diagnoses within their cultural background. The ICNP may offer a solution to this as it is not only a classification of nursing diagnoses, interventions and outcomes, but also a unifying framework for the parallel efforts of existing classifications [18]. However, Hogston [12] believes to the contrary, indicating that cross-referencing and mapping, while solving the problem of cultural differences, would result in diversification as opposed to unification. Ultimately, participation is required by many scholars and clinicians in the global nursing community to take the initiative and move away from relying on medical interventions and outcomes. In not doing so, the impact of nursing care will remain largely undocumented, unmeasured and invisible.

Although it is difficult to attribute particular patient outcomes exclusively to the intervention of one member of the health care team, the structure that is brought to nursing care through the use of classification systems demonstrates the role of nursing to other health professionals and so may enhance collegial relationships and lessen tension between nursing and other disciplines [19]. Furthermore, one could argue that improved communication and understanding between nurses themselves enhances the structure of their work together, so making it more visible. Improved communication, understanding and recognition from both within and witout the nursing profession may impact positively on morale and recruitment.

Although Hyslop [20] criticised the classification because of their obscure format, others have argued that classification systems have specifically adopted this to allow diagnoses to be easily altered depending on whether they are actual, potential, limitations, excesses or deficits by merely altering the wording and so preserving the diagnosis intact [21]. Such standardisation will add to the sum of knowledge as problems of ambiguity and communication are overcome allowing nurses to compare outcomes across populations, settings and caregivers [22] promoting shared understanding [5].

Shared understanding and enhanced communication is also essential between nurses and patients and one could suggest that the unwieldy nature of established classification systems would compromise their incorporation into care plans aimed at sharing information with patients and involving them in their care. Furthermore, the extent to which a standardised classification system can meet the needs of each and every individual patient can be questioned. Indeed, some of the most distressing patient problems are not acknowledged within classification systems [21]. This apparent lack of recognition of patients' perceptions may jeopardise the inherent quality that characterises nurse-patient relationships. Nurses must seriously consider this potential problem before unconditionally accepting specific classification systems.

Despite its tremendous responsibility, to date nursing has little acknowledged power. Miller [23] described power as the ability to influence and change the behaviour of others and make decisions regarding care. Optimistically, through organising knowledge, providing a structure for development of nursing standards and defining patient outcomes, classification systems empower nurses by making nursing more 'visible'. This empowerment offered by classification systems in making nursing visible could also extend into the realms of measuring workload. Halloran [24] illustrated that variation in nursing workload was better explained by the patients' nursing conditions, through the use of classification systems, as opposed to medical conditions. This suggests that despite criticisms regarding a lack of sensitivity of classification systems, nursing care time is better predicted by patients' nursing conditions or problems. Indeed, costing care according to nursing classification systems takes into consideration nursing's unique knowledge and expertise and identifies specific contributions of nurses to patient care [19]. Additionally workload measurement and management systems organised around nursing classification systems will illustrate the value of nursing services that treat health problems differently from medical diagnoses, identify nursing staff needed to provide care and assist with nursing budgets [19].

However, the very role of the nurse as a diagnostician remains a contentious issue in contemporary health care. The term 'diagnosis' remains inseparable in some minds from medicine and ill health. The implementation of nursing diagnoses in the USA brought a strong backlash from medical staff who feared nurses were overstepping the boundaries of traditional medical responsibilities [21]. Indeed, NANDA's focus on symptomatology and strong physiological base mimic the traditional medical model [21]. Nurses must surely strive to ensure that all facets of life, physiological, psychological, social, spiritual and economic, are incorporated within classification systems.

Despite these known advantages and disadvantages of established classification systems and the variety of health vocabularies with which to communicate, it was acknowledged that to successfully accomplish the project's aims, a systematic approach was essential for gathering clinical information. Three reasons can be given for the need of this systematic approach.

- Integration of IT into cancer nursing to collect clinical information in itself required an element of categorisation and standardisation.
- Facilitation of comparisons between Clinical Sites and populations called for a universal standardised language to ensure successful communication.
- Identification of the unique contribution of nurses would be facilitated through a systematic approach to organising care.

5   The Use of Classification Systems within the WISECARE Project

Despite acknowledging the benefits of standardisation of classification systems, personnel involved in the project appreciated that classification systems are highly dependent on their purpose: why and how they will be used. Noting that the system for the WISECARE project would have to be of value for nursing, they concluded that it must meet the two criteria of being useful and usable. Firstly, to be useful it must be relevant to the task and contain relevant features in a form appropriate for the intended task. Secondly, to be usable, it must match the capacity of its users to use it, support processing by allowing its manipulation and match the context of its use, for example, by being usable on available media, supporting an appropriate level of error and not being too time-consuming.

Consequently, established classification systems such as NANDA or ICNP, were inappropriate for implementation within the project. It was believed that their lack of specificity and inherent rigidity would compromise the focus of the project and be neither particularly useful or usable for the nurses involved. Consequently, three established questionnaires with set responses were utilised to obtain both useful and usable information. One could argue, as suggested earlier, that they provided classification systems from which a useful classification tool was constructed that facilitated the aim of the project to enhanced communication between Clinical Sites to compare data and so improve practice.

The original tools selected were:
- The Oral Assessment Guide (OAG) [25] which is a concise, clinically useful tool comprising of 8 questions, developed through clinical expertise and literature review, to record and communicate oral cavity status and determine changes expected with stomatotoxic treatments. See annex 1.
- The Piper Fatigue Scale (PFS) [26] which is composed of 22 numerically-scaled items (0-10) which measure 4 dimensions of subjective fatigue, behavioural/severity, affective/meaning, sensory and cognitive/mood. Both subscales and total fatigue scores can be calculated. See annex 2.

- The European Organisation for Research and Treatment of Cancer Quality of Life Questionnaire (EORTC QLQ-C30) [27] which is a modular approach for evaluating quality of life. It incorporates 9 multi-item scales: 5 functional scales (physical, role, cognitive, emotional and social), 3 symptom scales (fatigue, pain, nausea and vomiting) and a global health and quality of life scale. Several single-item symptom measures are also included. The questionnaire takes, on average, 11 minutes to complete and patients generally require no assistance. See annex 3.

However, following a period of data collection it became apparent that these questionnaires were unwieldy and inappropriately lengthy for use in routine clinical practice. Poor patient compliance and clinical nurses resistance, coupled with a drive from data managers who believed only a small amount of information was being extrapolated from the data generated, forced alterations to the classification system in practice. While the OAG was left intact, the PFS was dropped from use and 7 specific questions that reflected the symptoms of pain, fatigue and nausea and vomiting were developed from the EORTC QLQ-C30 questionnaire. These alterations increased the focus of the project on specific patient problems while keeping intact the standardised nature of the language used. Using these standardised tools to develop a classification system for specific patient problems has provided nurses in each of the Clinical Sites with a common language in which to collect information in a standardised manner regarding specific patient problems. This has led to successful communication between Clinical Sites, avoiding the pitfalls of ambiguity and culture, with the aim being the generation of empirical data to describe nursing practice across Clinical Sites, patient populations, geographical areas and time. The screen below, Figure 1, illustrates the standardised format used to collect patient information and develop individual and global patient scores.

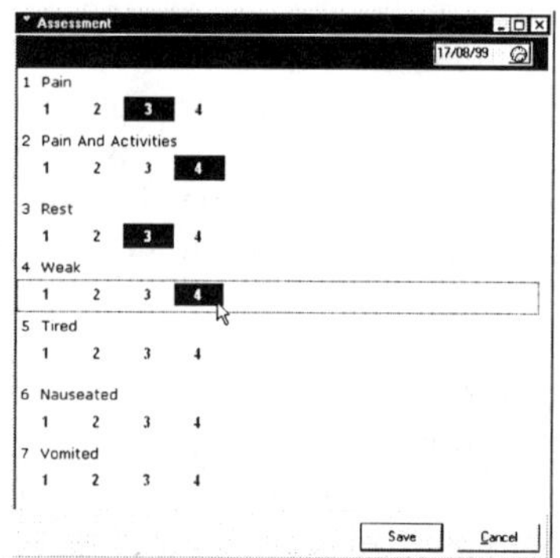

Figure 1   Standardised Data Collection Process

Utilising these tools as a type of classification has offered nurses involved in the WISECARE project the opportunity to develop a structure for the delivery of their nursing care regarding these specific patient problems. Focusing on the specific nursing domains of oral care, fatigue pain and nausea and vomiting will enable a link between identifying patient problems, implementing nursing interventions and evaluating patient outcomes to be made. Organising care in this systematic, structured way will allow nursing to become more 'visible'. The process of data collection, with the integral feature of 'instant feedback' facilitates the demonstration of the impact of nursing interventions on individual patient outcomes, going some way to prove the tangible difference that nursing interventions confer to patient outcomes. As can be seen below in Figure 2, the instant feedback graph is available for each of the specific patient problems, allowing nursing staff to:

- identify when a symptom is becoming problematic for patients
- implement nursing interventions accordingly
- systematically evaluate their impact.

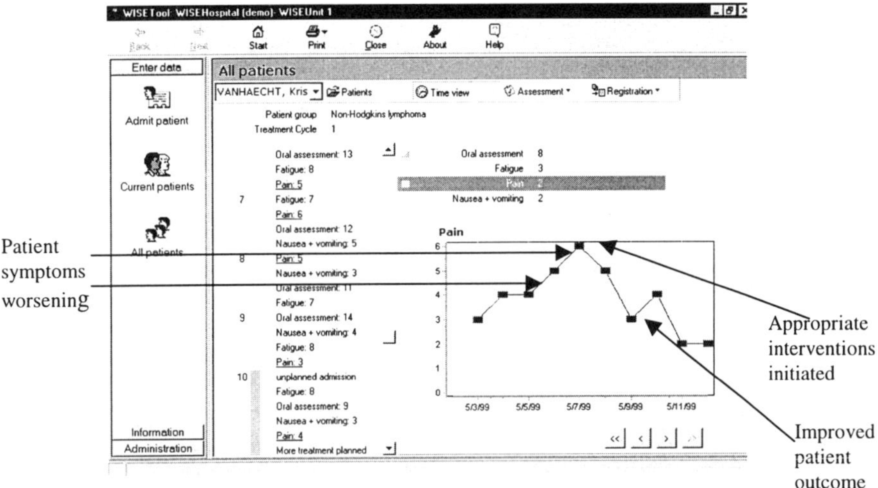

Patient symptoms worsening

Appropriate interventions initiated

Improved patient outcome

Figure 2   Instant Feedback Graph

Exercising this level of control over their nursing, empowers nurses to prove the value of their care. In addition, the use of these tools as a classification system has improved the communication between nurses and patients. Comments from patients have illustrated that their participation in the project has allowed them to be important contributors in their care, as opposed to passive recipients. They perceive that their feelings and experiences have been increasingly considered in the treatment plan. Completing the standard questionnaires would appear to have given patients a vehicle and a common language that allows them to express feelings or concerns that they may otherwise have found difficult to raise with members of the health care team, emphasising the importance of enhanced communication. Indeed, this enhanced communication has stretched beyond the problems specifically addressed within the WISECARE project, extending into specific areas of concern for individual patients. One potential explanation for this may be that the patient problems specifically addressed within the project, identified initially by clinically based nursing staff, reflect patients' primary concerns. See Chapter 1, Information Needs of Oncology Nurses. While standard classification systems, such as NANDA and ICNP, have been criticised for their lack of relevance to patients, tailoring the classification system used within the WISECARE project allowed the development of a system appropriate to both patients' and nurses' needs.

Standard established classification systems have been criticised for their medicalisation of nursing. However, the development of a specific structured system within the WISECARE project that focussed on established patient problems, amenable to nursing interventions, maintained the nursing focus throughout the project. Organising patient data through the use of standardised collection process has allowed nurses across each Site to increase their understanding of the importance of these problems to patients and highlight the importance of their subsequent nursing interventions. The use of a universal language has facilitated the comparison of patient outcomes across individual Sites and encouraged communication between countries regarding nursing interventions for specific patient problems. As a result, nurses importance as providers within contemporary health care has increased.

Thus, in relation to the WISECARE project, the classification systems used have been broad enough to serve the multiple purposes required by the different countries involved, simple enough to be regarded by nursing practitioners as a meaningful description of practice and a useful means of structuring practice, consistent with a conceptual framework but not dependent upon a theoretical framework and useable in a complementary or integrated way with existing nursing documentation. Based on these specific experiences of the WISECARE project, we can draw specific generalisations regarding the applicability of classification systems in meeting the needs of oncology nurses.

6   General Applicability of Classification Systems to the Needs of Oncology Nurses

To establish the relevance of classification systems in meeting the needs of oncology nurses, it is important to define exactly what these needs are. Across Europe, the impact of nursing on the quality of patient outcomes is rarely formally scrutinised [28]. However, in this era of cost-containment nurses must develop methods through which they can demonstrate their unique contribution to patient outcomes, highlighting the tangible effects of specific nursing interventions. The use of classification systems may provide a vehicle to allow nurses to do just that. Through a process of standardisation, classification systems provide nursing with a structure and process that fosters a specific, identifiable quality of care while also providing nurses with the means to evaluate the product of their care, that is, patient outcomes. Ultimately, nursing can be made more 'visible' and so professionally valuable. Establishing the link between nursing care and patient outcomes provides nursing with ammunition with which to justify its required resources.

Clark and Lang [3] succinctly describe the situation in nursing whereby, if we cannot name it, we cannot control it, finance it, teach it, research it or put it into public policy. The standardisation of language so necessary for classification systems is essential for oncology nurses. Kearney et al [28] have reflected on McVie's [29] proposition that highlighted the importance of greater dissemination of information and access to clinical and technical expertise in preventing many deaths from cancer across Europe. They contend that using clinical information and incorporating research findings in practice could harmonise the knowledge and expertise of cancer nurses across Europe and so enhance patients' experience of nursing care. Such harmonisation is essential when one considers the rapid pace of advances in cancer treatment and care. Utilising classification systems could enhance this process of harmonisation through addressing the problems of culture, language and geography. The use of a universal language would make explicit the nursing knowledge embedded in clinical practice and enhance communication and collaboration across boundaries.

Consequently, nurses are faced with the situation of demonstrating the effects and effectiveness of nursing [30] and it would seem that utilising a classification system may facilitate this. Based on the experience from the WISECARE project, one could argue that the systematic approach to nursing care, integral to the implementation of a classification system, is beneficial for effective provision, organisation and evaluation of nursing interventions and care. Using classification systems makes care measurable and evaluable, so ultimately visible. In making nursing visible, one can justify not only its existence but also its necessity within contemporary health care. However, while classification systems have their place and advantages, nurses should be cautioned against accepting them wholeheartedly into their practice. The disadvantages they bring such as rigidity, lack of relevance and specificity to patients and medicalisation of nursing make their unconditional acceptance into nursing practice questionable. Based on the experience of the WISECARE project, implementing the theory of classification into practice is beneficial for structuring, organising and evaluating nursing care, however developing a standardised system specifically tailored to the needs of the population that it aims to serve is essential. This leads the authors to recommend classification systems that meet the need for detail, flexibility and richly related concepts and yet still support analysis based on taxonomic hierarchy. The model for data collection and feedback is an example of such a classification system. Such a model should be regarded as software: complex representations that are processed by computers, underpinning well-designed interfaces, to facilitate the implementation of useful and usable classification systems.

7   Conclusion

The need to organise information systematically by grouping data according to common features and distinguish groups according to commonalties is intrinsic to the human mind [3]. If nursing is to grow, it must be orientated towards identifying its unique contribution to patient outcomes which in turn will empower the discipline. Classification systems, with their strength of communication, comparison and evaluation may provide the means by which the tangible effects of nursing can be proven. While their standardisation should be welcomed as nursing strives to prove itself within health care systems across Europe whose resources are undoubtedly stretched, the extent of the helpfulness of standardisation must be considered. Individualised care, the hallmark of quality nursing care, may be lost in the process of standardisation. Through the experience gained from the WISECARE project, the authors contend that although standardisation is necessary for developing and maintaining links across the boundaries of Europe, the complexity of human nature, the culture bound nature of nursing and the specificity required by each individual nursing speciality means that classification systems should be tailored in a way that makes their implementation clinically meaningful. The classification system inherent within the WISETool incorporates each of the dimensions whilst maintaining the capacity to deliver individualised patient care.

References

[1]   Briody ME, Carpenito LJ, Jones DA & Fitzpatrick JJ. Towards further understanding of nursing diagnosis: an interpretation *Nursing Diagnosis* 1992; **3**(3): 124-129.
[2]   Antrobus S. An analysis of nursing in context: the effects of current health policy *Journal of Advanced Nursing* 1997; **25**: 447-453.
[3]   Clark J & Lang N Nursing's next advance: an international classification for nursing practice *International Nursing Reviews* 1992; **39**(4) 109-112.
[4]   Gebbie KM & Lavin MA. Classification of nursing diagnosis: proceedings of the first national conference St Louis: Mosby, 1975.
[5]   North American Nursing Diagnosis Association NANDA definition. *Nursing Diagnosis* 1990; **1**(2):50.
[6]   Martin K & Scheet N. The Omaha System: applications for community health nursing. WB Saunders: Philadelphia, 1992.
[7]   Moorhead SA, McCloskey J & Bulechek G. Nursing intervention classifications: a comparison with the Omaha and Home Healthcare classification. *Journal of Nursing Administration* 1993;**23**(10): 23-29.
[8]   Saba V. The classification of Home Healthcare nursing: diagnoses and interventions. *Caring* 1992; **11**(3): 50-57.

[9]   Clark J How nurses can participate in the development of the ICNP. *International Nursing Review* 1995; **43**(6): 2171-2174.

[10]   Carnevali DL & Thomas MD. Nursing diagnosis and treatment decision making: complex but learnable tasks In Diagnostic reasoning and treatment decision making in nursing JB Lippincott Company, Philadelphia 1993.

[11]   Ingenerf J. Taxonomic vocabularies in medicine. The intention of usage determines different established structures. Presented at Proceedings of the 8th World Congress on Medical Informatics, Amsterdam: North Holland, 1995.

[12]   Hogston R.   Nursing diagnosis and classification systems: a position paper *Journal of Advanced Nursing* 1997; **26**: 496-500.

[13]   Mason G & Webb C. Nursing diagnosis: a review of the literature *Journal of Clinical Nursing* 1993.

[14]   Matz MR, Green PT, Johnson S & Smith J. Nursing diagnosis: a mark of nursing's place in health care *Pennsylvania Nurse* 1998; **53** (6)10, 13.

[15]   Geissler EM. Nursing diagnosis of culturally diverse patients *International Nursing Review* 1991; **38** (5) 150-152.

[16]   Wake M, Murphy M, Affara FA, Lang NM, Clark J & Mortensen R. Towards and international classification for nursing practice: a literature review and survey *International Nursing Review* 1993; **40** (3) 77-80.

[17]   Buenza I, Boulton N, Ferguson C et al. Diversity and commonality in international nursing. *International Nursing Review* 1994; **41**(2): 47-56.

[18]   Wake M &Coenen A. Nursing diagnosis in the International Classification for Nursing Practice (ICNP). Nursing Diagnosis: *the Journal of Nursing Language and Classification* 1998; **9**(3): 111-118.

[19]   Roberts SL (1990) Achieving professional autonomy through nursing diagnosis and nursing DGRs *Nursing Administration Quarterly* **14**(4): 54-60.

[20]   Hyslop A. Are programs intelligent? Nursing Times 1987**; 83**(8) :56-58.

[21]   Webb C. ...Or two steps back *Nursing Times,* 1992; **88**(7): 33-34.

[22]   McCloskey & J Bulechek G. Nursing Interventions Classification Mosby, St Louis, 1992.

[23]   Miller JF. Coping with chronic illness: overcoming powerlessness FA Davis, Philadelphia, 1983.

[24]   Halloran EJ. Nursing workload, medical diagnosis related groups and nursing diagnoses Research in Health and Nursing 1985; **8**: 421-433.

[25]   Eilers J, Berger AM & Peterson MC. Development, testing and application of the oral assessment guide. *Oncology Nursing Forum* 1988; **15**(3): 325-330.

[26]   Piper BF, Lindsey AM, Dodd MJ, Ferketich S, Paul SM & Weller S. The development of an instrument to measure the subjective dimension of fatigue. In management of Pain, Nausea and Fatigue Funk SG Torniquist EM Champagne MT Copp LA Wiese RA (Eds) Springer Publishing Company: New York,1989.

[27]   Aaronson N, Ahnedzai S, Bergman B, Bullinger M, Cull A, Duez N, Fiiberti A, Fletcher H, Fleischman S, de Haes J, Kaasa S, Klee M, Osoba D, Razari D, Rofe P, Schraube S, Sneeuw K, Sullivan M & Takdea F. The European Organisation for the Research and Treatment of Cancer QLQ-C30: a quality of life instrument for use in clinical trials in oncology. *Journal of the National Cancer Institute* 1993; **85**(5): 365-376.

[28]   Kearney N, Campbell S & Sermeus W Practising for the future: utilising information technology in cancer nursing practice European *Journal of Oncology Nursing* 1998; **2** No 3, 169-175.

[29]   McVie JG Current areas of treatment. *Seminars in Oncology* 1996; **23** Supp 1: 1-3.

[30]   Bond S & Thomas L. Issues in measuring outcomes of nursing *Journal of Advanced Nursing* 1992; **16** 1492-1502.

Organisation of the Database

Derek Hoy

1 Introduction

This section describes the design of the database, which formed the WISECARE 'data-warehouse'. That is, the database, which held the data, collected from the WISECARE sites, supported the analysis phase, and subsequently the feedback tools. This database held data describing: patient characteristics, patient care activity, and resources.

The design of the database did not include data item definitions because the choice of what data would be collected was to be flexible, but *types of data item* were defined. The design did not depend on any particular classifications, but relied on use of a coded clinical vocabulary, which would allow classifications, to be used where required.

2 Design Goals

The method used in designing the WISECARE data warehouse is described in Kimball [1] and represented best practice to meet the project requirements. The steps were:
- identify the key business processes to be supported;
- identify the level of detail required by each process;
- design the 'fact table' for each process; and
- design the dimension tables which will support analysis.

The main clinical focus of WISECARE has been oncology. However, one validation site included a surgical unit, and other clinical areas may be involved in further work. It was a prime goal of the database design (and all the WISECARE tools) that they would be applicable across any area of health care.

2.1 Supporting Service Processes

The term 'business' is regarded with distrust by some health service staff, so we might talk instead about *'service processes'*. These are the key activities done by WISECARE users that we expected our tools to influence.

From the preliminary statement of user requirements, we identified three key processes:
- clinical care of the individual patient,
- monitoring the service to groups of patients and
- resource management.

2.2 Clinical Care

'Elsie Stork is a 32 year old woman who has been admitted to the oncology department for high-dose chemotherapy. Following chemotherapy, her white blood cell count falls indicating neutropenia. Two days later she has pain in her mouth and shows other signs of

a mouth infection. Treatment is started to resolve it... '

This small piece of a clinical care scenario is typical in being very rich in information. Sub-processes might include; assessment, problem identification (diagnosis), goal setting, planning of interventions, and evaluation. It includes data describing:

- the person receiving care,
- the people giving it,
- where and when it happened,
- clinical facts (signs, symptoms, observations, and measurements, for example 'white cell count', ' pain in her mouth'),
- professional judgements (diagnoses, evaluations of outcome, for example 'neutropenia', 'mouth infection', 'mouth infection resolved'),
- care or treatment given; and
- the sequence of events.

2.3 Monitoring the service

'The nurses in the unit are reviewing their care of patients having severe mouth problems. A new anti-bacterial mouthwash product is available, and they want to consider the possible benefits if mouth infections could be resolved quicker. They want to know the incidence of mouth problems over the last 12 months, and any relation between type and severity of mouth problem, different forms of treatment, and prolonged length of stay in hospital...'

The expectation was that this kind of process could be supported through aggregation of data collected during clinical care, so that staff would not need to collect any extra data. Other data would be useful, for example patient episode data would describe length of stay.

2.4 Resource management

'The department management team are planning for next year, and want to see if changes in the case mix require some re-allocation of the budget. There seems to be some variation within the case-mix of patients, and there is some interest in whether nursing data might explain this. If so, it could lead to more accurate indicators of cost, and might suggest a change in the nursing skill mix, and implications for continuing education...'

This process would require additional data describing unit staffing levels, staff demographics (such as grade or educational qualifications), DRG, costing data.

3   The Data Warehouse: the 'Star' of the Show

Anyone familiar with the complex data models used in relational database systems will know the difficulties they present when it comes to analysis of the data. To build a query requires 'joins' across many tables, a process which requires a considerable level of skill for anything other than a trivial analysis.

Other natural ways of looking at data are not well supported: for example 'show me the percentage of patients who had mouth problems in our unit over the last three months' would require the entry of a range of dates rather than selecting 'second quarter 1997'.

Data-warehouses for large commercial enterprises often use a star schema. The term 'star' is used because the design involves central 'fact tables' with a number of 'dimension tables' linked to them (Figure 1).

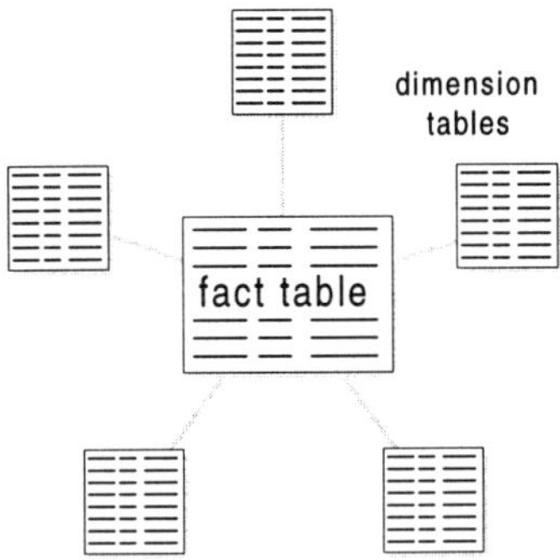

Figure 1   The star Schema used in a Data Warehouse

3.1 The Fact Table

The fact table is the hub of the data warehouse. The level of detail in the facts decides the lowest level of detail in the analysis. The aim here is to define a level of detail (the 'granularity' of the data) that is detailed enough, but no more than necessary.

For example, a clinical fact might include a description of a patient characteristic, or patient care characteristic, for a particular patient, made by a nurse, in a unit, at a certain time. To make that a little clearer, Table 1shows a simplified example.

Table 1   An Example of a Clinical Fact Table

Fact attribute	Example data	Note
Patient characteristic	'Red gums'	As above.
Patient	Patient number	See later section on confidentiality.
Nurse	Nurse number	As above.
Unit	Unit code	This would be unique for each unit, so would identify the hospital.
Time	Time code	See dimension table example below

3.2 Dimensions

The dimension tables form the constraints that will be used to query the fact table. They are likely to hold data which would be considered 'redundant' in an operational relational database, but which is included to make analysis easier and faster.

Time is a very common dimension. In the example above, why was there a time code and not just a time/date field? Frequently, queries on data are of the form: '*Show me the monthly totals of patients with red gums for the last year*'.

The calendar month can be calculated as part of the query, but this is not always practical so we could use a time dimension as described in Table2.

Using this, it becomes much simpler to make a query which joins the fact table and time dimension table on the time code attribute, and includes the month attribute from the dimension. An SQL[1] 'group by' month would give the required answer.

Using the example time dimension, we could query the incidence of mouth problems on public holidays, or weekends, if anyone was interested in such data.

---

[1] SQL is *Structured Query Language*, a standard for retrieving or manipulating data in relational database management systems.

Table 2 Time Dimension Table

Dimension attribute	Example data	Note
Time code	221	If the granularity of the fact table is to one day, then each day would have a time code.
Date	10/08/1998	
Day of the week	'Monday'	
Weekend	False	
Month	August	
Public holiday	True	This day is a public holiday!
Quarter	3	
Year	1998	

4   Proposed Design

4.1 Fact Tables

Three types of data were identified: patient descriptors; clinical activity; and resources. Patient descriptors included observation data and clinical judgements. This gave the data-warehouse greater flexibility. For example, measurement of outcomes could be done by analysis of assessment data (*'mouth pain-free'*, *'no inflammation'*), or by explicit evaluations (*'mouth infection resolved'*). Table 3 shows examples of these types of clinical data.

Table 3 Types of Data

Data type		Examples
Patient descriptors	Assessments, measurements, or observations + Judgements, diagnoses, goals, or evaluations	*Lack of energy* *Inflamed gums* *White Cell Count 4.2 $x10^9$/L* *Pain from suture line* *Infected wound* *Neutropenia* *Mouth infection not resolved* *Moderate fatigue*
Clinical activity		*Anti-bacterial mouthwash* *Mastectomy* *Chemotherapy*
Resources		*Nurse Andersen's 7.5 hours*

These three types of data are best reflected in three separate fact tables. The definitions follow.

4.2 Patient descriptors

Data might be collected in three formats:
- free text;
- single concepts; and
- compositional concepts.

Although free text is best avoided if data is to be aggregated for analysis, it may be necessary on occasion. For example, at the beginning of the project, the Piper Fatigue Scale was used. This is a 27-item measure, which uses scales (0-10) for most of its items. However, it has 4 open questions at the end, which had to be recorded as free text if this data was to be collected.

A 'single concept' is a term that is represented by one unique code in the WISECARE clinical vocabulary (described below).

Compositional concepts are coded and stored in parts, such as 'attribute' and 'value'. For example, 'White Cell Count' and '4.2 x10^9/L'. Numeric data otherwise requires a coded concept for each possible value, which is not realistic unless they cover a very restricted and predictable range.

Compositional representations add some complexity to the data, however they have advantages also:

- fit with structured data: Piper Fatigue Scale item 22 could be *'PFS22: able to remember'* (attribute) and *'3'* (value),

- helping analysis: all the scores (values) of *'PFS22: able to remember'* can be easily found, otherwise a search would have to compare each database record against a list of 11 codes representing all the possible scores and the results would require processed to extract the numeric scores,

- meeting standards: regarding electronic patient record structure and vocabulary[2].

A further attribute was added to support more complex compositional data: *'description_context'*. This allowed hierarchical nesting of records, for example, a Mouth Care Scale and score could be recorded. If it had a *description_key* of 362, then all the item scores entered could have *description_context* attribute of 362, allowing all the scores to be grouped together for subsequent processing.

There are a variety of data types that could be stored as values in this table. While WISECARE has used relational database technology, this needed to be dealt with explicitly. A common approach is to use a 'data type' field and use separate tables to hold the data, with one table for each data type.

An alternative simpler (though not very elegant) approach was used, with an explicit value field for each data type. This was used because: we could reduce the data types to three (free text, coded, and numeric); and we wanted to simplify the database and avoid the use of multiple tables and joins. Table 4 shows the design of the clinical fact table.

Table 4 Clinical Fact Table

Attribute name	Data type	Constraints	Note
description_key	integer	primary key not null	System Assigned Number (SAN)
description_attribute	char(12)	foreign key not null	
coded_value	char(12)	foreign key check (numeric_value is null and text_value is null)	Only one value attribute can be used
numeric_value	decimal(8,2)	check (coded_value is null and text_value is null)	Only one value attribute can be used. Standardised units are required.
text_value	char(255)	check (coded_value is null and numeric_value is null)	Only one value attribute can be used
time_code	integer	foreign key not null	
clinical_time_code	integer	foreign key not null	
staff_code	integer	foreign key not null	
unit_code	integer	foreign key not null	
patient_code	integer	foreign key not null	
episode	integer	foreign key not null	
description_context	integer	foreign key	

Some items that might be derived from patient episode data taken from validation site systems could be stored in this table rather than the episode dimension table (defined below), e.g. principal medical diagnosis, surgical procedure or DRG. The inclusion of this data in episode summaries is usually related to convenience for coding data sets for some central collection. It could be managed more flexibly by storing it in this fact table, where it could always be reunited with the episode details if required.

An important addition during the second phase of the project was the idea of 'clinical time'. To measure the significance of patient data items, it is necessary to relate them to some point in time. To do this, the project agreed that certain data items, e.g. chemotherapy, represented important clinical events. All clinical facts are therefore identified with the number of days since the last event for that patient. So an oral assessment score might be recorded as 4 days after the start of the last chemotherapy.

4.3 Clinical activity

This table is very similar to the previous, as it records activities done by a particular practitioner, to a particular patient, in a unit, at a particular time. The comments in the previous section apply equally here. Table 5 shows the design.

These activities are attributed to the patient, and there is no link between specific problems and interventions. This would be essential for an electronic patient record database, but for WISECARE it is not considered necessary: it is sufficient to know that an activity occurred at a particular time for this patient. Should this requirement change, an attribute would be added to this table linking records to the patient descriptor table using a '*description_key*'.

It should be noted that changes to the project protocols meant that activity data was not collected.

Table 5 Clinical Activity Table

Attribute name	Data type	Constraints	Note
activity_key	integer	primary key not null	System Assigned Number (SAN)
activity_attribute	char(12)	foreign key not null	
coded_value	char(12)	foreign key check (numeric_value is null and text_value is null)	Only one value attribute can be used
numeric_value	decimal(8,2)	check (coded_value is null and text_value is null)	Only one value attribute can be used
text_value	char(255)	Check (coded_value is null and numeric_value is null)	Only one value attribute can be used
time_code	integer	foreign key not null	
staff_code	integer	foreign key not null	
unit_code	integer	foreign key not null	
patient_code	integer	foreign key not null	
episode	integer	foreign key not null	
activity_context	integer	foreign key	

4.4 Resources

For WISECARE purposes, this is primarily concerned with the general nursing resource. An important distinction is between resource, which is patient-specific, which would be recorded in the activity table, and that which is not, and would be recorded as a general 'resource'.

This fits well with a flexible approach to costing. Deriving costing by analysis of resources used by a particular patient has the advantage of being based on more detailed data reflecting diversity of patient needs and service response. Whilst it is very attractive, it has serious limitations:

- nurses are 'multi-tasking', doing more than one thing at a time, and adding up all the activities may not be accurate;
- activities may appear more than once as they relate to more than one patient problem, so double-counting can occur; and
- either it relies on using data from the care plan, which may not be the care actually given; or
- the practitioner must keep updating the system to record what has been done.

This can be considered a 'bottom-up' approach, by adding up all the detailed use of resources to produce a total. An alternative is to use a 'top-down' approach, where the total costs (which are usually known with some accuracy) such as nursing staff costs are divided up in some way. The bottom-up data might be used to apportion the top-down costs.

The main requirement therefore was to record the variability in nursing staffing levels. The proposed design could record the hours worked by a particular staff member, for a unit, for a particular day. Data describing each member of staff could be stored in a separate dimension table, described below.

The inclusion of the *coded_value* attribute allows other resource types to have non-numeric values attached to them. The *resource_code* key can be used to join to the staff dimension table, or to other resource dimensions, providing the keys do not overlap. Table 6 describes the initial design.

Table 6 Resource Table

Attribute name	Data type	Constraints	Note
resource_key	integer	primary key not null	System Assigned Number (SAN)
resource_code	integer	foreign key not null	This would be a staff_code to record nursing hours
coded_value	char(12)	foreign key check (numeric_value is null and text_value is null)	Only one value attribute can be used
numeric_value	decimal(8,2)	check (coded_value is null and text_value is null)	Only one value attribute can be used
text_value	char(255)	Check (coded_value is null and numeric_value is null)	Only one value attribute can be used
time_code	integer	foreign key not null	
unit	integer	foreign key not null	

Table 7 Nursing Time Table

Attribute name	Data type	Constraints	Note
unit	integer	foreign key not null	
day	integer	foreign key not null	
hours24	integer	check (hours24 >= 0 and hours24 <= 24)	hours worked by nurse in previous 24 hours
nurse_level	integer	Check (nurse_level >= 1 and nurse_level <= 4)	4 levels of nurse are defined in the WISECARE data manual

As WISECARE progressed to collecting resource data, a protocol was designed which was based on nursing time and a patient acuity measure. See annex 5-6. The database design was modified to use two tables for these specific data items, rather than the more generic first design. Table 7 and Table 8 describe the designs actually used.

Table 8 Moffitt Scores Table

Attribute name	Data type	Constraints	Note
unit	integer	foreign key not null	
day	integer	foreign key not null	
hours24	integer	check (hours24 >= 0 and hours24 <= 24)	hours patient is in unit in previous 24 hours
WCPatient	boolean		is patient registered in WISECARE?
MoffittIndex	integer		
MoffittGrade	integer		

4.5 Dimensions

The three fact tables have key attributes for the following dimension tables:

- time;
- clinical time;
- patient;
- staff member;
- unit;
- episode; and
- clinical vocabulary.

The following tables describe each dimension.

Table 9 Time Dimension Table

Attribute name	Data type	Constraints	Note
time_code	integer	primary key not null	System Assigned Number (SAN)
time_code_date	date	not null	
day_of_the_week	integer	not null check (day_of_the_week between 1 and 7)	Integer number used to avoid having to put in days of week in several languages. Day 1 = Monday.
weekend	boolean	not null	True if day_of_the_week is 6 or 7.
month	integer	not null check (month between 1 and 12)	Integer number used to avoid having to put in months of year in several languages. 1 = January.
public holiday	boolean	not null	Need to be two records for any day that is a public holiday at *any* validation site.
quarter	integer	not null check (quarter between 1 and 4)	
year	integer	not null	

Table 10 Clinical Time Dimension Table

Attribute name	Data type	Constraints	Note
clinical_time_code	integer	primary key not null	System Assigned Number (SAN)
eventid	integer	foreign key not null	concept ID for last clinical event for a patient
event_days	integer	not null	number of days since last clinical event 0= no previous event

Table 11   Patient Dimension Table

Attribute name	Data type	Constraints	Note
patient_code	integer	primary key not null	System Assigned Number (SAN)
date_of_birth	date	not null	
sex	char(1)	not null check (sex in ('M','F'))	

Table 12   Staff Dimension Table

Attribute name	Data type	Constraints	Note
staff_code	integer	primary key not null	System Assigned Number (SAN)
date_of_birth	date	not null	
sex	char(1)	not null check sex in ('M','F')	
general_education	char(32)		not used
registration _code	char(32)		not used
post_registration_code	char(32)		not used
continuing_code	char(32)		not used

Table 13   Unit Dimension Table

Attribute name	Data type	Constraints	Note
unit_code	integer	primary key not null	System Assigned Number (SAN)
unit_name	char(255)	not null	
number_of_beds	integer	not null	
specialty_code	char(255)	not null	
validation_unit	boolean	not null	Used to distinguish between WISECARE validation units and later additional units
site_name	char(255)	not null	
country_code	char(2)	not null check (country_code in ('FI','UK','NL','SE'))	Uses 2 character ISO country codes

Table 14   Episode Dimension Table

Attribute name	Data type	Constraints	Note
episode_code	integer	primary key not null	System Assigned Number (SAN)
start_date	date	not null	
end_date	date	not null	Only completed episodes will be added to the data-warehouse
admission_type	char(32)		

4.6 Clinical vocabulary

WISECARE started with a requirement for 4 languages. The data-warehouse therefore used language-independent concepts, and data was stored using the concept codes. For display, a rubric was shown in the user's language. To achieve this, we could have used a set of tables: one table for each language. However, the maintenance of different tables would have been greater than just one.

We could also have stored multiple records in the table, with a 'language' attribute to allow the selection of the appropriate rubric. However, if the language attribute was not included in a query on the data, then multiple matches would result: one for each language. A less flexible approach was taken, with an attribute for each language, but this offered less chance of mistakes.

It was still possible to add other languages by replacing the entire vocabulary table as it was standard across WISECARE project sites. Classification attributes were not included in this table as standard. See section below for how this can be managed.

The addition of Slovenian and Greek required that all WISECARE software must handle alternative character sets.

Table 15   Lexicon Dimension Table

Attribute name	Data type	Constraints	Note
concept_code	char(12)	primary key not null	
ConceptName	char(128)	not null	default text identifier (based on English rubric)
FI_rubric	char(128)	not null	Finnish
NL_rubric	char(128)	not null	Dutch
SE_rubric	char(128)	not null	Swedish
UK_rubric	char(128)	not null	English
FR_Rubric	char(128)	not null	French (added later)
DA_Rubric	char(128)	not null	Danish (added later)
SL_Rubric	char(128)	not null	Slovenian (added later)
GR_Rubric	char(128)	not null	Greek (added later)

4.7 Treatment risks

During the second phase of the project, clinical indicators were added (fatigue, pain, nausea and vomiting, and mucositis). An important aspect of the work was to look at how risk of problems might be predicted. As treatments contributed greatly to variations in risk (e.g. chemotherapy treatments) a *treatment risks* dimension was added. This allowed analysis to group patients into risk-adjusted groups, dependant on their treatments. The Leuven Risk Assessment Scale is described in Chapter 2, Risk Assessment.

Table 16   Treatment Risk Dimension Table

Attribute name	Data type	Constraints	Note
concept_code	char(12)	primary key not null	
ConceptName	char(128)	not null	default text identifier (based on English rubric)
nv_risk	integer	check (null or (risk>=1 and risk<=3))	1= low, 2=medium, 3=high
oral_risk	integer	check (null or (risk>=1 and risk<=3))	1= low, 2=medium, 3=high
fatigue_risk	integer	check (null or (risk>=1 and risk<=3))	1= low, 2=medium, 3=high
pain_risk	integer	check (null or (risk>=1 and risk<=3))	1= low, 2=medium, 3=high

5   Other issues

5.1 Confidentiality

WISECARE had the following requirements for patient-related data:
- data must be attributed to an individual person;
- data regarding an individual must be linkable across repeated admissions to a WISECARE unit; and
- data sent to the WISECARE data warehouse must be able to be returned to a site if there are errors.

To achieve this it was necessary to have a patient identifier consistent across all admissions for the duration of the project. The danger was that the WISECARE data warehouse would then hold confidential data regarding individuals. To deal with this, it was made impossible to identify any individual from the data in the WISECARE data warehouse. The sensitive data items were: *patient name, local ID, WISECARE ID* and *date of birth.*

Patient name and *local ID* were only present on local data, on paper forms or a computer screen. They were used only to allow local staff to identify patients or data in a more user-friendly manner. They were removed from any data taken from the local WISECARE unit.

WISECARE ID was generated on first registration, by WISECARE system software, and was unique across all the WISECARE sites. It was used to identify a patient in the data warehouse. The WISECARE ID could not be used to access data in local clinical systems.

As the *date of birth* can be used to identify a patient, the day part of the date was removed. The date of birth was only used by WISECARE to calculate patient age, so accuracy to the nearest month was adequate. Removing the day makes this data much less likely to identify an individual

Discussion on confidentiality is usually focussed (rightly) on the patient. However, staff must have their confidentiality considered. When clinical data was recorded, a staff identifier was attached to ensure accountability. This identifier was confidential to the project. Staff identifiable data was only available to local staff, and following discussion and agreement regarding access control.

All local databases were encrypted, and encryption was also used when data was exported to the data-warehouse. Feedback tools also addressed the issue of confidentiality in accessing data from the data-warehouse.

Local WISECARE project members were responsible for ensuring that their sites met locally-accepted standards for security and confidentiality.

5.2 Populating the data warehouse

Data from the local WISETool installations was sent to Glasgow Caledonian University (GCU) and processed for addition to the data-warehouse before analysis at the Katholieke Universiteit Leuven (KUL).

5.3 Integrity

The unprocessed data provided by the sites, and the data-warehouse itself, was archived to ensure a backup was available should any data loss occur. Quality assurance was done by some automated cross-checking by queries on the data-warehouse.

5.4 Classification

Dimension tables can be customised to meet changing requirements. One use for this is to support heterogeneous data. For example, if WISECARE had needed to record more detailed data regarding an activity, such as medication administration, a modified clinical vocabulary could be used with added attributes to help analysis. This would leave the underlying fact tables holding the data unchanged.

In a similar way, classifications could be modelled using an added or modified dimension table. To aggregate data from detailed concepts to more general ones then the clinical vocabulary dimension table could be modified by adding a 'grouping' attribute. So if we needed to aggregate all mouth problems, then vocabulary entries such as '*gingivitis*', '*mouth infection*', '*glossitis*', '*oral thrush*' etc., could all have a grouping attribute set to '*mouth problem*'.

Standard classifications such as ICD10, the International Classification for Nursing Practice, North American Nursing Diagnosis Association diagnoses or the Belgian Nursing Minimum Data Set interventions could have been super-imposed on the data in this way.

5.5 Dependency on User Requirements

The data-warehouse was designed with flexibility as a high priority. WISECARE used an iterative approach to development. Inevitably, this led to an incremental definition of user requirements and modification was necessary over the course of the project. The design of the database supported all the required changes and was successful in its implementation.

References

[1]   Kimball R. The Data Warehouse Toolkit. John Wiley, New York, 1996.

[2]   CEN/TC251. Electronic Health care Record Architecture: Final draft 2. European Committee for Standardisation, Brussels, 1995.

Data Collection Manual

Nora Kearney, Morven Miller

1 Purpose of this Manual

The aim of this manual is to ensure the standardisation and smooth collection of data from both Validation and Demonstration Sites and will provide specific guidelines and instructions for data collection. Adhering to these guidelines as far as possible will ensure a successful final six months of data collection. Consequently, the feedback received will be meaningful and relevant to all participating Sites.

2 Aims of the Project

The final six months of data collection should see the following goals being achieved:
- The structured collection of focussed data from WISECARE patients using specific questions concerning pain, fatigue and nausea and oral status using the Oral Assessment Guide. The organised collection of data regarding patient acuity levels using the Moffitt tool and nursing resources.
- The meaningful feedback of data collected to date including: individual patients, all patients within each Validation Site and between Validation Sites. This feedback will be both ongoing and updated throughout this final six months of data collection.
- The successful communication and sharing of information between all Validation Sites using the WiseTool regarding their specific nursing interventions regarding the patient problems of pain, fatigue, nausea and vomiting and oral care. Review of feedback and comparison of patient outcomes across Sites will motivate nurses to compare and contrast nursing interventions across Sites.
- Access to all nursing staff involved in the project to up-to-date literature reviews and best practice guidelines regarding the patient problems of pain, nausea and vomiting, oral care and fatigue, via the WiseTool.

3 Data Collection

3.1 Clinical Data Collection

3.1.1 Patient Data Collection

This will focus specifically on the clinical indicators of pain, fatigue, nausea and vomiting and oral care. The three clinical indicators of pain, fatigue and nausea and vomiting will be assessed using only 7 questions, which focus on these patient problems. Patients will be asked to complete the questionnaires *once daily for 10 consecutive days* (day 1 being the start of treatment). This has been shown to be simple for patients to remember and has resulted in an increase in patient compliance

The Oral Assessment Guide (OAG) will be used to assess the fourth clinical indicator of oral status. It will be *completed prior to treatment and once daily from days 1-10* (day 1 being the start of treatment). Although designed to be completed by nursing staff, patients will be encouraged to complete the OAG as they will be required to do this following discharge until day 10 post-treatment.

To facilitate the comparison of data between Validation and Demonstration Sites, the questionnaire presented to patients must be standardised across all the Sites. Accordingly, the questionnaire that will be administered to patients can be found in annex 6. The introduction need only be used on the first occasion of each admission. On discharge patients will be given the remaining questionnaires to be completed and will be asked to return them in due course (e.g. when attending for next treatment). Again, to ensure standardisation across all Sites, the same Patient Prompt Sheet (see annex 7) should be given to all patients in all Validation and Demonstration Sites.

Feedback to the individual Sites regarding both the data already collected and subsequent data collected will be available during the following months. Two types of feedback will be available. Instant feedback will allow the generation of individual patient data regarding each clinical indicator in graph form whenever the data is entered to the WiseTool. Global feedback will be given on a regular basis following submission of data from each Site and will allow the comparison of patient outcomes for each of the clinical indicators across all clinical Sites. Specific dates have been allocated for clinical Sites to submit data for global feedback, however, if a Site submits data on more than these occasions, feedback will follow accordingly.

3.1.2   Nursing Resource Data Collection

This remaining data collection will include the collection of data regarding patient acuity via the Moffitt Tool, a validated oncology patient classification tool, and nursing resource data. The dates for this data collection have been randomly selected (Table 1). Data collection should occur at roughly the same time of day and be performed by the same member of staff if possible to ensure consistency in data generated.

Table 1   Dates for the Collection of Data

July	August	September	October	November	December
Fri 2nd	Thurs 5th	Thurs 2nd	Wed 6th	Fri 5th	Thurs 2nd
Tues 6th	Mon 9th	Fri 10th	Tues 12th	Fri 12th	Tues 8th
Mon 12th	Wed 18th	Fri 18th	Thurs 21st	Mon 15th	Thurs 16th
Fri 23rd	Tues 24th	Tues 21st	Mon 25th	Wed 24th	Tues 21st
Wed 28th		Mon 27th			Wed 29th

3.2 Nursing Interventions

Prior discussions have highlighted a strong need to keep the project focussed on nursing to maintain staff enthusiasm and patient participation in the project. Consequently communication and sharing of information is necessary between all Sites regarding their current nursing interventions for the specific patient problems of pain, fatigue, nausea and vomiting and oral care. Communication will be generated from the availability of data that compares patient outcomes between each Site that will be available to all Sites. Furthermore, recent comprehensive literature reviews with up-to-date best practice nursing interventions will be available to all nurses of the Sites via the WiseTool concerning each of the patient problems addressed within the project. Sharing knowledge in this way should result in the development of best practice guidelines and lead to the development of care packages.

4 Patient Groups and Sampling

A convenience sample of patients will be recruited over this final six-month period of data collection from each of the five Validation Sites and Demonstration Sites. The selected patient groups for WISECARE include:

- Lung cancer
- Osteosarcoma
- Non-Hodgkin's Lymphoma
- Breast Cancer
- Acute Lymphoblastic Leukaemia
- Acute Myeloid Leukaemia

5 Eligibility Criteria

Patient eligibility to WISECARE will be checked prior to registration.
Inclusion criteria:

- Patients of 17 years of age and older,
- Undergoing diagnostic surgery for either breast cancer, lung cancer, osteosarcoma or Non-Hodgkin's lymphoma,
- Pathologically confirmed diagnosis of: non-Hodgkin's lymphoma, breast cancer, osteosarcoma, lung cancer, acute lymphoblastic leukaemia or acute myeloid leukaemia,
- Admitted to a WISECARE unit for chemotherapy or surgery,
- Conscious and oriented (to allow completion of the questionnaires).

Table 2 Checklist of the Procedures to be performed when a Patient enters the Project

IS THE PATIENT REGISTERED WITH WISECARE?	
IF YES ↓	*IF NO* ↓
Patient WISECARE number will be marked on their nursing records ↓	Is the patient eligible (check eligibility criteria)? ↓
Patient will continue to be part of the project ↓	If yes does the patient give his/her informed consent (ensure the patient has received and had time to read the patient information sheet) ↓
Update admission details (e.g. treatment regimen, date of discharge etc)	Obtain written informed consent ↓
	Enter the patient's hospital number in order to register a new patient

6   Project Procedure

6.1 Patient Registration and Baseline Data

On the first admission to a WISECARE unit, a patient registration data set will be completed. This checklist shows the decisions to make on admission of a patient (Table 2).

Once registered the patient registration form will be completed. Additional information to be collected on admission and subsequent hospital admissions includes: Nursing interventions for oral care and questionnaire data regarding pain, fatigue and nausea and vomiting (both from previous and current admission).

Patient registration and baseline data will be entered in the electronic database. A WISECARE label should be attached to the nursing records in order to alert staff to a 'WISECARE' patient at subsequent hospital admissions.

6.2 Patient Data Collection

All patients recruited from each WISECARE unit will be asked to complete one assessment questionnaire days 1-10 of treatment, (day 1 being the start of treatment), consisting of the 7 questions from the sub-scales that address pain, fatigue and nausea and vomiting in the EORTC QLQ-C30 assessment tool and the OAG. Nurses must ensure that patients are thoroughly educated regarding the completion of the OAG.

Table 3 The Schedule for completing the Patient Assessment

	Fatigue, Nausea + Vomiting, Pain	Oral Care
On treatment	Days 1-10	Days 1-10

At each time point, the nursing staff prior to administering the questionnaire should complete the patient identification number and date of assessment. To prepare patients for completing the questionnaire following discharge until day 10, they should be encouraged to complete these independently during the time they are in-patients. In preparation for discharge, nursing staff should provide a package of the remaining questionnaires for completion with the relevant dates at the top. This package should be given to the patient on discharge following each routine hospital admission. In this way, standardisation of data collection across all Sites will be achieved.

Note that all questionnaires completed by patients should be kept in a designated filing case within each WISECARE unit and classified alphabetically.

6.3 Nursing Resource Data

6.3.1   Patient Acuity Assessment – Moffitt Tool

In order to assess the level of patient acuity in each Site, the Moffitt tool will be employed as a standardised assessment tool for patient classification. See annex 4-5. This will be completed weekly by a senior nurse in each of the units of the Sites. The same nurse should complete the tool to foster familiarity with the tool, so facilitating its speedy completion and reducing variability. The tool should always be completed around the same time of day and on the randomly dictated dates only. Moffitt data for each patient is best entered straight onto the WiseTool following the review of a paper copy of the Moffitt tool.

6.3.2　*Nurse Staffing Data*

In order to assess and evaluate nursing resources required to deliver care the following information will be collated from each of the WISECARE Validation Sites at the start of the resource data collection period:

- Staffing levels
- Education and experience of nursing staff
- Environment of care: Nurse/patient ratio
- Patient dependency
- Number of patients
- Management of care

The nursing resource form can be found from annex 9. Following the initial completion of this form, nursing resource data will be collected weekly at the same time as the Moffitt tool is completed. This data will be entered in the electronic database at the same time as the Moffitt tool data is being entered. The following information will be collected:

- *Education level of nurses*

Registered Specialist Cancer Nurse: possesses at least 5 years clinical experience within the speciality of oncology, has successfully completed a specialist cancer course rated at first degree level, is professionally accountable for his/her own nursing actions, is competent in patient care and possess theoretical knowledge to support clinical judgements

Registered Non-Specialist Nurse: successful completion of general nursing education, gaining clinical experience, providing professional patient care, professionally accountable for his/her own nursing actions

Unqualified nursing assistants: no professional nursing qualifications, provides general care to patients under the supervision of registered nurses

Student nurses: currently undertaking nursing qualifications, provides nursing care appropriate to his/her level of experience under the supervision of qualified nurses

- Hours worked in the last 24 hours

7　Patient Consent

In addition to verbal information, all patients will be provided with an information sheet prior to registration (example see annex 10). If needed along the guidelines of the hospital, all patients will be required to give written informed consent (see annex 11).

Risk Assessment

Jop Helleman, Kris Vanhaecht

1   Leuven Chemotherapy Risk Assessment Scale (LCRAS)

One of the main goals in the WISECARE project is the use of clinical feedback on four clinical indicators: nausea & vomiting, pain, fatigue and oral care. These clinical indicators are side effects of the therapy, mainly chemotherapy. The Clinical Sites use different chemotherapy regimens and every chemotherapy treatment is a mixture of different chemotherapy products. Every chemotherapy product has a specific risk for these clinical indicators. In order to give meaningful feedback with respect to the chemotherapy side effects we chose to group the different chemotherapy treatments in specific risk categories.

The Leuven Chemotherapy Risk Assessment Scale (LCRAS) is a scale that shows the risk that 36 chemotherapy products can have on 47 clinical indicators.

In 1994 a group of Belgian nurses, pharmacists and doctors, in close co-operation with Glaxo Wellcome and the Flemish Oncology and Radiotherapy Society, developed the Nurses Cytostatic Compendium, Practical Guide For Nurses [1]. In this compendium information is given on 36 chemotherapy products. For every product one can find information on the product delivery, storage life, incompatibility, skin contamination, eye contamination, spilling, extravasation, excretion, some general remarks and the side effects.

The information on side effects is provided by clinical indicator and risk. When the product has a high risk, the clinical indicator is shown in bold, moderate risk is shown normal and a low risk in brackets. When the product has no risk or the risk is unknown, it is not mentioned.
We recoded this information in a score from 0 to 3.

Table 1   Recoding of risk indications

Codes by Dhaenekint et al. 1994	Leuven Chemotherapy Risk Assessment Scale
Bold = high risk	Risk 3
Normal = moderate risk	Risk 2
(in brackets) = low risk	Risk 1
Nothing mentioned or unknown	Risk 0

Within the WISECARE project we focused on the 4 clinical indicators: nausea and vomiting, pain, fatigue and oral care. For the WISECARE fatigue clinical indicator we used the information of these clinical indicators concerning fatigue and bone marrow transplantation from the Nurses Cytostatic Compendium to obtain a final risk score. When the risk for fatigue and bone marrow depression in Dhaenekint et al. [1] was not identical, we used the highest risk score in the Leuven Chemotherapy Risk Assessment Scale.

It resulted in a table with 36 chemotherapy products and 4 clinical indicators. For every product the risk (3, 2, 1 or 0) is shown for nausea & vomiting, oral care, pain and fatigue. This layout was chosen by the nurses of the Leuven Validation Site and is daily used for patient education and side effect risk assessment.

The whole LCRAS (see annex 12) will be revised by nurses, doctors and pharmacists from the University Hospitals Leuven to provide the latest information on new chemotherapy products and their side effects.

2 Groningen Breast cancer Risk Assessment Scale (GBRAS)

In order to develop a risk assessment scale for breast cancer surgery on pain, fatigue, nausea & vomiting and oral care, literature was reviewed. No relevant literature was found. A risk assessment scale (annex 12b) was developed, based on empirical evidence of the nurses working on the AZ Groningen ward for more than 2 years.

First all the different treatments which are most common in the surgical treatment of breast cancer were listed. A Delphi-technique was used to score risk factors. In a first round all nurses scored the risks factors. In a second round these individual scores were brought together and discussed among the nurses. In the third round agreement was reached for all the different treatments. High risk treatments received a risk 3, medium risk a score 2 and low risk surgical treatments received a score 1.

References

[1] Dhaenekint C. et al. Nurses Cytostatic Compendium, Practical Guide for nurses, Glaxo Wellcome, 1994.

The WISETool

Derek Hoy

1   Introduction

In section 3 of this chapter the context of the WISECARE tools was described. To summarise, the tools had to support that activity of clinical networking, from local data collection, to aggregation in the data warehouse, analysis, and finally feedback of new information. WISECARE supported processes of *formal* and *informal* communication within the project. *Formal* communication was based on agreed data sets, data collection protocols and analysis. *Informal* communication was based on interpersonal processes and information sharing, for example by email and the Website.

At each Site a tool was required which would support data collection, management and feedback of new information from the project, both from the formal and informal processes. Nurses used multiple languages, were not generally experienced in use of IT, and had poor systems support. The tool therefore had to be: very easy to use by nurses at the Sites; require minimal training; easy to install and maintain by non-IT professionals; secure and confidential; and support local customisation.

The agreed requirement was for a stand-alone PC-based software tool with minimal duplication with existing local systems. Further, there should only be one integrated tool for data collection and local feedback. The WISETool was developed to meet these requirements.

2   Technical Platform

The WISETool was developed for Windows 32bit operating systems (Windows 95/98/NT) using the Borland Delphi development environment. Delphi offered: support for stand-alone, client-server, or web-enabled applications; good control of user interface; rapid application development; flexible database links; support for Microsoft distributed computing technology (DCOM, COM, Activex, OLE, DDE...), and CORBA; and very good third party support.

A proprietary relational database was used which supported stand-alone, client-server and network operation. This was low cost, with no licence fees, and proved to be robust, fast enough in use, and simple to administer. It required exporting of data to allow use of 'open' tools.

Only one of the Validation Sites had very good local IT support, while the others had little or no support. Installation was therefore kept very simple: it could be downloaded from a Website, copied to two floppy disks, and installed by a non-expert user. Further support for problems or feedback was provided by email and telephone.

3   Architecture

The WISETool architecture involved three layers: user interface, application modules, and server modules.

3.1 User Interface

WISETool used one main window for most operations. The interface was similar to the familiar Microsoft Outlook style, with a *button bar* for common operations and *pages* holding *function icons* in related groupings (see Figure 1). This produced a simple, clean design, without complex multiple forms.

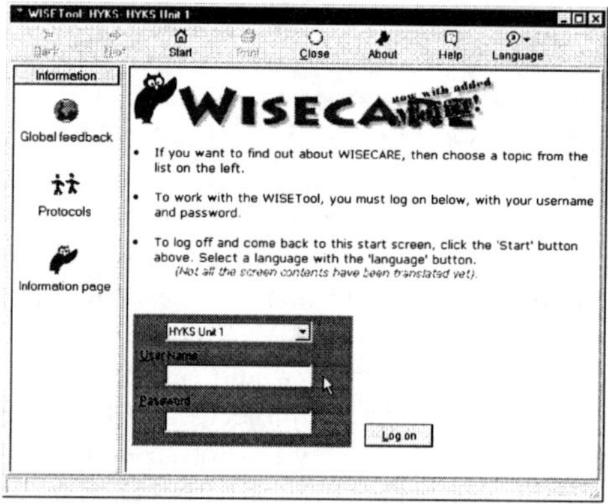

Figure 1   The WISETool User Interface

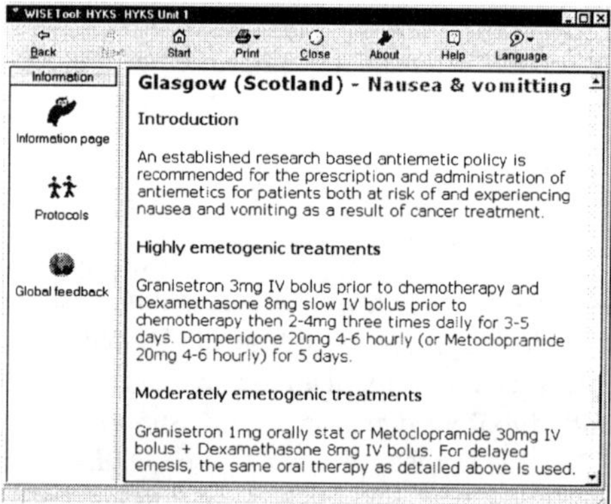

Figure 2   Example Information Page

3.2 Access Control

The start-up screen include a box for logging in, with user name and password. User access was in three levels:

- *General user* allowed only access to a page with information about the project, without any logging on being required (see Figure 2).
- *Clinical user* allowed access to the information page, and a clinical page for admitting

or discharging patients, review of existing records and data entry. This required a valid user name and password for access.

- *Administrative user* allowed access to both the above pages, and a third page with administrative functions, for example user maintenance, exporting data, resource data collection, and some simple system configuration.

3.3 Application Modules

Figure 3 illustrates how application modules are loaded into the main window area when the user selects a *function icon*. Examples of application modules are:

- Rich Text Format, which would load a file in RTF format produced by a word processor. This could be used, for example, to customise an information page with local information, in the local language.
- HTML (web page format), which allowed web pages to be linked into the WISETool, with hyperlinks and graphics.
- Data editors, which were generic modules, usually combined into larger data entry forms.
- Patient record modules, which allow selection of records, alternative views, and editing.
- Data export is done through a custom module, which is loaded if the user clicks the icon on the administration page.

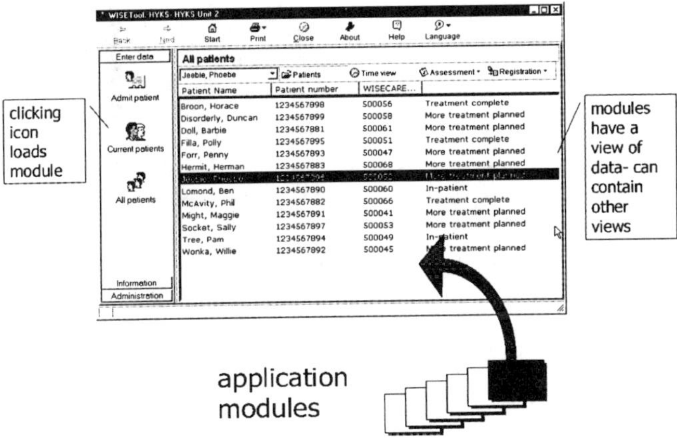

Figure 3   Application Modules

3.4 Server Modules

Server modules can be shared by *application modules* and provide common services across the whole application. For example, a data access module centralises all data access to a small set of generic functions, simplifying testing and maintenance of the system. It also allowed replacement of the database system as the WISETool moved from prototype to production versions.

A knowledge base server offers simple services including links to protocols (in HTML) and risk factors for treatments. Another server module manages links to other applications, with the first prototype link being to the HISCOM MIRADOR system by Windows Dynamic Data Exchange.

3.5 Terminology Server

In chapter 4 *Evaluation*, there is discussion about the role of the terminology model in WISECARE, which describes how the main requirement was for support of dialogue in the WISETool. These terminology and dialogue services were combined and delivered through one *terminology server* module.

This server used model files that were separate from the WISETool application to allow for flexibility in development and maintenance. One model file defined the concept space and semantic links within it. A separate lexicon file held the term labels for these concepts, with a set for each language required. Languages could be changed dynamically while the WISETool was running. Project team members at each Validation Site were able to translate terms using a simple spreadsheet (see Figure 4), which was then compiled into a lexicon file.

Within the model file were the links required to group concepts to meet dialogue requirements, for example the data items (including data types) for an assessment were modelled. WISETool could then query the terminology server for the data items for a particular assessment, and a form could be constructed from appropriate component editors according to information in the model.

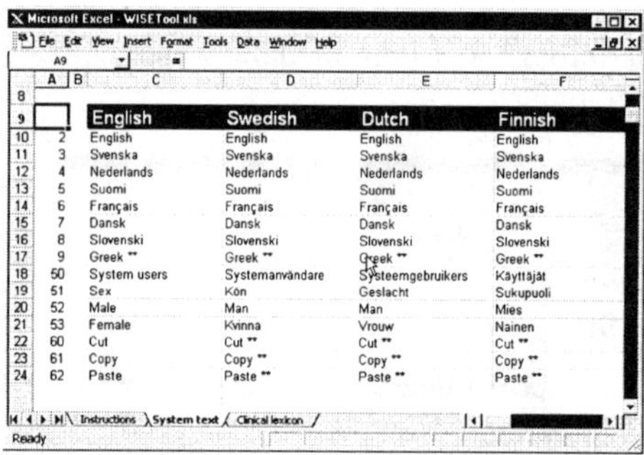

Figure 4   Using a Spreadsheet to manage Translations

4   Using the WISETool

The basic functionality of the WISETool was:

- manage patient registration;
- view and enter patient and resource data;
- correct errors in data (with restricted access and audit);
- export data for aggregation in the project data warehouse; and
- import feedback automatically.

While patient registration was achieved using simple standard data entry forms, a more flexible approach was needed for data entry to support needs for modification during the project and local customisation. For these reasons, data entry forms were generated dynamically using services provided by the terminology server to build forms from generic editors (see Figure 5).

4.1 Data View

Figure 6 shows the main patient record view. To the left is the *time line*, which shows a list of data items in an agenda format. Admissions, clinical events (for example, chemotherapy) and assessments are shown. Above this are some data items that change very slowly, such as *patient group*. Below are *indicator headings*, which show the current values of assessments for each indicator. The *feedback* graph shows the scores for selected indicators. Clicking on points on the graph selects that assessment on the *time line*, which can be double-clicked to open that assessment record for review. So, on seeing a high score, a user can quickly look at the assessment to see what was the cause. Clicking on the *protocols* button opens a window with protocols for the currently selected heading.

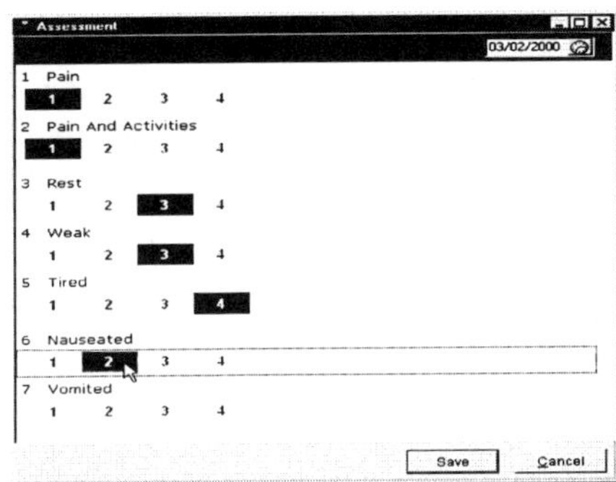

Figure 5   Dynamically generated Data Entry Form

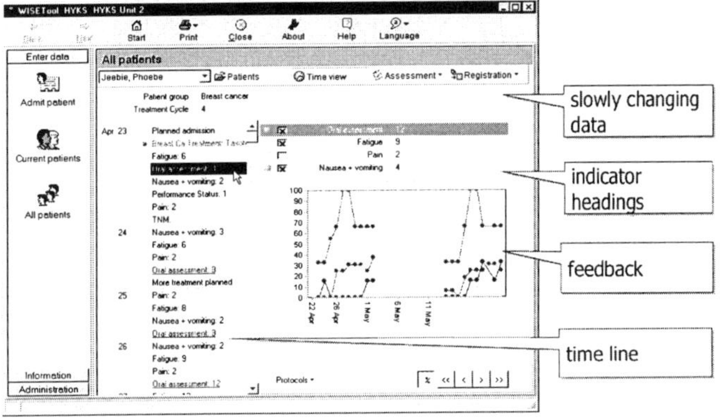

Figure 6   Patient Record View

4.2 Exporting Data

On the *administration* page, a user with administrator access can choose *export data*. A few simple options can be changed and then a button is clicked. After a few moments the user is informed that a data extract file has been successful.

This file has a snapshot of the current local database, but with patient and staff identifiers removed. The file is compressed and encrypted so it can be sent to the project data warehouse in a secure manner.

5   Future Development

The WISETool application will support follow-on projects by the WISECARE partners. The software is also being considered by a national nursing organisation for use as a standalone quality audit tool supporting national guideline implementation.

System suppliers are interested in integrating the tool in their systems. The current WISETool has a simple mechanism for tested with the MIRADOR system. Future developments include the ability to embed the core of WISETool within a commercial system.

6   Conclusion

The WISETool has proved itself as an easy to use, low cost, low maintenance, reliable and flexible software application. Within the constraints of the project, it has been continually developed over the course of the WISECARE project and now forms a useful basis for further development.

WISECARE WWW-Server

Petros Dounavis, Emily Karistinou, John Mantas

The WISECARE project has collected a variety of clinical data from the Validation Sites. Thus a communication channel between the participants was established not only for the exchange of information but also for the exchange of data. Here we describe the design of the Web server of the WISECARE project as well as the establishment of the BSCW-server (Basic Support for Cooperative Work), which was a file depository for the documents produced for the project.

1   Rationale

'Characterised by an unprecedented growth rate, *Internet* has started to influence a number of economic sectors, with the emergence of a fast-growing electronic-commerce economy… Internet is displacing traditional computer networks, and showing the first signs of how it may provide a platform which, over time, replaces traditional methods of trading' [1].

This section will describe the design and development of the World Wide Web server of the WISECARE project that was required to exploit and disseminate the project outcomes and to offer a communication mode. The WISECARE WWW Network supports the central information service, such as e-mail, FTP services. Everything that is produced by the WISECARE project will be available on the Internet with an easy to use, interactive interface which combines text, images, sounds and hypertext navigation facilities.

The idea of bridging distances and allowing individuals to exchange information on a global scale has been with us since the invention of the telephone and the telegraph dramatically extended the reach of mankind's traffic in information. But it wasn't until the last few decades that innovations in telecommunications took a quantum leap. This revolution in how information is stored, transmitted, and accessed has extremely important implications for the health sector, on primary care and disease prevention, health promotion and consumer education, in the context of service delivery guided by equity, quality, effectiveness and efficiency.

Consequently, the health sector must harness these new information tools if it is to fulfil its goals in the best and most efficient way possible. Internet is a case in point. The network's size, ubiquity and growth are staggering. It is anticipated that Internet may well link more than 400 million persons world-wide by the end of the century Internet's benefits to the health sector are without question. It already holds an impressive array of information on health-related topics, and this storehouse promises to increase in the future. Wider Internet use has the potential to radically transform health sciences research, education, patient care and health management practices [2].

Specifically, the objectives of the team responsible for networking in the WISECARE project are to:

- Set up a WWW-server by which oncology work flow information can be disseminated.
- Keep the WWW-server up-to-date meaning that local data have to be loaded.
- Provide tools for downloading benchmark data and the application software so that the local practice can be evaluated.

2   Website of the WISECARE Project

2.1 *Goals of the WISECARE Website*

The scope of this Website is to support the communication tasks between the partners in the WISECARE Project. It is also used in the dissemination process of oncology workflow information.

In more detail the Website has the following functions:

- To make known the WISECARE Project to the Internet society.
  The Website includes any information concerning the WISECARE Project such as a detailed description of the project, its objectives and how they will be accomplished, also the members of the project with their roles and their responsibilities.
- To provide a communication channel for the participants of the project.
  This is one of the most important objectives of the WWW server and of great importance also for the project itself. In this Website any information is available which the participants of the project need. There is a place for every group and member that is taking part in the project and in addition there are different access levels for each user of the WWW server. In this way general information is available for global access, but if someone wants to read or download documents which are dedicated for the partners then the system provides a prompt for a "username" and "password". By its Discussion Forum page it also gives the possibility to all external interested parties to exchange ideas.
- To provide a data repository.
  The Website is linked with a FTP site so that every document or binary file related to the project can be downloaded in the original form. This FTP site includes not only all the documents, which are going to be produced through the project (for example managerial paperwork), but also some of the deliverables to assist the dissemination process in the project.
- To provide a link with the other European Project in the Health Care domain
  It is very important for the success of the project that the outcomes are harmonised with other results coming from projects concerned with the training of health professionals.

2.2 *Structure and Information Content of the WISECARE Website*

The address of the WISECARE Website is: http://wisecare.dn.uoa.gr
The WWW site of the WISECARE project is organised in a way that will serve its main goals.

The information content of this site is divided into 3 main categories:

- General Information: A brief description of the project, including the objectives, outcomes and the members.

- Specific Information: Documents related to the members.
- Services: The Workplace server and the WISECARE Discussion Forum. (The BSCW system configured for the project, includes exchange of the documents, meetings and other goodies)

All these areas are available in the Home Page through the use of graphical buttons and text-links. The Home Page also includes a counter, which enables the user to see how many people have visited this page.

The Workplace Server acts as a communication platform for the members of the WISECARE project, it includes Meetings, Folders, Uploading and Downloading of documents combined with security access mechanisms. In order to use this service someone should Register him/herself to the system. After the registration he/she receives by email a personal login name that he/she uses in order to use the system.

The WISECARE Discussion Forum is a Bulletin Board System that can be used for easy and quick communication. The user can raise issues for discussion and gets replies from other users who use the WWW. Advanced features include: Email notification of replies, different ways of presenting the message index and several others.

- Feedback: All comments and suggestions about the project, the products and the Website are welcome.

- Related Links: The related projects are presented.

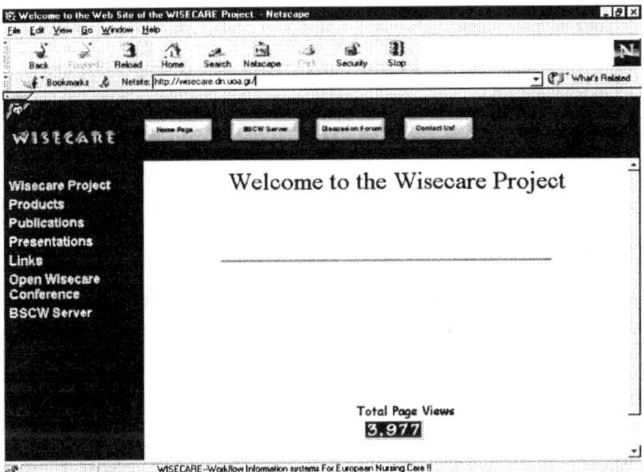

Figure 1   The Home Page

2.3 *Characteristics of the WISECARE Website*

The term "characteristics" is used in order to identify the style of a Website meaning the way it is constructed. As it was mentioned in the beginning, the difference between the World Wide Web service and other Internet Information Services is mainly the use of hyperlinks and graphics for the presentation of the information to the user. But there are some limits that must be kept in mind before creating a Web page and those are:

Network connection speed

This is measured in units of bits per second, which can be transferred through our network line. There is a floor of 28.8 kbits per second for services like Gopher, Telnet, Finger or WAIS but for WWW service at least 56 kbits per second is required. When the speed is fixed to for example 256 kbits per second then the communication speed between a server and a client in the WWW is proportional to the size of the information, which must be transferred between these two computers. If the information is presented only in text, the speed of transfer is quite high compared to the use of graphics because the size of a character is 8 bits and a full page of text 80*25 is equal to 16000 bits but a picture of a size 320*200 pixels with 16 colors is equal to 32000 bits.

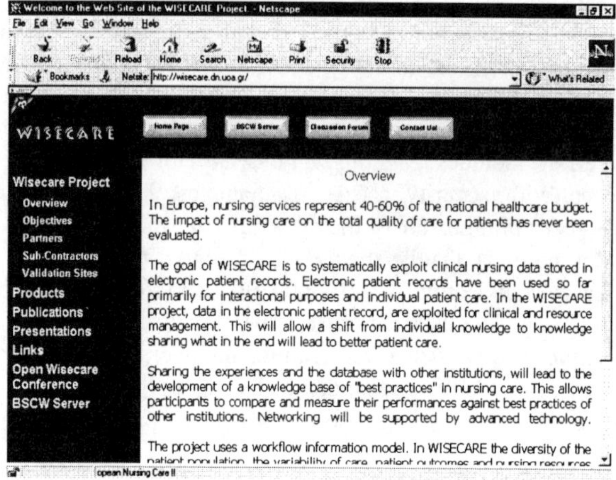

Figure 2   The Overview Page

Network load (Network traffic)

There are two sources of network traffic from information servers: queries sent to the server and the responses it sends in reply. This traffic determines the load of an Internet server, or in the case of the WWW, the load of a Web server. When the Web pages are filled only with text, the queries (and the replies) are quite small and this the load of the server is not big, but when the Web pages consist of a lot of pictures the load can be enormous.

So there must be a choice of "style", a Website with pages full of pictures but slow or a Website with pages consisting of a limited number of pictures, which are transmitted fast, but which are not so interesting.

The pages used in The WISECARE Project were created by the philosophy that although the transfer time is critical, the user-friendliness and the ease of use is of great importance. The use of graphics inside the text is done in such a way that the page is not overloaded but it helps the user to navigate with greater ease through the available information even if the user has no experience using an information service like the WWW. The screens of the site and the buttons are self-explanatory most of the time.

In order to make the User Interface (UI) as simple and flexible as possible even for the novice user the WWW server is built using HTML and JAVA extensions. The JAVA scripts are used in order to make the UI more active for example the buttons which define the different areas inside the Information Content (Overview, Objectives, etc.) are lightened when the mouse "rolls" over them, also informative messages are scrolling in the status bar in some pages.

2.4 Advanced Facilities of the WISECARE Website

The Web server of the WISECARE project is not just a simple way of presenting some information and making various documents available to the public. The challenge that this WWW server has to face is to support the dissemination of the outcomes of the project. This is done by including some advanced techniques such as the two-way communication between the user and the information server. This is one of the most interesting and powerful features of the WWW service because data can be collected from the user and then processed to suit various needs. For example a questionnaire can be published on the Web concerning the WISECARE project itself or the various services and the users give their feedback, so there is a direct way of evaluating the project and its outcomes.

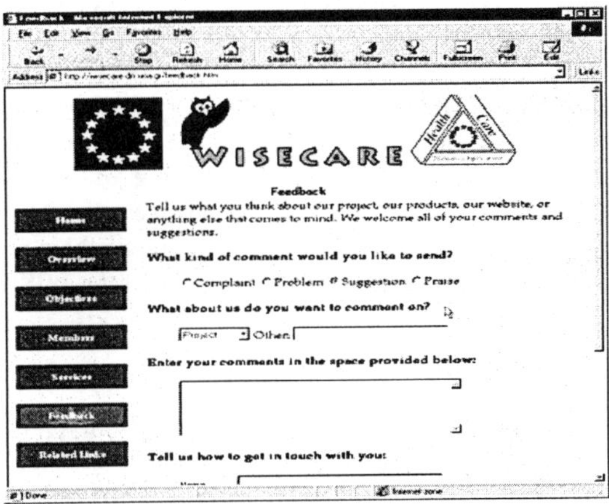

Figure 3   The Feedback Page

2.4.1   The "Search Engine"

The ability of obtaining input from the user also enables also another advanced feature and that is the "search engine". The "search engine" is used as a method for supplying specific information to the user about a subject of interest. It consists of a set of programs, which have the following functions:

- The indexing of the available information in a form that can be used by the "search engine"
- An interface for communicating with the user, and in which the user can "tell" the "search engine" which topics are of interest.
- The main "search engine" which is responsible for finding the appropriate information from the index files. The main function of the search program is to scan the index files in order to find where the needed information is.
- A screen in which the results are presented in a format which the user can understand.

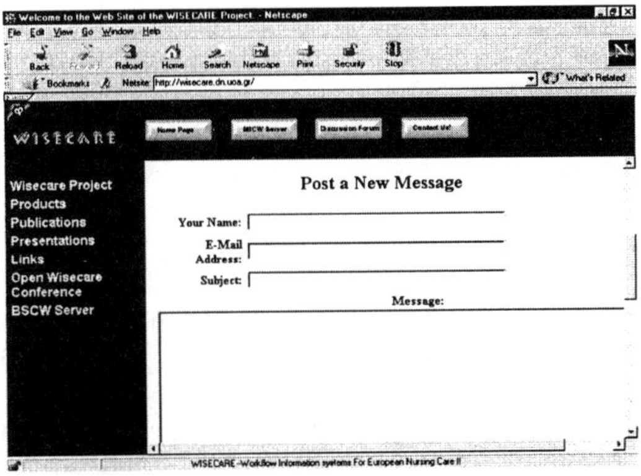

Figure 4   The WISECARE Discussion Forum

2.4.2   WISECARE Discussion Forum

Another advanced feature in the Web server of the WISECARE Project is the Discussion Forum, this is a service that provides a communication channel for the members of the WISECARE project as well as any other interested in the project.
The WISECARE DISCUSSION FORUM is developed using the PERL Programming Language and it is, as the name implies, a Web-based bulletin board.

It stores the messages as simple text files and creates HTML pages "on the fly". This means that the message index can be tailored by the user based on date and/or subject (via built-in keyword search capability), and can be viewed as either a chronological or a threaded list. In addition, it supports automatic quoting of message text and e-mail notification of those who want to know immediately when a new message has been posted.

The BSCW is another service upon the Web server, actually is a separate server, it is used as common working environment for the participants of the WISECARE.

2.4.3   What is BSCW?

BSCW (Basic Support for Cooperative Work) enables collaboration over the Web. BSCW is a 'shared workspace' system which supports document uploads, event notification, group management and much more. To access a workspace you only need a standard Web browser.

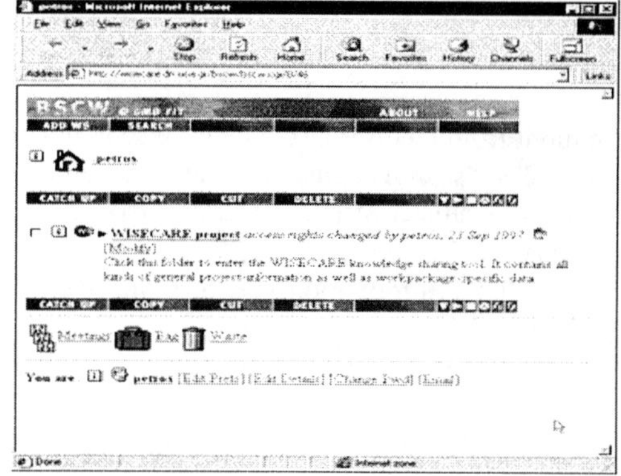

Figure 5   The BSCW Server

Overview of BSCW
The BSCW system supports collaboration by providing **shared workspaces** over the Internet. A shared workspace allows storage and retrieval of documents and sharing information within a group. This functionality is integrated with an event mechanism to provide each user with an awareness of the activities of others within the workspace. It comprises numerous features, e.g., support for threaded discussions, version management of documents, group management, search features and many more. The system is designed primarily to support self-organising groups.

Benefits of BSCW
BSCW supports asynchronous and synchronous co-operation with your partners over the Internet, in your Intranet or in a network with your business partners (Extranet).

For *asynchronous* (not simultaneous) co-operation, BSCW offers *shared workspaces* that groups can use to store documents, manage them, jointly edit and share them.
The essential *advantages*:

- With a BSCW workspace, workgroups can share documents — independent of the specific computer systems that the members use.
- You need not install any software before using BSCW. You only need a standard Web browser.
- You access BSCW workspaces, browse folders and download documents to your local system just like "normal" Web pages.
- BSCW keeps you informed of all relevant events in a shared workspace.
- You can upload documents to a shared workspace using any standard Web browser.

For *synchronous* (simultaneous) cooperation, BSCW provides tools for

- planning and organizing meetings,
- starting 'virtual' meetings on the basis of conferencing programs or by telephone,
- ad hoc communication with partners who are currently logged in to a shared workspace and therefore are likely to be working on a common task.

Security Issues

The BSCW supports registration of the users as a security measure for the operation of the service. The user is registered once as a user of the BSCW server. After a simple authentication procedure, the BSCW server "knows" a *registered user* as a combination of

- A user name with
- a current password and with at least
- one valid personal email address.

This combination is *mobile*:

Using a user name and password, the user can access his/her folders and shared workspaces from any computer with Internet access and a suitable Web browser.

Registering as a BSCW user

A BSCW server may — or may not — allow *self-registration* by prospective users. If a server has not been configured for self-registration, then only the BSCW administrator(s) can register new users and this is the case with the WISECARE BSCW server.

The key to the user's registration is his personal email address. The BSCW server will typically get it:

- from the user by means of the registration form — or
- from somebody who is already a registered user and who invites you to cooperate with him/her in a shared workspace.

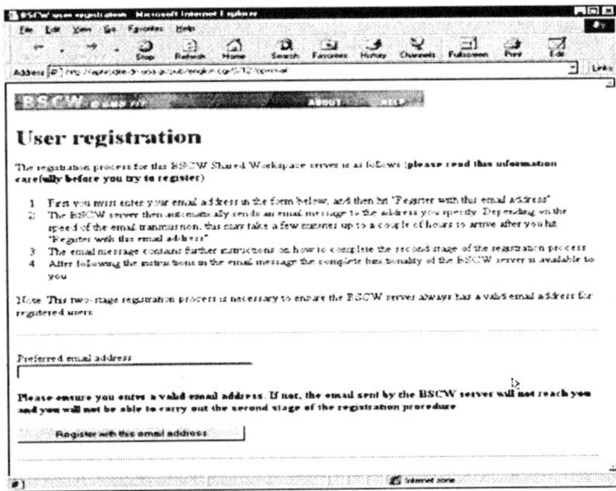

Figure 6　The User Registration

When the registration procedure is initiated by specifying the users email address, BSCW sends an email to that specified address. This email contains a special URL which the user should open in his/her Web browser.

Opening this URL (which can be used only once!) brings up a form to fill in a user name and an initial password.

When the form is submitted to the server, BSCW combines the information in the form with the email address, registers a user with the user name and is ready for the user's first log-in using this user name and the password that was specified.

Starting a BSCW session

A registered user logs into the BSCW server and identifies him *to begin each session.*

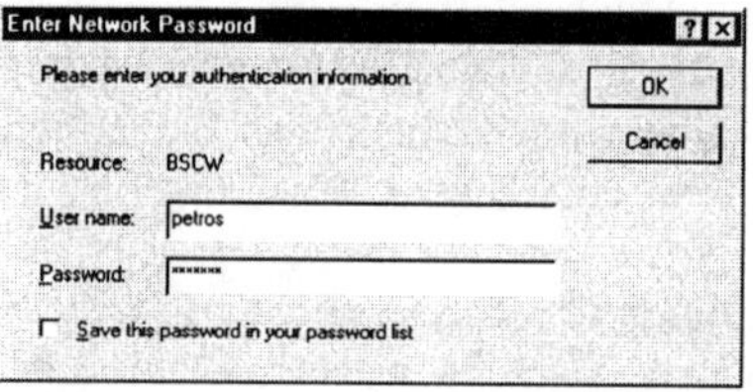

Figure 7 The Login Window

A session is initiated on a BSCW server when the user accesses an information object by

- opening the URL http://wisecare.dn.uoa.gr/bscw/bscw.cgi/
  (This link is currently available under Services section of the WISECARE project)
  BSCW will display the user's home folder, which contains his personal folders and the shared workspaces he is a member of, with all the BSCW objects they include.
- accessing an object in one of the user's folders or workspaces directly, using a URL, e.g., from his list of *bookmarks* or *favourites*.

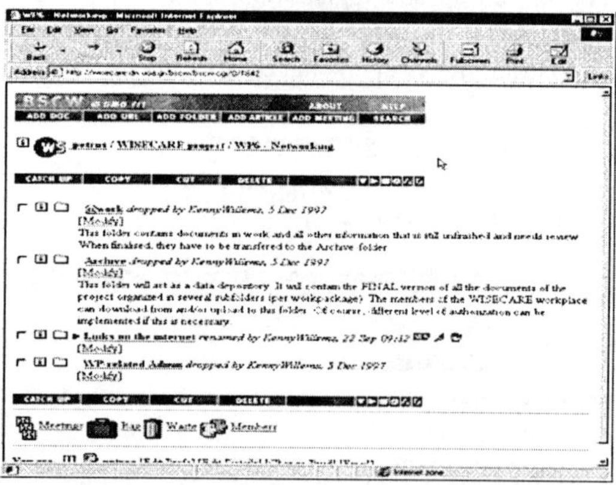

Figure 8 A Folder's Content

For login and identification, he has to submit his user name and his password. After verification, BSCW lets him access the Home folder of the user name he has specified. If he has accessed an object in a workspace directly by specifying a URL, BSCW will immediately take him to the content of this object. For instance, if somebody sends him the URL of a folder, he will see the contents of this folder immediately on logging in (provided he has suitable access rights).

Closing a BSCW session

A BSCW session is *closed* automatically when the user *terminates* the browser program on his local computer.

Until then the access rights granted to him under his user name remain in effect.

Parallel BSCW sessions

At any point in time, the user's Web browser can represent *only one user name* on any given BSCW server. Parallel sessions with different user names on one BSCW server are *not* possible.

However, most Web browsers will allow the user to have active sessions on several different BSCW servers simultaneously.

References

[1]   European Commission : Green Paper on the Convergence of the Telecommunications, Media and IT Sectors, and the implications for regulation, towards an Information Society Approach

[2]   Iudicissa S, Oliveri M, Gamboa N, Roberts C. (Eds): The Internet, Telematics and Health. Amsterdam, IOS-Press. 530 p. ISBN 90.5199.289.0. Vol. 36 of the Series Studies in Health Technology and Informatics 1997

WISECARE Technology Assessment Tool

Martin Steegh, Jacob Hofdijk

1 Introduction

1.1 Need for Technology Assessment

As information systems became mature and give operational support to the care process, the (cost) effectiveness of clinical IT systems became an important factor in the decision making process concerning investment in IT systems within health care institutions. The large investments both for the development and the use of telematics applications urged the rationalisation of decision making on the purchase and implementation of company wide IT systems. A small group of IT developers of health care applications began to create methods and tools to ensure the (cost) effective development and implementation of telematics systems.

Special focus has been given to the assessment of the impact of increasingly complex telematics applications on health care delivery. Much has been learned from medicine, which has a tradition of determining effectiveness of new technologies for diagnostics and treatment (*Technology Assessment*).

A useful definition of Medical Technology Assessment is the following:
Medical Technology Assessment denotes any process of examining and reporting properties of a medical technology used in health care, such as safety, efficacy, feasibility and indications for use, cost and cost-effectiveness, as well as social, economic and ethical consequences whether intended or unintended. [1]

A major problem however is that information systems are more than a device, which can be tested on its formal specifications, the IT systems have an impact on a living human organisation where it is implemented. It has an effect on the way people work and communicate. Therefore a successful assessment of information systems should have a strong focus on the human factor. The impact of information systems on an organisation should be measured by the potential of the system to change the organisation. How successful the system has supported the organisation to achieve its objectives should be measured. In the case of a hospital it relates to providing more effective patient care within limited available resources.

1.2 Technology Assessment and Nursing

In the late eighties HISCOM, then known as BAZIS, a foundation of a large group of Dutch hospitals for the development and support of information systems for hospitals started the development of an integrated nursing information system: the VISION Project. The aim was to support the work of nurses by providing an IT system, which could be used as close as possible to the "point of care", "the patient's bed". Extensive tests have been made with terminals at the bedside, in the patient's room or on the nursing desk. As data collection is the key to any system, ease of access is certainly a critical success factor for a nursing information system.

The VISION system is developed as an integrated part of the HISCOM Hospital Information System (HIS), thus providing direct access to all relevant patient data and to other services of the HIS. The VISION system focuses at the support of primary patient care. To be able to assess the impact of the implementation of the VISION system, HISCOM initiated a "technology assessment" process of the system in three hospitals.

2   Technology Assessment Approach in WISECARE

2.1 Introduction

The management of a hospital demands an increasing need for information about care delivered at nursing wards. The need to manage the ever-decreasing resources is growing day by day. "Nursing" has developed a growing interest in understanding its own "practice". This information is needed for educational purposes in addition to supporting nursing resource management. The latter requires objective information on the requirement of nursing staff to provide the services needed to care for a specific patient case load. So the need for reliable and real-time information on nursing practice is growing. The WISECARE project intends to stimulate the use of existing, and collection of missing, data to provide information about nursing practice. The process will build towards a continuous use of information for both individual nursing care and for nursing management.

As hospitals face a changing health care environment with an increasing intensity of the required delivery of care, the nursing society becomes aware of the increasing pressure on nurses. Meanwhile more proof is gathered of the positive impact of a more personal approach on the quality of care delivery to patients. Issues for the management of nursing resources and an intensive search for determining the most appropriate nursing activities for specific nursing problems and diagnoses is required. There is still no nursing parameter in the equation for determining the adequate budget for nursing resources. One thing is beyond discussion "Objective information is needed on the provision of nursing care".

The main objective of WISECARE is to assess the impact of more complete and adequate information on the nursing care process to support the "management of nursing care". This will be done both from the perspective of improving the delivery of nursing care to the individual patient and from the perspective of managing the scarce resources of a nursing department in any kind of hospital. As nursing care is closely related to the provision of clinical care, it is extremely important to establish a logical link between the management of the "clinical" and the "nursing" processes and resources.

During this process, optimal use should be made of the data collected in the information systems of the hospitals. The WISECARE project could ultimately stimulate the integrated approach of the care process of these two highly integrated professional dimensions. Furthermore, insight should be gained in the added value of nursing, as compared to the existing case-mix management systems that focus solely on the medical activities.

2.2 The Objectives

The main target of the WISECARE project is to enhance the use of information about "nursing" by nurses. The objective of the technology assessment is to measure the *impact* of the WISECARE project on nursing management in each of the five Validation Sites. To assess the impact of a more extensive use of information on nursing activities within the

WISECARE Sites and in order to compare the results between the Sites, common approach is mandatory. In the workpackage three areas of assessment are defined:
(1)　The eight "WISECARE questions".
(2)　The impact of the use of information by the nurse managers.
(3)　The market for the WISECARE approach in Europe.

To assess the impact of WISECARE we have to deal with a range of aspects of technology assessment. The eight WISECARE questions deal with resource management issues, the impact of organisational aspects on nursing care, the relation between medical treatment and nursing care, and the outcome of nursing care provided to oncological patients. To assess the WISECARE approach requires dealing with a wide range of aspects of the use of information technology.

The assessment of the use of information on the management is not restricted to the assessment of an information system. The emphasis is on the *process of change* of management in the department. WISECARE will stimulate this change process on different levels of nursing management. It will provide information on the best practice of nursing care process. It's effect ranges from the management of individual patient care to the management of nursing care of the oncological department.

2.3 WISECARE Questions

In WP5 verification and validation questions have been defined as criteria for success of a workflow information systems for nursing care. These questions are based on the notion that a workflow information system applied in a nursing environment should improve the management of the nursing department, i.e. the allocation of human resources and supplies, thereby improving the quality of care. The technology assessment study should determine if the following questions can be answered (better) with the aid of a workflow information system:

- To what extent is nursing care related to the aim of care (diagnostic, curative, palliative)?
- To what extent is the dependency level of the patient different according to the aim of care?
- To what extent is treatment influenced by the age of the patient?
- To what extent will the organisational structure (number of nursing staff, qualification level, care environment) influence nursing care?
- To what extent will the medical diagnoses and the medical treatment influence the nursing care?
- To what extent will the choice of treatment and nursing care influence the quality of life?
- To what extent is the quality of life influenced by the continuity of care and emotional support during the caring process?
- To what extent will the cost of treatment and the related expected quality of life influence the choice of treatment?

These questions defined in the technical annex of the proposal of the European Commission form the basis for the evaluation. Evaluation will establish the between medical care and nursing care aspects, as WISECARE attempts to bridge both worlds.

2.4 Nursing Management Information Issues

The management of the hospital has currently virtually no information available about care related activities at nursing wards to base the management of nursing resources on. The budgets for nursing care are defined primarily on historical grounds. However, the hospital is faced with a changing health care environment: amongst others a reduction in the length of stay, a changing patient population and advancements in the technological possibilities for diagnosis and treatment. As a result, the nursing workload is changing, which requires tuning of the budgets allocated to nursing. This tuning demands adequate information on the nursing resources required for the care process. Moreover, today's health care requests more insight into the primary process of care delivery. Research in developments in patient care and patient needs requires detailed information on nursing.

The object of a Workflow Information System in Nursing Care is to manage the availability of human resources and the supply of goods (drugs, bandages, etc.) from the moment a patient enters the hospital until the moment the patient is discharged. During the treatment of a patient with a specific medical and a range of nursing problems, data should be entered into the hospital information system about the care given. Based on these data information should be available on the necessary human resources, and the supply of goods for each of these problems. The original focus of the analysis was on measuring the impact of a continuous flow of information on the ward management. As the project shifted to a focus on a set of specific nursing problems the spotlight of the analysis changed as well. The WISECARE data collection was based on a formal protocol of the specific nursing problem, and it left the issue of identifying "missing nursing data" unanswered. The data collected however helped the clinical Sites with the process of identifying the information needed for management. The introduction of the confusing concept of "Clinical Time" was an example of the process of bridging nursing data collection with nursing management information. The positive conclusion is that the "Race is on".

2.5 The Approach

As the hospital is primarily interested in balancing case load and available financial and human resources, the emphasis in this project is on managing nursing resources at the ward level. In order to produce useful management information, underlying data must be complete and reliable. This demands that:

- Data registration should not require additional work of nurses. By preference, data should be registered automatically. In all cases it should be integrated in the nurses' daily work.
- There should be adequate feedback of the recorded information to the source to obtain correct and complete data. It should be clear to the nurses for what purpose data is collected and they should themselves make use of the data.

The WISECARE project is stimulating this approach at the Validation Sites. The technology assessment is focused at measuring the impact of the WISECARE approach on the management of the delivery of nursing care. The first step in the process is the assessment of the status quo at the beginning of the WISECARE process, i.e. the zero measurement. During the project additional assessment measurements will take place after each defined stage of data collection. These samples will provide information on the changing role of information during the WISECARE project. The assessment of the "management information practice" will be done by asking a set of relevant questions concerning the management of the nursing ward/department, the working conditions, patient outcome and satisfaction, recording of nursing data, the use of the information, etc. A software tool will be used for these assessments. This approach will make it much easier to process the results, to compare them for the different Validation Sites and to analyse them with statistical packages such as SPSS and SAS. The methodologies on which this tool is based and the features of the tool are described in section 3 of this article: "The WISECARE Technology Assessment Tool".

2.6 Evaluation Results

The project will be successful if the hospital management can be convinced that the hospital wide application of the WISECARE approach may provide the management information:

- to support the management of nursing care, at ward level, sector level and general hospital management level;
- to gain insight into the actual workload of nurses;
- to provide a quantitative basis for ward budgets for personnel and other resources;
- to support adequate response to trends in patient population and care developments based on quantitative and qualitative evidence.

3 The WISECARE Technology Assessment Tool

3.1 Introduction

The assessment of the WISECARE approach will be supported by an automated tool, which is called ComPass (computerised assessment). The tool is based on the assessment methodology developed by Rank Xerox to support the "total quality approach"[1]. The focus of that approach was on an assessment of the complete production chain, including the suppliers of the company. Rank Xerox wants to evaluate the management processes of their suppliers in the same way as they do within their organisation. The methodology has been implemented in a software tool, which is programmed within the Delphi application development environment [2]. The tool has been adapted to assess the WISECARE Validation Sites. The experiences of the VISTA project [3,4] and special Case Mix assessment [5] principles have been integrated in the system. The tool is designed to be used by different groups of users, such as hospital managers, nurse managers, head nurses etc. Each group is presented with a special set of questions. ComPass is basically a questionnaire tool which consists of a user interface were the questions are presented to the user and answers can be given on a one to five point scale (most questions have five answers, others three, four or two). This scaling makes it possible to compare the answers (in time and among the different Validation Sites) and to calculate scores by class of users and class of questions. A standard can be set for each of the issues and an evaluation can be based on these scores.

The questions are focused on the WISECARE issues and deal with the management of the hospital, the nursing department, the recording of data (patient demographics, nursing data and medical data) and the use of information. They have been discussed with two of the five Validation Sites (Leuven and Groningen). The automated technology assessment tool consists of the following kinds of questions:

- Questions about the management of the Hospital/Department/Ward (adapted from the EFQM assessment methodology)
- Questions on nursing aspects adapted from the VISTA research project (technology assessment of the VISION nursing information system)
- Questions on Case-mix aspects

---

[1] An Integrated Approach - Implementing Total Quality through Japanese 5-S and ISO 9000

- Questions on aspects of the hospital information system.

In section 3.4, "Description of the Tool" the user interface and the functionality of the tool are presented and described. Below the methodology is described on which the original tool is based.

3.2 EFQM Methodology

ComPass is based on the European Foundation of Quality Management (EFQM) Model [6] including Leadership, Human Resources, Policy & Strategy, Resources, Processes as the so-called *Enablers* and Employee Satisfaction, Customer Satisfaction, Impact on Society and Business Results as *Results*. ComPass represents a new classification process in which internal and external suppliers play an important and direct role in the strategic positioning of a large volume purchaser (= the assessor). Therefore these suppliers need to be assessed and evaluated on the competitive advantage they can offer the assessor on the short and long term.

ComPass is aiming to assess the suppliers by looking at their capacity to offer world class competitiveness, technical capabilities, management practices (including codes of conduct), research & development, manufacturing (including environmental care), services, integration ability and customer support.

The objective of ComPass is to provide Quality Assessors with a software tool according to a pre-defined Management Model, Business Framework, Functional Checklists or a Quality Model. Because of its flexible and multifunctional database engine and its easy maintenance program, ComPass can be adapted to every possible auditing environment, ranging from hospitals via rapid deployment forces to jet engines. The level of the assessment exceeds ISO 9000 and 14000 standards and can be enhanced with any other standard, like HACCP[2]. ComPass includes both a supplier self-assessment program and a final Site-assessment program, which makes it a very suitable tool for both external & internal auditing, reducing assessment & analysis time.

3.3 Other Methodologies

The questions have been obtained, as was already briefly mentioned, from various sources. The questions about the management of the Hospital/Department/Ward are adapted from the original (EFQM) tool. They have been re-written to make them suitable for the hospital environment. Questions on specific nursing aspects have been adapted from the VISTA research project, especially the instrument "quality co-ordination of care" proved very useful. These questions relate with the recording of nursing data, such as measurements, nursing diagnoses and interventions.

The case-mix aspects are obtained from an Australian study [9]. These are statements, e.g. "DRG derived information is an effective tool for evaluating the quality of patient care" to which the user can respond on a one to five scale (with answers varying from "I strongly disagree" to "I strongly agree").

The WISECARE team conceived the questions about the use and facilities of the hospital information system and the outcome of care. The draft of the assessment questions has been discussed with users at the University Hospitals of Leuven and Groningen. Based on these interviews the set has been adjusted and refined.

The users which have to answer the questions/statements are: the nursing staff of the pilot ward, i.e. a senior nurse and the headnurse, the nurse manager, the chief physician of

---

[2] see http://www.promega.com/qualitymonitoring/qmhaccp.html

the oncological department, the manager of the oncological department and the information manager of the hospital.

3.4 *Description of the Tool*

The user of the tool is first confronted with the "main screen" of the tool (see below) where he/she can browse through the different Validation Sites (with the browse buttons on the left part of the screen), and where the menu options File (Extract Self Assessment Data and Exit), Print (questions, score, overview) and Help (not functional) are presented. The buttons Assessment and Summary have the following functionality (the "Close" button closes the application): the Summary button gives an overview of the assessment results in a graphic way.

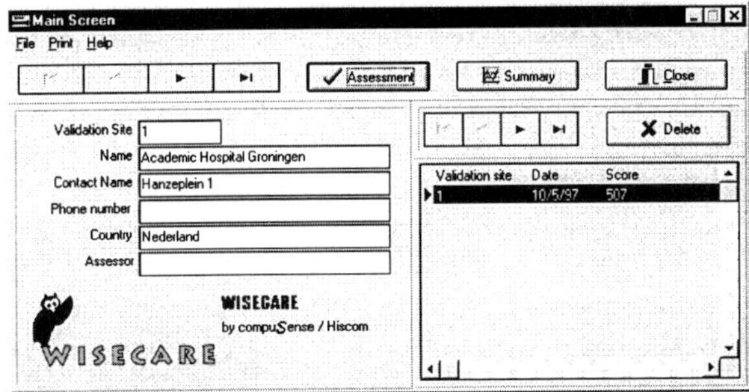

Figure 1   The main Screen of the Assessment Tool

When the user presses the Assessment button, the assessment window appears, which is the core of the tool (see below). Here the questions are presented to the user. The upper right pane shows the question, the one below shows the helptext (what is meant with the question) and the one below that shows a hint (how should the question be answered). Below these three panes the possible answers are shown. These answers are interpreted as scores and there are two (e.g. Yes and No), three, four or five possible answers, were 1 represents the lowest score and 5 the highest. At the bottom of the window are radio buttons that correspond with the answers. The user answers a question by clicking one of these radio buttons.

4 The Assessment Process

4.1 *Introduction*

The assessment of the WISECARE project focuses on the measurement of the effect of a better use of information at the five Validation Sites. The measurements will be done at different moments in time to assess the changes induced by the WISECARE process. The measurements will be done with the ComPass tool, which is to be used by the different users involved in the management of the nursing departments/wards of each of the Sites. The second part of the validation process will be the assessment of the "information potential" based on the existing data on clinical and nursing activities at the Validation Sites, this process will be part of workpackage 3. This will lead to fingerprints of the five Validation Sites, showing their clinical and nursing production based on current registrations.

Combining the information of these measurement tools to the nursing interventions helps to define the nursing impact on patient outcomes.

The last element of the Validation study is the assessment of the market potential of the WISECARE approach. The results of the assessments of the WISECARE approach of the Validation Sites will give a first impression of that potential. This lead will be followed in the next stages of the project. The Roll-out phase will provide additional information about the market potential of the WISECARE approach.

4.2   The use of the ComPass Tool in WISECARE

4.2.1   Start Measurement

The assessment tool was distributed to each of the Validation Sites in April 1998. A web based-training course was made available on the WISECARE Website to assist the Validation Sites with the use of the tool. The tool has been updated based on the first experience and has been demonstrated at the user conference which took place in Helsinki in June 1999.

The data collection took place three times during the verification and validation of the project. The first data collection was in March 1999 before the first global feedback, the second in May after the global feedback, and the third in September in the end of the validation phase. Two Demonstration Sites were able to join the last, i.e. the 3rd, WiseCompass data collection. The results have been used in the impact analysis.

4.2.2   The Method of Analysis

The three different assessment "tools" will all have a special method of analysis. The process of collecting and processing the data will be the same for all Validation Sites.

For each of the assessment studies data collected by the Validation Sites will be send to HISCOM. At HISCOM a database has been created containing the information gathered during the assessment stage. The evaluation will focus on the impact of the WISECARE approach on the use of information within the department. The main objective of the process is to evaluate the impact of the use of information in each of the five Validation Sites.

But even more important is the learning process of sharing experiences among the WISECARE partners. So an important aspect of the analysis will be the comparison of the Validation Sites. The famous WHO approach of the "Good Apples" will be applied. The result of the individual assessment provides examples of "good or even best practice". The results have been used to illustrate the effect of an improved use of IT. The WISECARE Validation Sites were stimulated to learn from the experience at other Sites.

4.2.3   The results of the assessment

The Results of the assessment have been gathered in steps and stages during the WISECARE project. The results have been presented at the WISECARE user group meetings. The results have been used to enhance the WISECARE technology assessment tools. The final results have been documented in the deliverables 5.2, 5.3 and 5.4

As the project made changes in the focus of the data collection and the original eight questions were put aside. The assessment has shifted from the impact of WISECARE on the use of information for the management of nursing to the assessment of the potential of the WISECARE approach for improving nursing care. The assessment of the outcome and patient satisfaction has been performed as planned. The results of the assessment have been integrated in the final WISECARE report and as far as relevant in the TA Tool. The objects of study were nursing care assessment, assessing the links between medical and nursing care and the use of the nursing information system for improving nurse management. These aspects have been studied within the framework chosen by the WISE nurses within the project. As the focus was on specific nursing issues for a limited number of clinical conditions the discussion on the assessment of WISECARE on nursing management in general has been excluded from the agenda. The main theme of the technology assessment process within WISECARE still was "Assessment by the Excitement of trying to be a WISE nurse with WISE tools".

References

[1]   Institute of Medicine (U.S.). Committee for Evaluating Medical Technologies in Clinical Use. Division of Health Science Policy. In *Assessing Medical Technologies*. National Academy Press, Washington, D.C, 1985.

[2]   See http://www.borland.com/delphi/

[3]   Eurlings F, van Asten A, Cozijn H, Klaassen-Leil C, Stokman R, van Valkenburg R, Van Gennip E. Effects of a Nursing Information System in 5 Dutch Hospitals. In: U. Gerdin et al (Eds.), Nursing Informatics: The impact of Nursing Knowledge on Health Care Informatics. Studies in Health Technology and Informatics, volume 46, pag. 50-55. (IOS Press, Ohmsha 1996).

[4]   Steegh M., Cost analysis in VISTA II. in *Proceedings VISTA II symposium* F. Eurlings (ed) (Leiden: HISCOM b.v., 1997), 59-67.

[5]   Degeling P, Black D, Palmer G & Walters J. A national survey of the knowledge and attitudes of hospital staff about casemix. Report no. 1. The centre for hospital management and information systems research, the University of New South Wales, Sydney, 1995.

[6]   See http://www.efqm.org/

Methodological Issues

Luc Delesie

1 Issues and Options

The purpose of WISECARE information management is to generate feedback for the management of the workflow derived from the WISECARE data. We will investigate what is meant by feedback. This feedback will demand some European standardized or WISECARE way. But foremost feedback requires:

- to aggregate data: operations of aggregation, levels of aggregation, summarizing data,
- the measurement issue: what do the indicators measure: Several list of 'criteria to evaluate the utility of indicators' exist. The most popular criteria are: reliability (consistency, dependability, stability, predictability, accuracy), validity (specificity) that differentiates between content validity (comprehensiveness, comparability, homogeneity), predictive validity and construct validity, precision, sensitivity, timeliness, cost-effectiveness, flexibility and acceptability.
- to benchmark data: the reference issue: to reference, mirror, benchmark, calibrate, normalize or standardize those indicators.

In order to arrive at these stages of aggregation and benchmarking, one has first to analyse and evaluate the available data and decide on the types of feedbacks one aims at.

2 Variables, (Electronic) Database and Experimental Design

The analysis and evaluation of the WISEHOOS database can be done on different levels. One implies clinical evaluation if the level is the individual patient or his episode of care. Note that no aggregation of the individual electronic nursing records is involved on this level: just retrieval of archived, and possibly sorted data. This is still the most common application of electronic data analysis. Most feedback applications in the nursing unit that are based upon data in the electronic patient record are geared towards short and long lists of data or cross-tabulations of elementary data in some sorted way: by patient, by date and time, by nursing unit, by nursing activity, by problem.

But one can also analyze and evaluate the data in the database on higher levels: a level where the data is always aggregated. The scope of objectives of this database analysis and feedback on the aggregate level is quite large. It can involve clinical objectives: more effective or more efficient care or better-managed, sequenced care. This is the domain of evidence based nursing care. Some selected data are collected using a standardized and controlled scientific protocol on a sample of some selected patients by way of some experimental design and analyzed by way of some inferential statistical techniques to test the statistical significance of some hypothesis with respect to some nursing care problem, procedure or care path.

This nicely controlled type of clinical experiment is not the first purpose of WISECARE. The WISEHOOS database may constitute in due time a database for a whole range of most interesting hypotheses with respect to nursing care problems and procedures. But as of now, other priorities still prevail in WISECARE information management.

The first purpose of WISECARE is a database on day to day nursing care activity to allow the generation of workflow information with a view to the management of resources. One can compare this with the database of customer sales in a retail chain or of client transactions in a large bank. This type of database is by definition huge and ever expanding. The sensible analysis of this type of database for management purposes is of another nature than the statistical analysis of some nicely sampled data in the framework of a scientific experimental design, research activity or publication [1]. Misinterpretations, data errors and missing data are common in those multivariate databases due to the large number of participants and the lack of feasibility of scientific and controlled protocols. The common transactional communication, which these databases serve usually, goes on without major interruption as the sender and receiver of the data or message usually have redundant multivariate information or just pick up the local phone. The analysis of a large multivariate database from some point that is far away from the working floor, e.g. European feedback, requires some special precautions and expertise.

Figure 1 summarises the type of variables that WISECARE uses, hence those that are available for the generation of feedback information. Several variables have been reshaped during the WISECARE project while some others have been added. See chapter 1, Information Needs of Oncology Nurses.

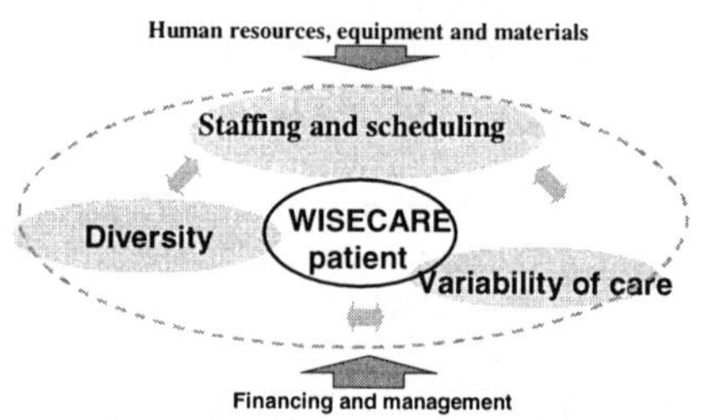

Figure 1   WISECARE Data

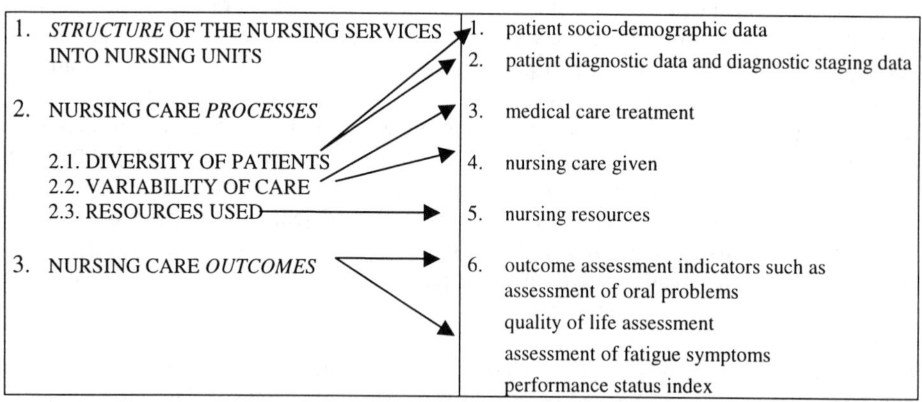

1. *STRUCTURE* OF THE NURSING SERVICES INTO NURSING UNITS	1. patient socio-demographic data
	2. patient diagnostic data and diagnostic staging data
2. NURSING CARE *PROCESSES*	3. medical care treatment
2.1. DIVERSITY OF PATIENTS	4. nursing care given
2.2. VARIABILITY OF CARE	
2.3. RESOURCES USED	5. nursing resources
3. NURSING CARE *OUTCOMES*	6. outcome assessment indicators such as assessment of oral problems
	quality of life assessment
	assessment of fatigue symptoms
	performance status index

Figure 2   WISECARE Variables

The data variables changed quite a lot during the course of the project to the following final variable definitions.

2.1 Patient Socio-Demographic Data

These data variables have stayed unchanged during the project. The feedback did not produce evidence one way or the other.

2.2 Patient Diagnostic Data and Diagnostic Staging Data

These variables were particularly inclined to be missing. Six diagnostic groups were chosen. The additional variables to describe their diversity in a more detailed way, e.g. severity, complications, … are predominantly missing and not retained for further analysis.

2.3 Medical Care Treatment

The medical care treatment variables have been thoroughly reshaped and expanded. As the classification of treatments became too lengthy to stay relevant, an aggregation became necessary that would be more relevant for nursing care. It has been developed. The reducing mapping implies that each treatment gets a risk category with respect to some nursing problems based upon the Leuven Chemotherapy Risk Assessment Scale (LCRAS).

A major change as a result of the first feedback was the inclusion of clinical time in the list of variables. This major addition was readily accepted by the clinically oriented nurses because of their natural propensity to think in clinical time terms with respect to every single patient. The time of the most important clinical events for the patients during their treatment is recorded as well as the time of care and the time for most data variables, including also the outcome variables.

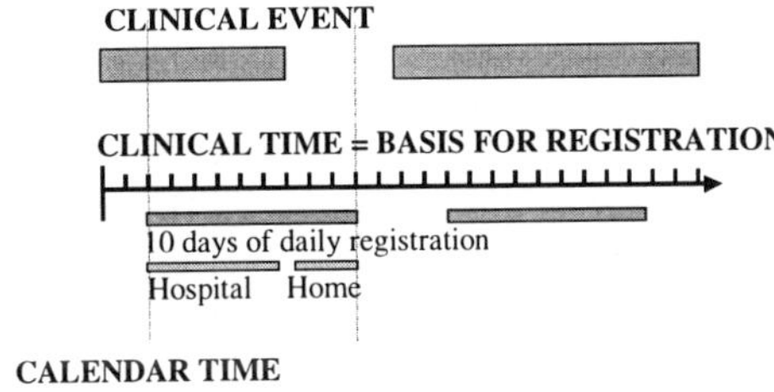

Figure 3   Clinical and Calendar Time

The introduction of clinical time helped the nurses in a major way to understand the whole project endeavour of which the data collection and registration is the most visible part to them.

2.4 Nursing Intensity

The measurement of nursing intensity was based on the nursing care given. A rather lengthy scale was introduced to classify the nursing care given into 4 ordinal categories. The Moffitt scale was used for this purpose. This scale was developed to provide one overall test of hypothesis in some scientific controlled experiments in oncology research and not at all for the daily management of individual patients. Nevertheless, the scale was well known and popular and hence was easily accepted. It was used not only for WISECARE patients but for other patients in the units as well.

2.5 Nursing Resources

Two variables measure the nursing resources:
- the number of hours of nursing per calendar day selected,
- the qualification level of the nurse: 4 ordinal qualification levels are identified.

Again the issue of time must be considered. The diversity of patients is of interest to epidemiology and a continuous calendar time perspective is advisable: the number of patients during the year, the number of new patients each semester. With respect to the relationship between the variability of care and the team however, a sampled time frame is advisable. To collect all data at all times, e.g. days of the year requires too big an effort.

2.6 Nursing Care Outcomes

The first feedback on these variables showed a lot of missing data and a major overhaul was required. Finally the following choices were made:
- Oral Care: the Oral Assessment Guide: the 8 original items were all retained.
- Pain: EORTC QLQ C-30 subscale: 2 questions were retained.
- Nausea & Vomiting: EORTC QLQ C-30 subscale: 2 questions were retained.
- Fatigue: EORTC QLQ C-30 subscale: 3 questions were retained.

The Piper Fatigue Scale was dropped. The scale was evaluated as too time-consuming for patients; the psychometric properties (reliability, consistency) have to be researched more profoundly. 23 of the original 30 EORTC QLQ C-30 items were not retained within the course of the project to prevent information overload.

Moreover although the Likert assumptions of the original scales were sufficient for overall hypothesis testing purposes, more research is needed for management purposes where every nurse expects a reliable score for every individual patient at any specific time. Hence the decision was made to continue temporarily the feedback based on these Likert assumptions and to wait for more data and experience before moving to a more refined and more sensible level of analysis. Hence the project version of the global feedback will use the following measurements:
- Oral care => likert score based upon AOG: score 8 to 24
- Nausea & Vomiting => likert score based upon EORTC: score 2 to 8
- Pain => likert score based upon EORTC: score 2 to 8
- Fatigue => likert score based upon EORTC: score 3 to 12

All scores were standardized between 0% and 100% by EORTC-data manual protocols [2].

3   Feedback

Feedback has many different meanings to many different people. To begin with, feedback as such is not a goal but a tool: a tool towards the achievement of some objectives. These objectives are specified in the project contract:

"The objective of the project is the evaluation of the impact of nursing care in the whole quality care for patients, through a systematic exploitation of data in electronic patient records, the definition of a model for integration of the nursing component in DRG-based systems and a development of a knowledge base of "best practices" in nursing care".

Objectives:
- A workflow information model to systematically exploit clinical nursing data, stored in electronic patient records, for clinical and resource management will be developed.

The diversity of the patient population, the variability of care, the patient outcomes and the nursing resources will be quantified using existing patient classification and coding systems. This information will be made visible using state-of-the-art data presentation techniques. Relations and links between the data will be analysed in a multivariate way, using state-of-the art statistical and analysis tools.

- A network of oncology care centres will be established by using network software (WWW, Lotus Notes) in which the clinical practice information will be shared. This will lead to *state-of-the art knowledge dissemination and sharing through the network partners.*

- The impact of the availability of information on the diversity of the patient population, the variability of care, patient outcomes and nursing resources that have been used and the links between these components, will be evaluated.

A core objective is "state-of-the-art knowledge dissemination and sharing through the network partners". What is knowledge? What is sharing? Figure 4 gives an overview of knowledge and sharing.

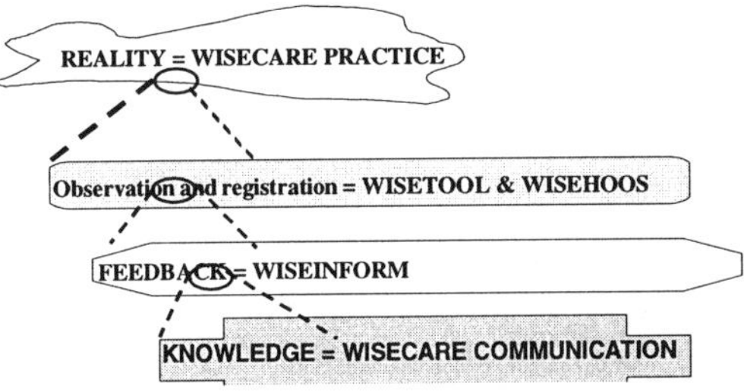

Figure 4   From Practice to Knowledge

Now starts the sensible data analysis to produce "information" which becomes knowledge through careful reading and sharing by way of communication: e-mail, web BSCW and meetings. The main goal of the feedback becomes the generation of information useful to the users; e.g. the nurses and nurse managers. They will use the feedback products in what is commonly known as their "decision cycle" (see Figure 5). The process of sensible data analysis is rather tricky [3]. The purpose however is clear: it has to foster communication among the nurses in order to improve their nursing practice. Most energy undoubtedly still goes to the collection, the registration, the storing and the communication of data. However, the main goal of all these efforts is to generate information that induces nurses to start thinking about their practice and to start a discussion among them in order to improve their nursing practice.

However, one has to realise that nursing care is primarily a clinical activity: the first objective of the nurse and the nursing care is the well-being of the patient. Once qualified, nurses start practising and will occasionally update their clinical knowledge. Though nurses spend at least 20% of their time recording things with respect to their patients on all types of order sheets and records, the main purpose of this data is the operational, daily, clinical management of the care for the patients that they are in charge of. Few of the enormous volumes of data that are stored in those order sheets and records are ever analysed with a view to better patient or more specifically, better nursing care. Evidence-based nursing is growing but still has a very long way to go in comparison to evidence-based medical care regarding publication of results, exchange of findings, meetings and congresses. A general investigative spirit and awareness still have to take root within the nurses group at large. This development is hampered by the fact that most patients respect the medical profession regarding their care and look at the nursing profession only as doctor's assistants. The public at large is unaware of the high cost of nursing care in comparison to medical care and of the specific contribution made by the nursing profession to patient care.

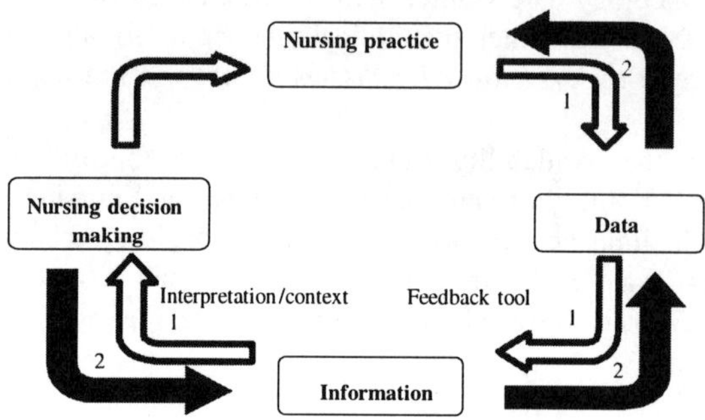

Figure 5   Nursing Decision Cycle

Moreover, though the project is meant to improve clinical nursing care, it is also meant to improve nursing resource management by the use of workflow information. The analysis of nursing care data with a view to a better management of nursing resources is even more limited than the clinical objectives. There is hardly any evidence-based information on the allocation of nursing staff for the care of oncological patients. We hardly even know how many nurses at all that are practising in European health care. Figures are mainly overall national figures on the number of nurses' diplomas, the number of nurses per bed or the number of qualified nurses by level of qualification.

The differences are due to:

- different health care systems, including differences in the capabilities of the nursing teams,
- differences in the processes of nursing care,
- differences in the outcomes of nursing care.

The real-life allocation of nurses in accordance with the needs of the patients is guesswork at best.

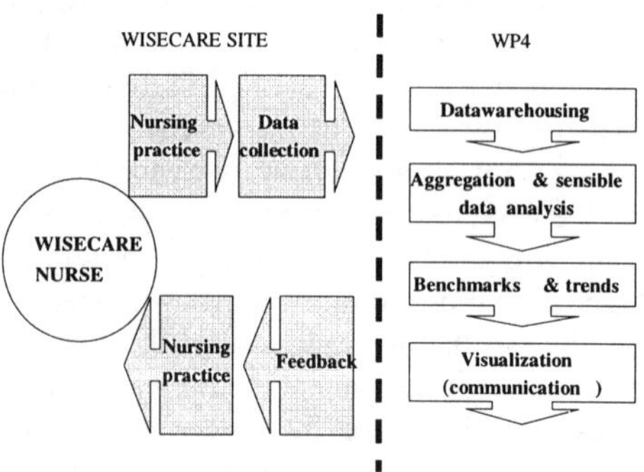

Figure 6   Feedback System

3.1 Feedback Possibilities

The project has already identified two types of feedback: the instant feedback and the global feedback. Many more feedback types are possible. This section explains the different types.

- In order to explain different feedback we want first define what feedback involves. Figure 6 shows the elements of the feedback. Few nurses have been confronted with feedback information beyond the level of the single individual patient. Three feedback problems emerge.
- What does aggregate data mean to the individual nurse?
- What does benchmarking mean? What is the difference between an absolute norm and a relative norm, e.g. how many nurses to deal with oral care problems? What does a trend mean?
- Once the feedback is produced in some way, be it a plain verbal story, tables or visualized data, what do you do with those things? On average, nurses have very little experience of how to reflect on their own nursing practice or to communicate and discuss their individual findings with her colleagues in order to improve the nursing practice on the unit.

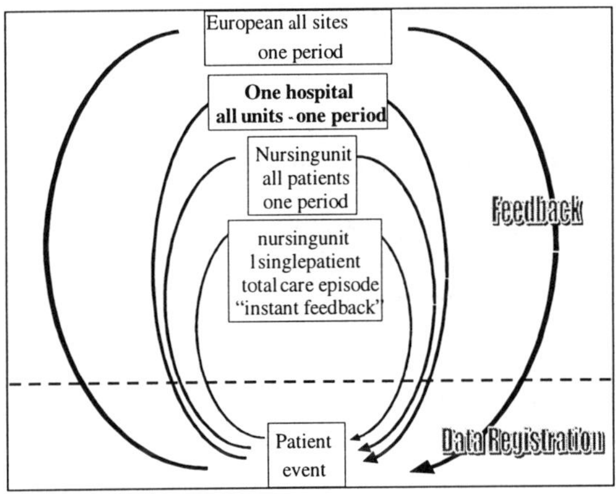

Figure 7   Feedback Levels

In order to solve these problems one more step was taken. Feedback and the feedback process can indeed be organized at several different levels of aggregation. Figure 7 gives the main levels. It was decided to separate the single patient – care episode feedback from all other levels of feedback. This single patient-care episode feedback is called instant feedback. It involves no benchmarking and no aggregation of patients. This instant feedback concentrates on the visualization of all the data that has been registered for the single WISECARE patient. Indeed this instant feedback amounts to something as a visualization of the data items in the "electronic" nurse patient record. It can be anticipated that this object of instant feedback would one day be incorporated into some basic electronic patient record alongside the medical elements and the administrative elements.

Experience showed that the nurses are quite happy with this instant feedback: Indeed it is easily recognized: no operation or abstraction is involved. The plain data as recorded are visualized.

As a result, what we will call the global feedback is reserved for any feedback that involves aggregation of patients and patient data and benchmarking.

3.2   Global Feedback Options

The first global feedback experience revealed a need to stick to the very basics and to start the communication about nursing practice from the very first step. Hence some reorientation of global feedback options became necessary.

The introduction of clinical time during the project put the solution of the time problem on the right tracks. However it was technically unfeasible to backtrack all WISECARE data already available and to amend it by way of including this clinical time. Hence it was decided to divide the WISECARE project and databank in two parts: the first part BCT (or Before Clinical Time Introduction) and the second part ACT (After Clinical Time).

The BCT-databank was further split up in two time periods for educational purposes only. BCT 1 goes from April 30 until December 30, 1998. BCT 2 goes from January 1, 1999 until April 15, 1999. ACT 2 goes from April 15, until September 30, 1999. ACT 2 is in process of analysing and goes from October 1 until December 31, 1999.

The introduction of a sampling time frame – see Figure 5 – put the solution towards the problem of resource management information on the right tracks. A uniform basically random sampling procedure of one random day per week was agreed upon to record nursing resources and their utilisation on the WISECARE unit. This sampling procedure allows investigating, analysing, aggregating and benchmarking the relationship between the variability of care – e.g. Moffitt scores – and the care team.

4   Levels of Aggregation and Benchmarking

Once the variables are understood and once the notion of global feedback explained, we can turn our attention to the methodological issues of aggregation and benchmarking: to aggregate and benchmark what, for what purpose.

This creates a problem, at this stage of WISECARE. The primary goal is to provide a frame of reference that is common to all participating nursing units. This frame of reference can only be developed after a global analysis of the data. As of 1999, data have been collected on some 300 patients involving some 600 episodes only. On the one hand it does not make sense to provide a local frame of reference when only 10 or 15 patients are involved. On the other hand some 300 patients is much too early for validity, precision and acceptability for many subgroups of patients.

Consequently, we conclude that:

- The feedback information should be as close to the user as technically feasible,
- For this, the feedback tools will run on a personal computer/Intel® with a Windows® operating system (windows 98®, windows NT®)
- Calibration will be done on the sideline using state-of-the-art methods and tools. The results, e.g. aggregating the multidimensional PFS item scores into a one single fatigue indicator, will have to be imported into the feedback tools later on and on an ongoing basis by way of conversion tables and sets of logical statistical operations
- The feedback should be highly graphical for the nurse users. The feedback data should only be available in background mode.
- Learning the feedback information language is not straightforward. The feedback information language is not a natural language. It is a man-made language in the same way as, e.g. the accounting language: yearly balance sheets, cost and income accounts. One cannot expect to understand the language after a few hours Berlitz-type

course. Some language learning and training will be necessary before the users will grasp the meaning and non-meaning of feedback indicators, ratios and graphs.

Hence, we focus on the issues, problems and solutions which we anticipate with respect to the local and global feedback once the project has reached cruising speed.

4.1 Time problem

The WISECARE clinical data aim at an epidemiological, incidental or longitudinal perspective of the selected oncological patients. The WISECARE resources data aim at a cross-sectional, prevalence analysis of the oncological patients at one particular moment or 'window' of time.

The clinical data aims at the tracing of specific patients through their care paths and their resulting status evolution. This makes sense. Indeed many WISECARE measurements, hence variables, change over time. Sex and diagnosis may stay the same, but many other measurements diagnostic stage, even age, but foremost all assessment variables, medical treatments, nursing care and resources change over time even if these changes are not always taken into account. The calendar time as such is of little value. One wants to pinpoint each measurement to a specific moment of time with respect to each patient, his diagnostic stage, and treatment progress. We call this the patient time or patient clinical time. Status, assessment and resources measurements highly depend on the clinical time of the patient's treatment. In order to monitor, evaluate, aggregate and benchmark the data one has to take into account this clinical time. It is however no easy task to keep track of this clinical time.

This demands the co-ordination not just of the variables that are recorded in the WISECARE project but also of the time of registration of these variables. Experience with patient and patient care databases that are used for management purposes demonstrates that it is no easy task to keep track of the patient's time. Moreover most managers are not yet interested in the patient time and leave this patient time to the clinicians. For example it is hardly relevant for financing purposes, when some activity took place in the context of the individual patient; it suffices to know that it took place. Indeed, most resources are not allocated on the basis of one individual patient but are allocated on the basis of the total workload that confronts a particular care team such as a nursing team on a nursing unit, at one particular moment in time, e.g. a specific day or a weekend. However, as WISECARE aims at workflow management, hence workflow information, with an emphasis on flow, it seems prerequisite to keep track of the patient's clinical time.

Some WISECARE participating Sites record the diagnosis and diagnostic stage at one moment of time only. This moment of time may be completely irrelevant to the nursing workflow, e. g. the diagnosis and diagnostic stage is recorded at the historic ambulatory contact of the patient with his physician when the oncological diagnosis was first confirmed. Some WISECARE participating Sites record particular variables at fixed time intervals unrelated to the patients' treatment on the patient's status.

As a result, some WISECARE variables are felt as a nuisance by the nurses. Hence, their recording becomes shaky and unreliable, for example Oral Assessment Guide. Oral problems may vary from day to day. As a result the Oral Assessment Guide is instructed to be recorded daily. However many days go by without any real oral problems at all. After a while, nurses start to "forget" or to keep track of oral assessment. This is a classical "crying wolf" situation: too much monitoring creates motivational problems and results in less reliable monitoring.

The WISECARE project solved this issue of time recording. Most Sites started to record clinical time manually. One Site solved this by going to a complete electronic patient record that keeps track of all patient episodes and interventions, hence clinical time automatically. This demanded a major investment in information technology and information education. It may be the direction of future development but to date little cost-benefit experience is available and in any case the other WISECARE Sites were not yet ready to take this step.

4.2 Aggregation problem

Feedback beyond the individual clinical level requires aggregation and benchmarking. We first focus on aggregation. Indeed if one wants to keep track of clinical indicators over clinical time, one needs very valid and precise aggregate indicators in able to monitor anything.   Any 60% reproducible scale [4] leads to statistical significance given a sufficient number of observations. Real-life management wants 99%!   If the 80% confidence interval for a particular score is, e.g. 15 plus or minus 6, one will no longer be able to determine if the next day's score of 12 plus or minus 6 really differs from the old score and if action is warranted. Reliable scales are prerequisite.

The WISECARE assessment scales are the cornerstones of the WISECARE project. These are inherently subjective. Not "evidence" but "consensus and control" are the important aspects for assessment scales. The scores are all the result of some operations of aggregation on the level of the patient. Items and gradations are recorded. The recorded data are aggregated. The most common operations of aggregation are plain sums and averages. These operations are perfectly correct with respect to a whole set of common life variables: age, temperature, and many cost data. On the other hand these operations become complete useless in some other situations.   E.g. WISECARE provides for 5 patient groups and a numerous list of medical treatments. Though one can easily add 3 breast cancers with 2 lung cancers, any calculator will do the trick, the sum becomes meaningless: 5 what?   The same holds for the many treatments. If one could map the treatments onto a common cost scale, one could still compare usefully the cost of treatment. But even if one could map the treatments upon one common ordinal scale of toxicity one can no longer continue adding: a treatment with toxicity category 2 plus one treatment with toxicity 1 does not equal to one treatment with toxicity 3. Notwithstanding the senselessness of this addition in several cases, several WISECARE variables, widely published and highly referenced in the literature, add up without any reflection or concern for the meaning or intelligence of the operation.

Aggregating data depends on the level of measurement of the data and on the distribution of the data[1] The WISECARE variables use three levels of measurement.

4.2.1 Nominal or categorical data

Diagnostic Data, Treatment Codes, Sex, Nursing Units
Nominal measurement results from the use of classifications. We take the ICD-International Statistical Classification of Diseases as an example. The different versions of the ICD, now at its 10th version, reflect our growing understanding of morbidity [3]. The 5-character ICD-10 code identifies some 14.000 different diseases and related health

---

[1] The next sections are basically derived from an existing non-WISECARE text. See: Delesie L, Considerations on Rates for hospital and health services development, World Health Organization, District Health Systems, Division of Strengthening of Health Services, Geneva 1998 (in print). The purpose of this copying is the elucidation of the points made.

problems at the finest level of detail. This allows for very precise measurement in the case by case or clinical approach but ends up with many zeros and many small numbers as soon as one moves to the group or management level: the epidemiological perspective. The number of different diagnoses or combinations of diagnoses is just enormous. Hence the temptation is very real to drastically reduce or aggregate this large number to a so-called "manageable number of diagnostic categories" such as the 27 Main diagnostic Categories, the original 467 Diagnostic Related Groups (DRG), the 619 AP-DRG-10.0's [5]. This simplification into a smaller number of main groups unfortunately covers up the fine shadings which were registered at great cost by the individual service providers. Diseases that are considered different at the more detailed level of classification become exactly alike at the higher or the less detailed level in the hierarchy of the classification.

The problem becomes what logical operations can be used on these ever-expanding databases to bridge the gap between the micro world of the clinicians and the macro world of the managers. The numerical operations in use nowadays to produce these management summaries, are most frequently sums and averages. Weights are also easy to understand and have become most popular: a relative cost index by diagnosis, a national nursing care value by DRG or procedure. This simple operation of a weighted sum or average provides for a synthesis but, by the same token, conceals very much the variability and the highly skewed distributions of nursing care within the patient groups under consideration.

Recently methods are becoming available to display the information hidden in the ever-expanding databases in an accessible and meaningful way. These methods rely on modern descriptive statistical techniques, computers and graphical interfaces. These methods demand some sophistication. A fictitious example illustrates this. Suppose we want to look at the treatment codes for Lung Cancer and Breast Cancer patients. One can look at the patient groups by way of their treatment profile or the vector of the treatment codes by patient group: see Table 1. It is important to understand that the vectors of care demand different "units of measurement" on the different levels of decision-making. This is true to such extent that what may look identical at one level of observation may be completely different on a more detailed, zoomed-in, level of observation. The two treatment classifications or levels of observation are of course hierarchically related. The number in the cells of the Tables 1 and 2 give the number of patients in each of the two patient groups who received the particular treatment as indicated by the column.

Fictitious example: Patient group Lung Cancer and patient group Breast Cancer: the first table assumes that there exists 8 major categories of treatments.

Table 1 'Treatment Code' 8 Major Treatment Codes

Lung Cancer	83	65	17	9	5	2	1	1
Breast Cancer	83	65	17	9	5	2	1	1

However, suppose now that each of the 8 major categories of treatments can be subdivided into 2 more detailed, so-called minor categories of treatments. This results in a total of 16 minor treatment categories. The previous table now looks like:

Table 2 'Treatment Code' 16 Minor Treatment Codes

Lung Cancer	83	0	65	0	17	0	9	0	5	0	2	0	1	0	1	0
Breast Cancer	0	83	0	65	0	17	0	9	0	5	0	2	0	1	0	1

Everybody agrees that the two patient groups are exactly alike with respect to their treatment profile when both vectors of care have exactly the same number of observations in each category. Everybody agrees that the two patient groups completely differ with respect to their treatment profile when the vector of one patient group has observations, only in those categories where the other vector has no observations, and conversely. On the basis of the 8 major treatment code categories, patient group Lung Cancer completely resembles patient category Breast Cancer. At the same time, on the basis of the 16 minor treatment code categories, patient group Lung Cancer is completely different from patient category Breast Cancer.

The filtering process into a manageable number of treatment code categories and the subsequent comparison of patient groups on the basis of vectors of care or treatment code categories profile invoke quite a few fundamental measurement problems.

Within the WISECARE project, the limited number of data does not allow yet to skip the issue of aggregation by turning immediately to benchmarking: feedback for every possible combination of patient type and sequence of treatment codes.

The WISECARE project does not yet aggregate or benchmark nominal data: no aggregate patient profiles (the diversity of patients) nor care vectors (the variability of medical and nursing care) are yet established on the level of the different Sites.

4.2.2   Rates For Ordinal Data

Illness Stage, Performance Status, Quality Of Life Assessment, Oral Assessment Guide, Piper Fatigue Scale
The use of ordinal measurements in health and hospital care is expanding and the WISECARE shows numerous examples. Obtaining an item-by-item measurement is a common exercise. The problem arises as soon as one wants to aggregate the ordinal data to obtain one single rate or indicator on the level one patient, let alone on the level of a group of patients. Rule of thumbs and simplifications prevail and even the statistical literature states that the violation of the statistical assumptions can be considered a minor problem. The most used operation of aggregation is a weighted sum. Consider however the EORTC Quality of Life assessment scale QLQ-C30 (version 3). The scale has 28 items and each item has four categories of ordinal scores: I, II, III and IV. One illustrative example (Table 3) is selected:

Table 3   EORTC QLQ C-30 Selection

Do you have any trouble taking a long walk?	1- Not at all 2- a little 3- quite a bit 4- very much
Do you have any trouble taking a short walk outside of the house?	1- Not at all 2- a little 3- quite a bit 4- very much

It must be clear that the sum score can hardly already be obtained.
- First fact: a score of (short walk = very much = 4) is unlikely to be combined with (long walk = not at all=1).
- Second fact: what does a sum with a value of 5 means? (Short walk = very much) + (Long walk = not at all), (Long walk = very much) + (short walk = not at all), (Long walk = quite a bit) + (short walk = a little) all sum up to 5 even though every scoring combination measures quite divergent situations! Just summing these scores to one overall number is meaningless.

If the operations of aggregation imply nonsense, the aggregate assessment scores become unvalid, unprecise and useless for monitoring purposes. As these ordinal assessment scales are central in the WISECARE project, we will show in a next section how the available data allow already aggregating the Oral Assessment data in a more reliable, valid and precise way.

The small example of the 2 items shown indicates that the EORTC Quality of Life assessment scale QLQ-C30 (version 3) is at least partially a Guttman scale or an hierarchical ordered scale which takes into account that every item contributes to an overall score in its item specific way. Most probably the EORTC Quality of Life assessment scale QLQ-C30 (version 3) scale is a mixed type scale (Likert + Guttman type) which demands for its proper gauging, taking into account the cultural and translation problems of each WISECARE Site. The other scales, the Oral Assessment Guide and the Piper Fatigue Scale are just the same. Just a look at the Piper Fatigue Scale (Table 4).

Table 4 PFS Selection

To what degree is the fatigue you are feeling interfering your ability to visit or socialize with your friends?	0 no distress 10 a great deal of distress
To what degree is the fatigue you are feeling interfering with your ability to engage in sexual activity?	0 no distress 10 a great deal of distress

One WISECARE participant explicitly wondered how one dares to assume that these 2 items contribute equally to an overall score. He could only imagine so if 'socializing with your friends' implied 'sexual activity' and conversely!

The Piper Fatigue Scale also asks for how long the patient has been feeling fatigue. The actual responses vary between minutes and 'two years'. How can 'one sum' possibly aggregate these two scores in a sensible way? The available database does not yet contain sufficient data to start gauging the different scales in a reasonably accurate way.

Can we just 'weight' the patient scores? Though weighted sums and averages are popular operations of aggregation, this hocus pocus with weights can really run out of hand and provoke much friction. The error in this construction is logical and very basic: the weights assume or impose an absolute measurement where only a relative measurement exists. To obtain an aggregate measurement, one can only obtain a relative value by way of e.g. a Wilcoxon type score such as a rank score or a ridit [6]. This aggregate score will demand for calibration and continuous monitoring [7]. Examples illustrate how any result can be manipulated with the popular simplification of weights, leading to distrust of nurses, managers and policy-makers when confronted with scores in this new expanding area of ordinal measurements on severity of case-mix, intensity of care and outcome measurements such as quality of services and health performance status. The statistical sophistication that is necessary to deal with these ordinal rates in some acceptable, reliable and routine way is unfortunately not yet widely available.

4.2.3 Rates For Metric Data

Age, Duration of Episode

Metric data such as the WISECARE variables age and duration of episode are best known, most easily understood and fortunately, demand readily available expertise only. The common operation to arrive at the group rate or the aggregation for management purposes, is the (weighted) sum or average: average cost, average length of stay. The common problem with these linear operations of average, correlation and analysis of variance on which many rates are based, is that the underlying assumption of normal distributions of the measurements (cost, length of stay) is very frequently overlooked. Unfortunately, highly skewed, non-symmetric distributions often prevail in the hospital services: more complex, more severe, high risk cases are (by definition!) a small minority. Moreover, and again quite unfortunately, these more complex, more severe, high risk cases are exactly the ones that need or consume most resources. The "law of large numbers" that alleviates this aggregation problem for large populations, does not work anymore with limited groups, the ones that managers have to deal with.

The database gives some nice examples. The Oral Assessment Guide varies between 8 (the minimum score) and 24 (the maximum score). The distribution of this score will very much depend on the recording habits of the nursing unit. Scores everyday for all patients will result in a lot of "value 8 scores" and a few scores of higher value. An average score value may be 8,5. But this makes as much sense as an average score of 2,5 heart transplants yearly by hospital. Most hospitals do not have any heart transplants and only a few hospitals have them. Hence how to aggregate? Do we leave out all the value 8 scores? But then why should they be recorded in the first place? The problem of choosing the right denominator is very much present in the WISECARE project.

Indeed the whole health care sector is very skewed: less than 10% of the population consumes more than 90% of all resources, e.g. 20% of all oncological cases use more than 80% of all oncological hospital resources: what does a decrease in an average length of stay for an episode of hospitalization mean? Are all types of patients discharged one day earlier? Are bigger readmission risks taken for the more severe patients? Are more less severe cases (with short lengths of stay) admitted? As stated, no sound nursing manager would anymore dare to base his decision-making, e.g. the allocation of budgets, staff, on averages alone. This complicates the development of resources: the old "average" based rates that were sufficient in the period of expansion or allocation of resources, are no longer suited to finetune resource re-allocation in the age of 'closed budgets'. Though non-linear statistical techniques that look beyond the common average and the common variance or standard deviation are becoming more and more available, they are only slowly diffused as they require some more advanced course. Undoubtedly, the wide-market distribution of statistical software that is now taking place in the path of personal computers and international networks will foster the diffusion of fine-tuned rates for management purposes but even the most sophisticated computer tool requires a competent professional to use them.

4.3 Benchmarking Problem

The second feedback problem is benchmarking. In shorthand this means that if one nurse looks at the feedback in one WISECARE Site she has read and understand the same things as another nurse in another WISECARE Site. Feedback indeed requires a common frame of reference in order to foster communication about nursing care, workflow information and resource management. Older or less fashionable words for benchmarking are standardizing, normalizing, mirror data reference points, calibrating data.

The WISEHOOS allows to benchmark in different ways: one frame of reference by WISECARE Site, e.g. instant feedback; one frame of reference for all WISECARE Sites, e.g. global feedback, one frame of reference by patient group across WISECARE Sites, one frame of reference by patient and by treatment code across WISECARE Sites.

The sequence of WISECARE variables (diagnosis, stage, treatment, age, sex, clinical time…) to arrive at homogeneous WISECARE patient groups suitable for benchmarking can be quite lengthy. Also, the number of combinations of these variables, hence the number of feasible sequences is limitless. Given that the database is still in its infancy with some 300 patients and some 600 episodes, it will take more time before it contains enough data to arrive at a reasonable number of patients by WISECARE defined homogeneous patient groups.

The alternative is just to map all patients into one single, all encompassing, list of a manageable number of, so-called, homogeneous patient groups. This approach is very popular, as it is very easy to explain and is easily understood by most care providers. A nice example is the Diagnostic Related Groups: one single list of 619 different patient groups (version AP-DRG 10,0). The problem of this benchmarking approach however is that these groups are assumed to be homogeneous but that they often are not. These groups assume that the average age characterizes the group, while in fact the distribution of age is quite large; they assume that all members of the group receive the same 'standard' package of care, but a closer look often reveals quite variable care activities; the groups assume that the average length of stay characterizes the group, while in fact the length varies from e.g. 5 to 50 days. Moreover, a closer look at the distributions themselves often reveal that they are hardly 'normal' or Gauss. As a result the use of an average and standard deviation, which assume a normal distribution, as overall, synthesis indicators of the distributions is questionable.

The feedback process found a common ground between those extreme positions. The second benchmarking problem is the number of intervals by variable e.g. the age variable, one wants to cluster the variable into some limited number of contiguous age groups. The number of clusters/intervals and the choice of clusters will however very much depend on the problem of investigation: one cannot cluster in a sensible way before some analysis of the data.

In order to arrive at some sensible clustering for benchmarking purposes, a preliminary data analysis is necessary. This data analysis will involve at least some reasonable number of observations: 300 observations is too little to arrive yet at a sensible benchmark.

It is also quite possible to arrive at some relevant age clusters with respect to e.g. the Piper Fatigue Scale that differ from the age clusters that are relevant with respect to some other variable such as, e.g. EORTC QLQ-C30.

5   More refined Calibration of the WISECARE Assessment Scales

5.1 Introduction

Each type of measurement demands for its proper and valid, logical, mathematical and statistical operations. E.g. one can not in a valid way "sum" 2 measurements on diagnosis. The "sum" of 5 breast cancers plus 3 lung cancers has no meaning. Nevertheless it is still common practice to sum the response data on individual items to arrive at one outcome indicator score. This sum operation is easily understood and the sum score is most likely highly correlated with the true outcome assessment. Although inherently invalid, this sum score is good enough for many statistical applications but as indicated already it often leads to useless scores for clinical monotoring purposes or management information.

- Does one pair of patients with 1 patient with response 1 and 1 patient with response 2, equal 1 patient with response 3? In any case, the "sums" are equal.
- It can easily be the case that a moderate problem with teeth is perceived by the patient or the nurse as a bigger problem than a major problem with lips.
- How do we manage the data when one item has not been scored?
- Are all the items interchangeable or are there different subgroups of items?

By way of introduction, the Oral Assessment Score already analysed more thoroughly. This exercise goes through the different steps and presents the evidence from the WISECARE database. Some unfamiliar and complex data analysis software and algorithms are used along the way. Unfortunately, sensible data analysis is a profession that demands its proper training. There is no quick "60 minutes" course in data analysis. Final results only are presented.

5.2 Problem Formulation

The items and their individual response categories are copied from the Oral Assessment Guide (Table 5).

Table 5 OAG Score sheet

Item	Response categories		
Voice	Normal =1	Deep or Raspy =2	Difficulty talking/painful =3
Swallow	Normal swallow =1	Some pain on swallow =2	Unable to swallow =3
Mucous Membranes	Pink and moist =1	Reddened or coated without ulceration =2	Ulceration with or without bleeding =3
Tongue	Pink and moist and papillae present =1	Coated or loss of papillae with shinny appearance with or without bleeding=2	Blistered or cracked =3
Lips	Smooth and pink and moist =1	Dry and cracked =2	Ulcerated or bleeding =3
Gingiva	Pink and stippled and firm =1	Oedematous with or without redness =2	Spontaneous bleeding or bleeding with pressure =3
Teeth & Dentures	Clean and no debris =1	Plaque or debris in localised area =2	Plaques or debris in generalised along gum line or denture bearing area =3
Saliva	Watery =1	Thick or ropy =2	Absent =3

How can we meaningfully assign one single score, one number, in this case an outcome assessment indicator, for the aggregate of all items on oral problems, to each WISECARE patient, at each moment of clinical time during his treatment? This is called the *scaling* problem. We will go through different steps or procedures and apply different operations on the original item responses to arrive at our OAG score.
After cleaning the data, 2172 observations are retained (Table 6).

Table 6 Number of observations by category

	Response categories			
	Missing	1	2	3
Gingiva	0	1900	251	21
Lips	0	1737	429	6
Mucous_M	0	1735	330	107
Saliva	0	1797	309	66
Swallow	2	1944	218	8
Teeth_And	1	1757	404	10
Tongue	0	1556	574	42
Voice	0	1858	300	14

Notwithstanding our thorough preliminary cleaning, some missings still show up. We drop the 3 observations as we assume that they will not influence the logic of our analysis.
We first investigate if all the OAG items measure the same thing or if some items measure different things. We therefore look at the well-known matrix of correlation

coefficients. As the variables under investigation are ordinal, we use the Kendall tau-B rank order correlation coefficients.

Table 7 Correlation measurement

Correlations

Kendall's tau_b			Gingiva	Lips	Mucous Membran es	Saliva	Swallow	Teeth and dentures	Tongue	Voice
	Gingiva	Correlation Coefficient		.000	.000	.000	.000	.000	.000	.000
		Sig. (2-tailed)	.	.000	.000	.000	.000	.000	.000	.000
		N	2169	2169	2169	2169	2169	2169	2169	2169
	Lips	Correlation Coefficient	.284	1.000	.244	.274	.186	.098	.306	.183
		Sig. (2-tailed)	.000	.	.000	.000	.000	.000	.000	.000
		N	2169	2169	2169	2169	2169	2169	2169	2169
	Mucous Membranes	Correlation Coefficient	.418	.244	1.000	.323	.215	.166	.393	.128
		Sig. (2-tailed)	.000	.000	.	.000	.000	.000	.000	.000
		N	2169	2169	2169	2169	2169	2169	2169	2169
	Saliva	Correlation Coefficient	.349	.274	.323	1.000	.399	.030	.372	.183
		Sig. (2-tailed)	.000	.000	.000	.	.000	.161	.000	.000
		N	2169	2169	2169	2169	2169	2169	2169	2169
	Swallow	Correlation Coefficient	.266	.186	.215	.399	1.000	-.021	.237	.256
		Sig. (2-tailed)	.000	.000	.000	.000	.	.333	.000	.000
		N	2169	2169	2169	2169	2169	2169	2169	2169
	Teeth and dentures	Correlation Coefficient	.171	.098	.166	.030	-.021	1.000	.095	.059
		Sig. (2-tailed)	.000	.000	.000	.161	.333	.	.000	.006
		N	2169	2169	2169	2169	2169	2169	2169	2169
	Tongue	Correlation Coefficient	.312	.306	.393	.372	.237	.095	1.000	.169
		Sig. (2-tailed)	.000	.000	.000	.000	.000	.000	.	.000
		N	2169	2169	2169	2169	2169	2169	2169	2169
	Voice	Correlation Coefficient	.203	.183	.128	.183	.256	.059	.169	1.000
		Sig. (2-tailed)	.000	.000	.000	.000	.000	.006	.000	.
		N	2169	2169	2169	2169	2169	2169	2169	2169

The table shows that most coefficients have pretty small values: with one exception, they are all smaller than 0.400. One coefficient is even negative, though not significant. These results point already in the direction that the items as such do not overwhelmingly point in the same direction. The items "Teeth and dentures" and "Swallow" even point in opposite direction. These are pretty strong signals that the items can not simply be summed as the published literature suggests. The evidence suggests to consider the item "Teeth & dentures" as different from the other items with respect to an indicator of oral problems. At this stage already we can state that there will be at least 2 oral assessment indicators: one based on "teeth & denture" problems and the other one or others ones - we will see - based on the other items. The formal scientific expression is that the 8 original items are not "summative" or Likert scale type or cannot be arrived at by summing the item responses.

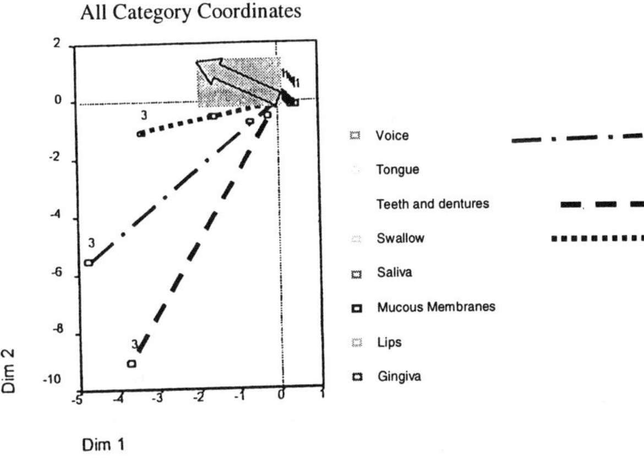

Figure 8   Dimensionality Problem

5.3 How many assessment indicators out of the 8 OAG items?

We now investigate the possible number of final OAG indicators. We know that "teeth and dentures" is a very strong candidate for one assessment indicator but what about the remaining 7 items? Do we end up with 1, 2, 3, ... knowing that the maximum is 7? This problem is called the *dimensionality problem.* (Figure 8) explains the dimensionality problem.

How far can we aggregate the original number of items into a smaller number of indicators? We prefer to end up with 1 or one overall OAG assessment indicator, but does the evidence support this aggregation. It could be that we have to settle with 2 or 3. Keep in mind that aggregate indicators or dimensions are not the same as their original items: one says that the aggregation is more than the sum of its parts. New concepts will have to be defined based on clinical and data analysis competence. Statistical algorithms are commercially available, some of which are called multidimensional scaling-MDS algorithms that allow to investigate and discover the number of dimensions that are hidden in the data. Figure 8 shows the MDS result for all 8 original items. Lines through 0 represent directions. The original response categories are represented on the lines by the points 1, 2 and 3. Correlation coefficients between items are represented by angles between the lines: Lines that coincide means that the correlation between the items concerns equals 1 or that the items measure the same thing. Orthogonality means correlation equals 0. To start with, the graph shows immediately the special character of the item "Teeth & dentures". This confirms our previous finding. Subsequently we see a direction for the item "Voice" and the item "Swallow". All remaining 5 items or directions are grouped into the arrow as they run very much parallel to each other.

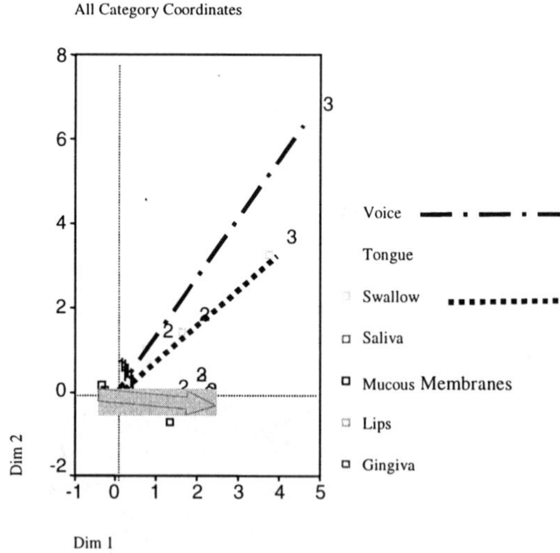

Figure 9   Directions of Dimensions

This MDS result points into the direction of no more than 4 dimensions for the 8 original items. One dimension is for sure: "Teeth & dentures".

We continue our investigation by zooming in on the remaining 7 items. The figure shows 3 directions: "Voice", "Swallow" and one direction for the 5 remaining items: "Tongue", "Gingiva", "Mucous Membranes", "Lips" and "Saliva". A nurse remarked that this result made clinical sense: all the blood organs, in which we include with some leniency the item "saliva", respond very similarly to chemotherapy which in fact is carried by the bloodstream. It makes sense that oral problems show up in all blood organs in the mouth area at the same time. In conclusion of this dimensionality search, the decision three directions with respect to our thorough analysis of mouth problems is represented in Figure 9.

In search of oral assessment indicators based on response data on the 8 items selected in the Oral Assessment Guide, we arrive at two aggregate indicators:

- The first aggregate oral assessment indicator deals with "Teeth & dentures"
- The second aggregate oral assessment indicator deals with the blood organs in the mouth area such as Tongue, Mucous Membranes, Lips, Gingiva, and Saliva but also includes, for reasons of simplicity, Voice and Swallow.

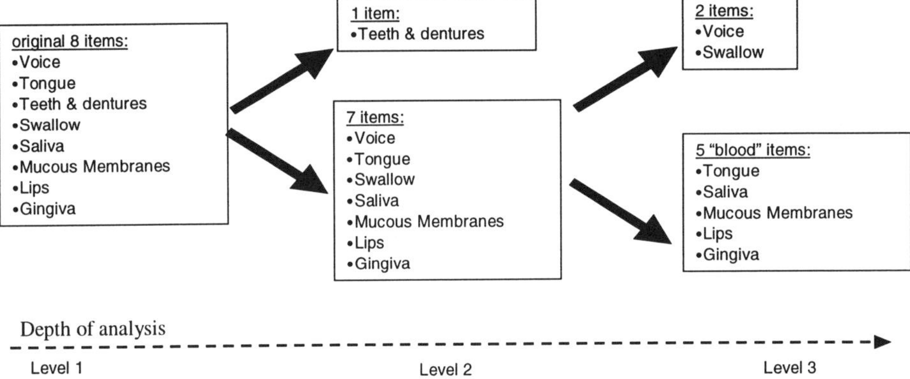

Figure 10 Aggregated Indicators

As the purpose of this exercise is only to show how outcome assessment scores will be more accurately be investigated in the future, we decide yet to stop at level 2.

5.4 How to aggregate the Item Category Responses to arrive at one Oral Assessment Indicator?

Now that we have decided on 2 outcome assessment indicators, the final problem is how to map/relate the original response categories into some value, point, category or interval on those 2 indicators. Each of these indicators is uni-dimensional or measures one direction as explained. Basically, there exist 2 prototype methods to do this. The first one is called a Likert or "summative" scale. This is the easy one to explain as it amounts to the commonly understood and easy operation of addition or summing of the item categories. It assumes that all items are interchangeable: all items contribute in the same amount to the assessment indicator. It also assumes that each category has the same impact independent of the item or in plain language: e.g. category 2 means the same thing on each item. Consequently, all items have to be linear and very highly correlated with each other.

The other prototype approach is called a Guttman, "cumulative" scale or scalogram analysis. This one is somehow more difficult to explain. Basically, it involves a hierarchy or progression in the responses on the items. With ordinal items there is always some hierarchy or progression present: e.g. on every single item a major problem presupposes the existence of at least a moderate problem. Guttman scale analysis goes one step further and is based on a hierarchy or progression among all item response categories as indicated in the figure. A progression or hierarchy implies an order or sequence of items and response categories. An example of such order is: e.g. one must have reached category 2 (= moderate problem) for item "Swallow" before one can reach category 2 (= moderate problem) for item "Mucous Membranes". This order also means that category 2 (= moderate problem) for item "Mucous Membranes" is perceived by the patients and nurses as a bigger problem than category 2 (= moderate problem) for item "Swallow" (Figure 11).

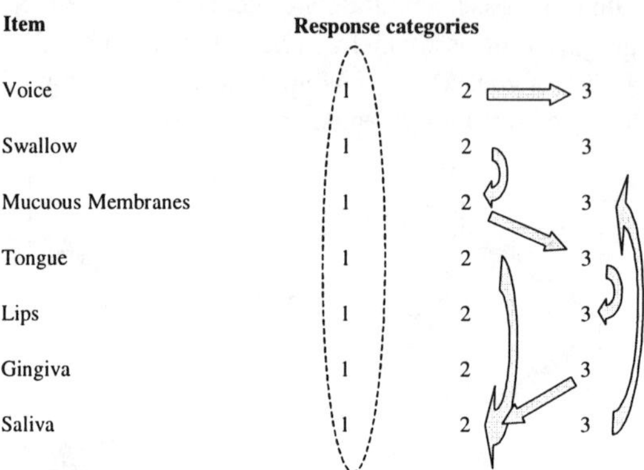

Figure 11 Guttman Scale Analysis

Of course there is no difference between the 7 "no problem" categories. Hence, we group all 1=no problem into 1 single category "no problems": the zero, null or minimum point of our assessment indicator. There are 7 x 2 or 14 item categories left for which we have to discover the most likely sequence of items and categories. An example of such sequence is given in Figure 12.

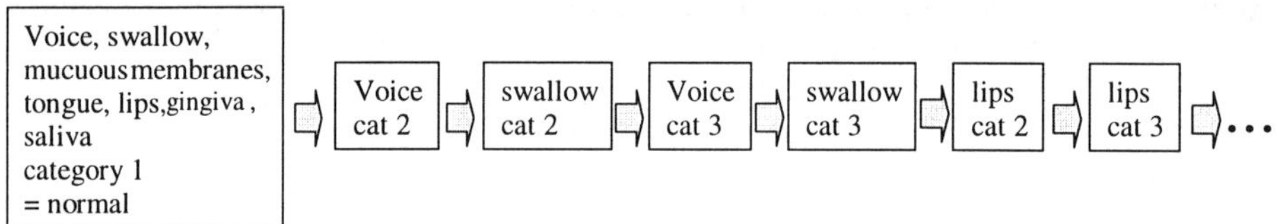

Figure 12 Sequence of Items

We do this by looking at all possible pairs of item-category responses. Voice 2 and Swallow 2, Voice 2 and Swallow 3, Voice 2 and Lips 2 and so on. As mentioned, pairs of item response categories of the same item are always ordered: voice 2 always comes before voice 3. Actually there are (14 x 13)/ 2 or 91 pairs left to investigate with respect to most likely order: e.g. does Tongue 2 comes before Lips 3 or is it the other way around?

To check the order between any pair of item categories, we just look at the evidence:

- The number of WISECARE patients for whom Tongue 2 is scored while Lips 3 is not scored:

Tongue 2	Lips 3
1	0

- The number of WISECARE patients for whom Lips 3 is scored while Tongue 2 is not scored:

Tongue 2	Lips 3
0	1

If there are more patients present in the WISECARE DATABASE where we find the first possibility (1) - in the ideal case all patients - we will conclude that the order is: "Tongue 2 comes before Lips 3".

If there are more patients in the WISECARE DATABASE where the second possibility (2) is found - again, in the ideal case all patients - we will conclude that the order is: "Lips 3 comes before Tongue 2".

We proceed with all possible pairs to end up with a final complete ordering of all item category responses. In our case this would mean an assessment indicator with 1 plus 14 or 15 shadings or ordered categories from minimum to maximum: from no problems on all 7 oral problem items to major problems on all 7 oral problem items.

In real-life a prototype Likert scale is as rare as a prototype Guttman scale. Most scoring instruments are a mixture of Likert and Guttman. The OAG with the 7 items is no exception. There is evidence of Likert characteristics: 5 of the 7 items point into the same direction and hence are somehow interchangeable. There is also evidence of Guttman characteristics. In the table of number of observations by item response categories, we do already observe that major problems (=3) with item "mucous membranes" are much more frequent, 107 observations, than major problems (=3) with item "lips", 6 observations only. This indeed implies that a patient will most likely have major problems with "mucous membranes" before he develops major problems with "lips".

5.5 Final oral assessment indicators

As there is only one item for the oral assessment indicator "teeth & dentures", we do not have to aggregate and can use the original item categories responses. We now aggregate the 7 remaining items by assuming a Guttman scale and will test this hypothesis.

We use statistical algorithms that we developed for this purpose. These give the best ordering of all the original item response categories. This order and the number of observations for the 15 original item response categories are represented in Figure 13.

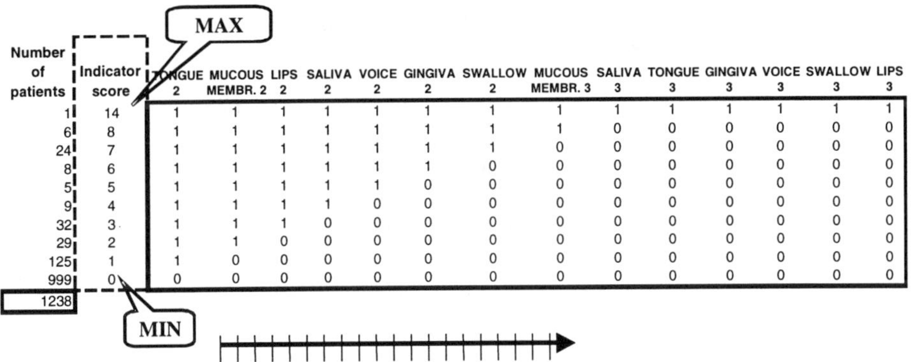

Number of patients	Indicator score	TONGUE 2	MUCOUS MEMBR. 2	LIPS 2	SALIVA 2	VOICE 2	GINGIVA 2	SWALLOW 2	MUCOUS MEMBR. 3	SALIVA 3	TONGUE 3	GINGIVA 3	VOICE 3	SWALLOW 3	LIPS 3
1	14	1	1	1	1	1	1	1	1	1	1	1	1	1	1
6	8	1	1	1	1	1	1	1	1	0	0	0	0	0	0
24	7	1	1	1	1	1	1	1	0	0	0	0	0	0	0
8	6	1	1	1	1	1	1	0	0	0	0	0	0	0	0
5	5	1	1	1	1	1	0	0	0	0	0	0	0	0	0
9	4	1	1	1	1	0	0	0	0	0	0	0	0	0	0
32	3	1	1	1	0	0	0	0	0	0	0	0	0	0	0
29	2	1	1	0	0	0	0	0	0	0	0	0	0	0	0
125	1	1	0	0	0	0	0	0	0	0	0	0	0	0	0
999	0	0	0	0	0	0	0	0	0	0	0	0	0	0	0
1238															

Figure 13 All Perfect Scores

1238 or 57% of the 2187 WISECARE patients perfectly score this best order. There were no patients with a score of 9, 10, ... 13 in the WISECARE DATA and only 1 patient scored major problems for all items of the OAG. This single observation already looks suspicious.

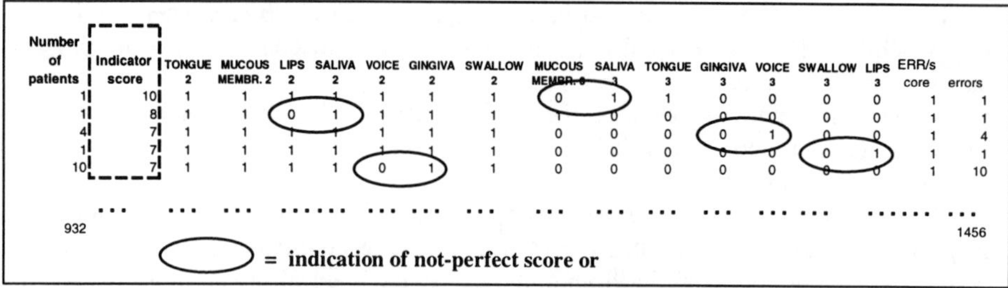

Figure 14 Selection of 5 of the 166 not-Perfect Scores

However perfection is a rare thing. Figure 14 shows a *selection* of the 166 response patterns that show deviations or errors with respect to this best order. 932 patients, a minority, are involved. Remark that one patient can have 1, 2 or more errors. The figure shows all errors present in the selection. According to the best order of original item response categories, a total of 1456 such errors are present in the OAG database available.

How do we find this best order and how good is the best order found. To find the best order special computer algorithms are needed. Indeed there are 1*2*3*4...*14 or 14! or 87,178,291,200 possible orders. Only 1 of these 87,178,291,200 possible orders is the best. To select this best order we look at the errors. Some examples are given in the table of Figure 17. We count these errors in a specific way for every single order of the 87,178,291,200 possible orders. Obviously, we select this order with the least errors and call this order the best order. The literature mentions different ways of counting errors [8]. Two techniques are rather popular: the Guttman technique and the Goodenough_Edwards technique. We use a variant of the Guttman technique.

When the best order is found, the question arises how good is this order or in other words how good is the scale, e.g. the OAG global assessment indicator, found. Again criteria exist. The percentage of perfect scores, in our case 57%, gives already some indication. Another measure of goodness for the Guttman scale is the probability of hurting the same best order or sequence of response categories in any random pair of two OAG items for any random patient: this measure is called the Guttman reproducibility coefficient. The value of this coefficient is 0.9514. Guttmann himself suggests that values larger than 0.90 are necessary for a good scale [9]. Hence, according to Guttman, we are all right. More measures exist. In this case, for instance, the hypothesis of a Guttman scale is highly statistically significant: p < 0.0001.

Notwithstanding these acceptable results already, we still want to improve the validity and reliability of the scale. We still think that the global OAG assessment indicator that is based on 7 of the 8 original OAG items can still be improved. Indeed the level of detail, 15 ordered categories, is too refined for daily clinical nursing practice.

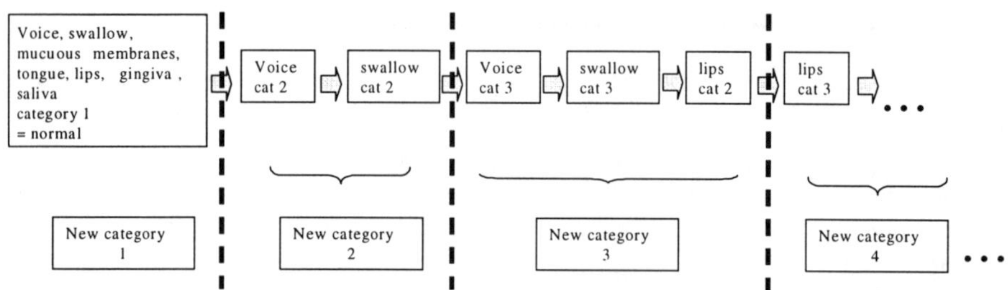

Figure 15 Original adjacent Categories

Hence, we will zoom out and develop a less detailed or refined scale that however will prove to be still more reliable. We zoom out by taking some of the original adjacent categories together (Figure 15).

After several attempts we arrive at the following final proposition for an ORAL assessment indicator based on the WISECARE database till September 1999.

number of patients	indicator score	SALIVA2_T ONGUE2_V OICE2	LIPS2_ MUCOUS MEMBR.2	GINGIVA2_S WALLOW2	MUCOUS MEMBR.3	SALIVA3	TONGUE 3	GINGIVA3	VOICE3	SWALLOW3	LIPS3
1	10	1	1	1	1	1	1	1	1	1	1
21	4	1	1	1	1	0	0	0	0	0	0
166	3	1	1	1	0	0	0	0	0	0	0
184	2	1	1	0	0	0	0	0	0	0	0
302	1	1	0	0	0	0	0	0	0	0	0
999	0	0	0	0	0	0	0	0	0	0	0
1673											

Figure 16 All perfect Scores – final (reduced) Oral Assessment Indicator

Actually, we reduce the 14 (non 1) original item categories to 10 new categories. E.g. a patient scores the new category LIPS2_MUCOUS MEMBRANES2 if he scores either LIPS2 to or MUCOUS MEMBRANES2. This simplifies the final scale by reducing the number of scale categories: from 1+14 (of which only 10 are present) to 1+10 (of which only 6 are present). Also, the number of patients with perfect scores increases from 57% to 76%. Of course, the number of errors decreases. The Guttman reproducibility coefficient improves to 0.9728. At most 2.7% of all pairwise OAG measurements do not follow our best order (Figure 17).

number of patients	indicator score	SALIVA2 ONGUE2 OICE	LIPS2 MUCOU MEMBR.	GINGIVA2 WALLO	MUCOU MEMBR	SALIVA3	TONGU 3	GINGIV	VOICE	SWALLO	LIPS	err/ case	errors
12	4	1	1	0	1	0	0	0	0	0	0	1	12
21	3	0	1	1	0	0	0	0	0	0	0	1	21
86	3	1	0	1	0	0	0	0	0	0	0	1	86
154	2	0	1	0	0	0	0	0	0	0	0	1	154
19	2	1	1	0	0	1	0	0	0	0	0	1	19
21	1	1	0	0	0	1	0	0	0	0	0	1	21
52	0	0	0	1	0	0	0	0	0	0	0	1	52
13	6	1	1	0	1	0	1	0	0	0	0	2	26
40	4	0	1	0	1	0	0	0	0	0	0	2	80
418 shown												shown	**471**
514 in total												in total	**595**

Figure 17 Final Oral Assessment Indicator - Selection of main not-perfect Scores

5.6 Conclusion with Respect to a global OAG Assessment Indicator

In conclusion we check the different options with respect to aggregating the 8 original OAG item categories. The options are represented in Figure 18.

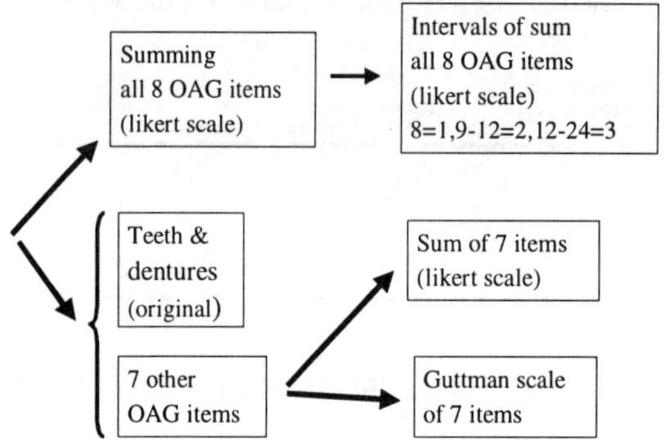

Figure 18 Options for Aggregation

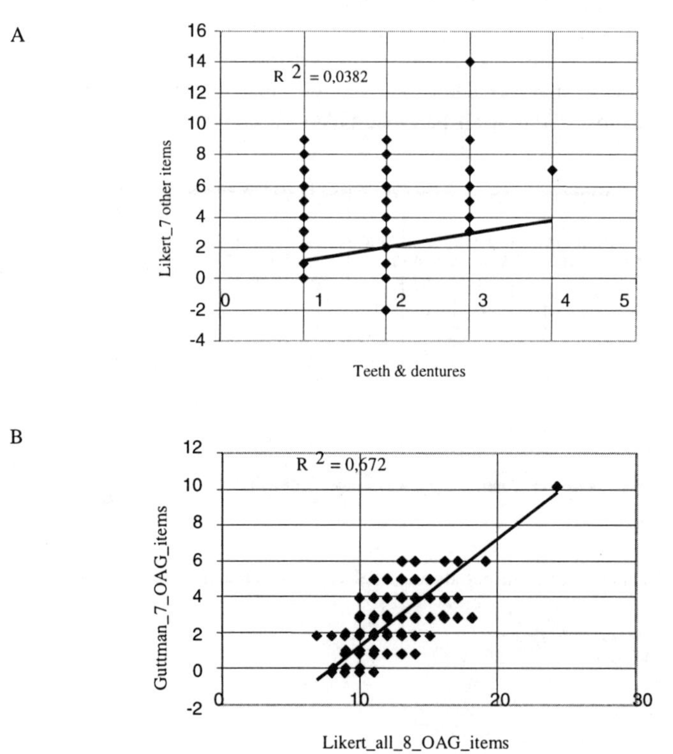

Figure 19 (a and b) Relationship between the two different OAG Assessment Indicators

The above graphs visualise the relationships between the different OAG assessment indicators. The first figure (Figure 19a) shows that the common way of summing all OAG original item categories makes no sense at all. There is little or no relation (R^2= 0,038) between a patient score on the item "teeth & dentures" and his score, in the figure a plain

Likert sum score on the other OAG items. The item "teeth & dentures" is one of the 8 original OAG items that demands its proper assessment indicator independent from all other 7 OAG items.

The next figure (19b) visualises to what extent the Likert, plain sum, assessment indicator and the Guttman assessment indicators, that we developed, converge or diverge. The figure shows a correlation coefficient of 0.672. At first sight, this indicates that it actually makes little difference if we use the Likert sum scale or the Guttman type indicator. But… a large correlation coefficient only implies that some general hypothesis will most likely be statistically significant. An example of such general hypothesis is: "older patients have higher OAG scores than younger patients". Unfortunately, this is not what the nurse wants with respect to an assessment score to monitor her nursing care for her individual patients. A nurse wants that if she scores e.g. 14 today and 16 tomorrow, that then, the higher score implies that the patient's situation is actually worse and that she has to take special precautions with respect to her nursing care. But look at the scattergram in the figure. The sum scores – if all the items are recorded - are all between 8 and 24. But a sum score of 14 can mean any Guttman score between 1 and 6. A sum score of 16 can be a Guttman score of 3, 4 or 6. How will a nurse react when she finds out that her score is untrustworthy or unreliable? Even a large correlation coefficient still implies a lot of uncertainty with respect to the meaning and interpretation of a Likert type sum score on the level of an individual patient. The assessment indicator may be sufficient for testing of hypothesis purposes but becomes unreliable for piloting her nursing care for her individual patient in daily nursing practice.

We started out looking for good, reliable and robust assessment indicators. We explained how aggregating for feedback implies on the one hand good measurements and on the other hand measurements that can be interpreted without to much uncertainty and error in daily nursing practice. The example of the OAG assessment indicator shows that this is no easy matter. The WISECARE database of some 2187 OAG measurements already allowed us to arrive at some conclusions. It is sure that further and periodic data are necessary to guarantee good reliable and robust indicators over time.

References

[1]   Hand D, Data Mining: Statistics and More?, The American Statistician, 1998, Vol 52(2): 112-118

[2]   Fayers P. et al. EORTC QLQ-C30 Scoring Manual, 1997

[3]   Hand DJ Intelligent Data Analysis: Issues and Opportunities. In Xiaohui L., Cohen P & Berthold M. (Eds), Advances in Intelligent Data Analysis: Reasoning about Data, Berlin: Springer, 1997: 1-14.

[4]   World Health Organization, History of the development of the ICD. In: World Health Organization. ICD-10, International Statistical Classification of Diseases and Related Health Problems, Tenth Revision, Volume 2. Geneva: The Organization, 1987: 139-151.

[5]   3M Health Information Systems, All Patient Refined Diagnosis Related Groups (APR-DRGs), Version 12.0, 3M Health Information Systems, Wallingford, CT (USA), 1995.

[6]   Ralphs V Zimmerman H. Scores: ordinal data with few categories - How should they be analyzed?. Drug Information Journal, Vol. **27**, 1993: 1227-1240.

[7]   Sermeus W & Delesie L. Ridit analysis on ordinal data. Western Journal of Nursing Research, Vol. **18**, 1996: 351-359.

[8]   Swanborn PG. Schaaltechnieken. Boom, Amsterdam, 1993.

[9]   McIver JP, Carmines EG,.Unidimensional Scaling. Sage Publications – Sage University Papers - Quantitative Applications in the Social Sciences, Beverly Hills, CA, 1981: 48.

Part III

Results

Global Feedback on Clinical Management

Luc Delesie, Walter Sermeus, Kris Vanhaecht, Lieve Goossens

1   Introduction

WISECARE feedback is no evaluation of the care given. The feedback benchmarks a nursing site against all other sites for each indicator. The feedback does not indicate good or bad, but only low or high. It is up to every Validation Site to give meaning and to interpret a low or high score.

Before the feedback, there was only limited knowledge about low or high. Based on global feedback, every Validation Site gets a first indication of its position. A lot of variables influence these different positions: patient characteristics, way of data collection, organisation of care, nursing care priorities.

The feedback will become more meaningful when there is systematic feedback available over a longer period. This can show information about the stability and variability of the score. For the nurses working on the unit it can give an idea of some trend (higher, lower) in the direction in which they work.

The feedback will only be meaningful when it is used as a tool for communication within the nursing team. The main focus is to see (what is our position?), to understand (why we are here?) and.... carefully.... to say where you want to be. However be careful not to evaluate too quickly. The feedback is a starting point for communication.

This feedback is not perfect. Feedback will however never be perfect. Awareness of the limitations in the feedback leads to carefulness in interpretation. Feedback is a mainly learning process.

2   WISECARE Data Collection

The WISECARE data used for this feedback were recorded at the 5 oncology nursing Validation Sites (7 nursing units) in 5 European countries. They were recorded over the period April 1998 to September 1999. As WISECARE data variables, definitions and registration practices changed over this period 3 time periods are identified:

- April 1998 – December 1998,
- January 1999 – April 14, 1999,
- April 15, 1999 – September 1999.

The outcome assessment indicators were redefined for the period April 1999 to September 1999. The definitions and score item finally retained are:

- EORTC Quality of Life assessment scale – QLQ-C30 (version 3). These subscales (7 questions) are retained from the original 9 multi-item and 3 symptom subscales and several single item symptom subscales of EORTC QLQ-C30 (28 questions). The possible range of scores varies from 2-8 for nausea and vomiting and pain, and from 3 - 12 for fatigue. These results are transformed 0 to 100 according EORTC-scoring manual rules [1]. Each of the 28 items of the QLQ C-30 has four categories of ordinal scores: I (Not at all), II (a little), III (quite a bit) and IV (very much):

Fatigue:	*3 items*
Nausea & Vomiting:	*2 items*
Pain:	*2 items*

- ORAL ASSESSMENT GUIDE. The scale has 8 items and each item has three categories of ordinal scores: I (No problem), II (Minor problem), III (Major problem). The possible range of scores varies from 8-24. These results are transformed to a 0-100 scale.

3   Description of the Sample

Table 1 shows the total number of WISECARE patients and the distribution by diagnosis and by Validation Site. The majority of the included patients do have breast cancer (46%). Five of the 7 Validation Sites have included these type of patients. The diagnosis group with the lowest numbers are patients with hematological disorders: ALL (3%) and AML (5%). Also the osteosarcoma group (6%) is only represented in 2 Sites. Near a quarter of all patients (24%) are lung cancer patients. Non-Hodgkin's Lymphoma patients represent 16% of all patients. The dispersion of all patients over the Sites varies from 15-62 (average = 38). Site A and D included only breast cancer patients while Site C only included lung cancer patients. Site E and F seem to be hematological Sites. Site B and G have include patient belonging to different diagnosis groups.

Table 1 WISECARE Patients by Diagnosis and Site

Site Code	Non-Hodgkin's Lymphoma	ALL	Breast Cancer	Osteo Sarcoma	Lung Cancer	AML	Total
A			57				57
B	28		17	11	4		60
C					18		18
D			26				26
E	4	7				4	15
F	9	1	2			10	22
G			18	5	39		62
Total	41	8	120	16	61	14	260

(missing: N=22)

Table 2 shows the distribution by sex of all WISECARE patients for every Validation Site. The majority of the patients were breast cancer patients, which explains the representation of 62% women and 38% men in the WISECARE sample.

Table 2 WISECARE Patients by Sex and Site

Site Code	Male	Female	Total
A	0	59	59
B	41	23	64
C	10	8	18
D	0	26	26
E	10	6	16
F	13	15	28
G	31	34	65
Total	105	171	276

(missing: N=6)

Table 3 gives the distribution by age of all WISECARE patients for every Validation Site. More than half of all WISECARE patients (55%) is between 40-64 year. Age seems to be normally distributed. Site A seems to be the surgical ward, which included three patients above 85 years. The younger patients (less than 20 year) are included at a hematological site.

Table 3 WISECARE Patients by Age and Site

Site Code	<20	20-39	40-64	65-84	85 plus	Total
A		13	33	10	3	59
B		15	29	20		64
C		1	15	2		18
D		3	23			26
E	2	5	9			16
F		6	14	8		28
G		19	31	15		65
Total	2	67	155	55	3	282

Every admission for administration of chemotherapy or surgery is called a 'Treatment Episode' (TE). Table 4 shows the total number of 'treatment episodes' for all WISECARE patients and the distribution by Site along the number of treatment episodes. Table 4 shows that Site A, B, E and F are hospitalisation wards, and Site C is a one-day hospitalisation ward. Most of the patients (70%) have been admitted 1, 2 or 3 times. 30% of all WISECARE patients have been admitted more than 4 times.

Table 4 Number of Treatment Episodes by Site

Site Code	1 TE	2 TE	3 TE	4 TE	5 TE	6 TE	7 TE	8 to 11 TE	12 to 15 TE	>15 TE	sum
A	59	9						0	0	0	68
B	29	17	8	5	3	2	1	1	0	0	66
C	44	38	32	28	25	17	12	23	12	6	237
E	16	13	9	7	6	4	3	11	1	0	70
F	28	13	7	2	2	1	1	0	0	0	54
G	65	15	8	5	1	1		0	0	0	95
sum	241	105	64	47	37	25	17	35	13	6	590

4   Impact on Clinical Management

For every clinical indicator a feedback form is developed.

- The scores on pain, fatigue, nausea and vomiting and oral problems are represented for every risk category for all patients.
- The feedback shows clinical time (until ten days after a clinical event) in relation to the different identified time periods. A clinical event can be (1) the administration of chemotherapy or (2) surgery.
- Every Validation Site is positioned against general benchmarks.

4.1 All Patients

Figure 1 gives the average day-to-day pain score for all patients of the Validation Sites during the first 10 days after a clinical event with N= total number of patient assessments. It shows that the pain score for the risk 0-group (N= 2209) is low (10%) and is almost constant during the 10 days. The pain score for the risk 3-group (N= 337) is high (50%) and stay constant during 5 days and decreases from day 6-9. From the data it is obvious that risk group 1 (N= 589) and 2 (N= 2116) does not differentiate according to pain scores.

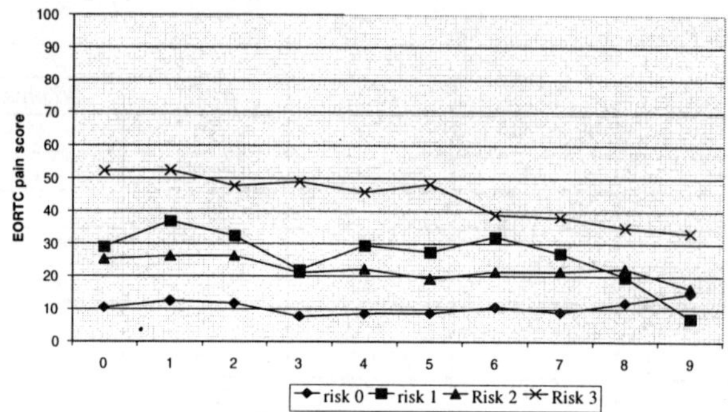

Figure 1   Pain profile per risk category per day (all WISECARE Patients)

Figure 2 shows the average day-to-day fatigue score for all patients of the Validation Sites during the 10 first days after a clinical event. Regarding the different risk factors, the trend is decreasing for the risk group 1 (N=589) and 3 (N= 337) over the ten days.

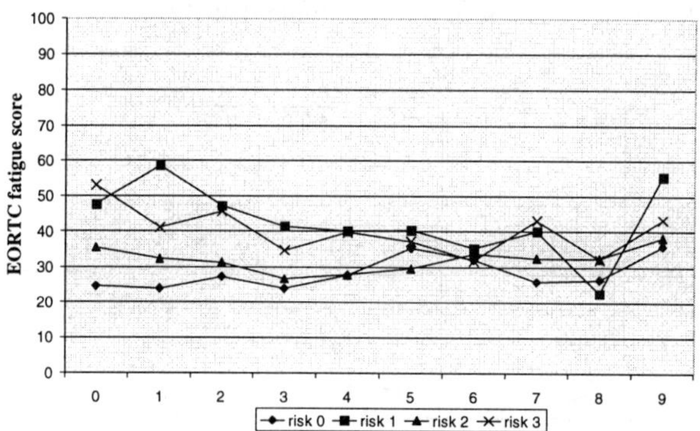

Figure 2   Fatigue profile per risk category per day (all WISECARE Patients)

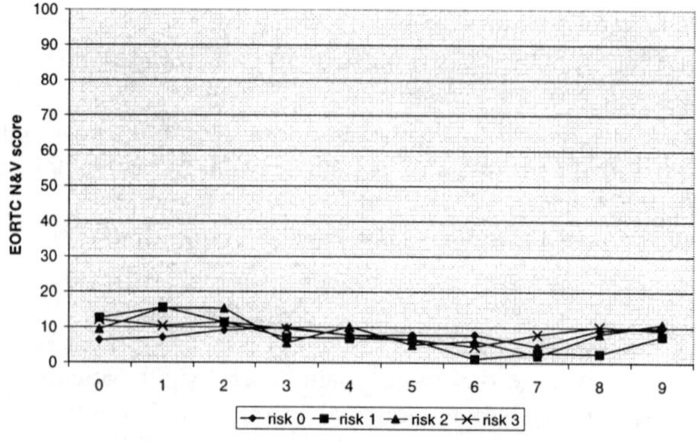

Figure 3   Nausea and Vomiting profile per risk category per day (all WISECARE Patients)

A clear change is noticed on 10th day. More close evaluation is needed to understand why the average pattern scores are going up at day 10. This indicates that measurement after 10 days might be interesting. The fatigue scores in the risk group 0 (N= 2209) and 2 (N= 2116) are similar.

Figure 3 gives the average day-to-day nausea and vomiting score for all patients of the Validation Sites during the first 10 days after a clinical event. The scores are low and constant very similar over the 10 days. The first two days the scores are somewhat higher. The risk category (risk 0 (N= 1150), risk 1 (N= 1614), risk 2 (N= 1027) and risk 3 (N= 857)) does not seem to determine nausea and vomiting scores.

Figure 4 shows the average day-to-day oral problems score for all patients of the Validation Sites during the 10 first days. Oral problem scores are similar for all risk factors: risk 0 (N= 578), risk 1 (N= 702), risk 2 (N= 460) and risk 3 (N= 394). They are low and show almost no variation. There is a possible need for measurement beyond 10 first day period because a slight tendency is visible that the scores become higher after one week.

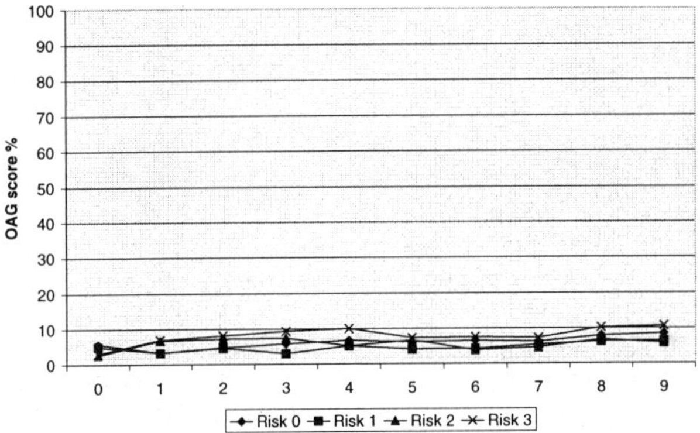

Figure 4   Oral problem profile per risk category per day (all WISECARE Patients)

4.2 All Time Periods

In the following examples, the clinical indicators are given for a defined risk factors with respect to the 3 defined periods of WISECARE data registration.

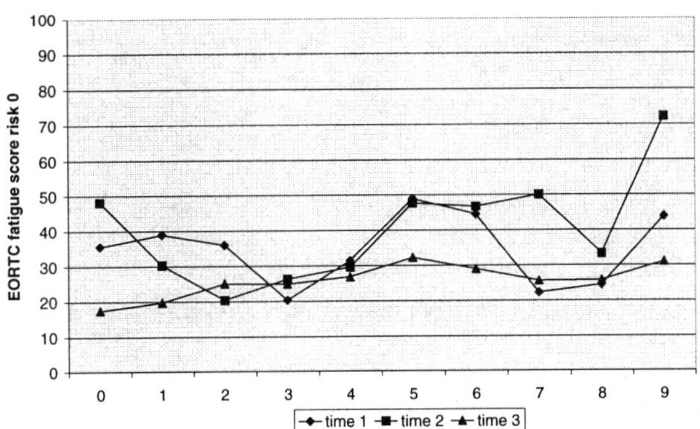

Figure 5   Fatigue scores (risk 0) over the 3 WISECARE Periods

Figure 5 shows the average day-to-day fatigue score for all patients of the Validation Sites within the risk group 0 for fatigue during the 10 first days after the clinical event.

The fatigue scores at time 1 (N=97) and 2 (N=74) show some variability and are high at the 10th day after the clinical event. The scores of the third period (N=472) show less variation.

Figure 6 gives the average day-to-day fatigue score for all patients of the Validation Sites during the first 10 days after a clinical event. It shows for the patients of the *risk 1-group* differences between the three WISECARE time periods.

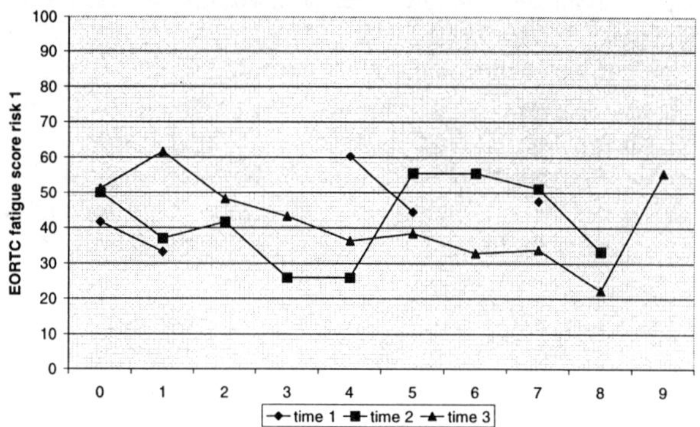

Figure 6   Fatigue scores (risk 0) over the 3 WISECARE Periods

In the first (N=40) and second period (N=33) the scores are fluctuating while in the last period (N=228) the fatigue scores are more stable. However 10 days after the clinical event an increase of the score is visible. The scores in the first time period are not daily recorded.

Figure 7 gives the average day-to-day fatigue score for all patients of the Validation Sites during the first 10 days after a clinical event. It shows the differences between the three WISECARE time periods for the patients of the *risk-2 group*.

The scores for time period 1 (N=143) and 2 (N=143) show again high variability while the third period (N=692) seems to be stable with a slight increase on day 10.

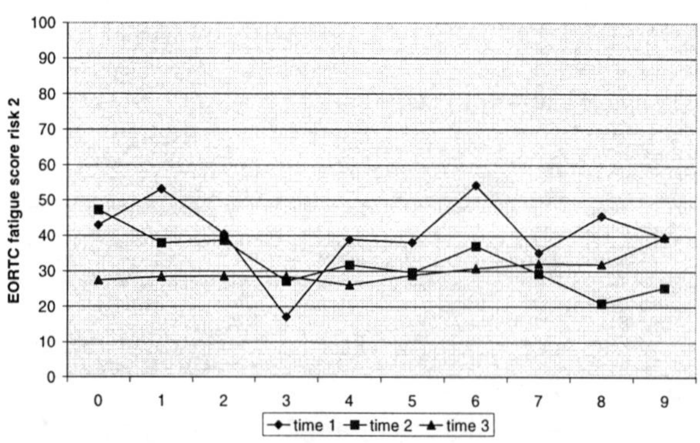

Figure 7   Fatigue scores (Risk 2) over the 3 WISECARE Periods

Figure 8 gives the average day-to-day fatigue score for all patients of the Validation Sites within the *risk 3-group* during the first 10 days after a clinical event. The first two time periods (period 1 (N=40), period 2 (N=18)) show large variation. In the third period (N=187) the scores are more constant. There is a slight decrease in average fatigue score in the third period during the 10 day period. Again there is a tendency to increase at the end of the 10 days of measurements.

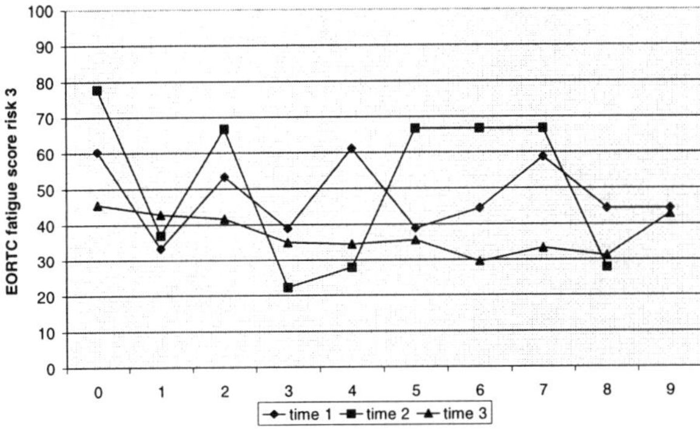

Figure 8   Fatigue scores (risk 3) over the 3 WISECARE Periods

4.3   All Validation Sites

For the feedback by Site, results from nausea and vomiting are chosen as an example representing the different Sites with respect to the risk factors. Figure 9 gives the average day-to-day nausea and vomiting score for all patients of the Validation Sites during the first 10 days after a clinical event. It shows for the patient group with *risk 0* for nausea and vomiting the differences between the Validation Sites. The figure shows that Site A seems to have no measurements for nausea and vomiting risk 0. Site B (N=81) has the most variability in its scores.

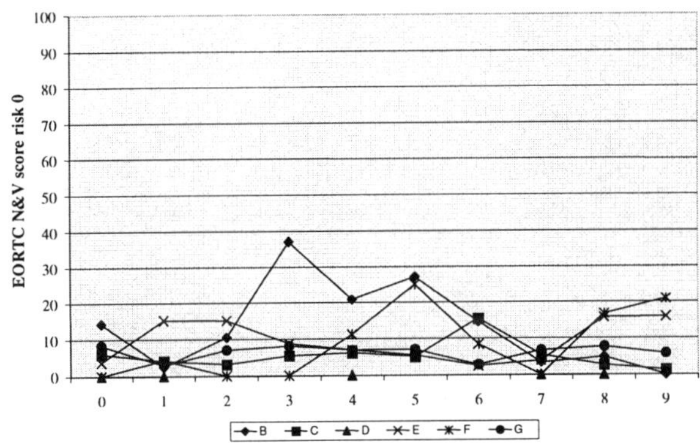

Figure 9   Nausea and Vomiting Score for Risk 0 (all Validation Sites)

The figure shows a higher average score from day 3 till day 6 after the clinical event. A same pattern is visible for Site F (N=27) except that this Site also has increased scores at the end of the 10-days measurements. This higher scores at the end of the period of measurement is also viewed in Site E (N=366). A longer measurement time could be interesting for these Sites. Site D (N=38) misses scores for some days, however the available scores reveal no problems. The scores of Site G (N=349) stay low and stable over the total period.

Figure 10 gives the average day-to-day nausea and vomiting score during the first 10 days after a clinical event. It shows for the patient group with *risk 1* the differences between the Validation Sites. The figure shows that Site A (N=370) has high scores the first two days after the clinical event, Thereafter the scores decrease from day to day. Site B (N=20) have low nausea and vomiting figures except a slight increase at day 4 and 5.

Site G (N=76) and Site C (N=84) are mostly at the baseline. Site E(N=83) has more variability in its scores. Especially on day 8 and 9 higher average scores are obtained.

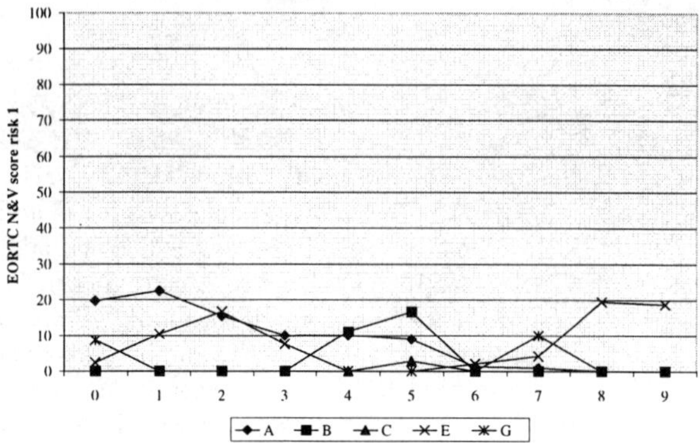

Figure 10 Nausea and Vomiting Score for Risk 1 (all Validation Sites)

Figure 11 gives the average day-to-day fatigue score for all patients of the Validation Sites during the first 10 days after a clinical event. It shows for the patient group with *risk 2*, for nausea and vomiting, the differences between the Validation Sites. Figure 11 reveals that Site A (N=66) has high scores the first two days after the clinical event. Thereafter scores seems to be lower. Site B (N=92), D (N=116) and E (N=99) are quite similar in variability, but there is a slight increase of the nausea and vomiting scores at the end of the 10 day period. Site F (N=27) seems to have high scores from day 3 to 5 whereafter the scores decrease again.

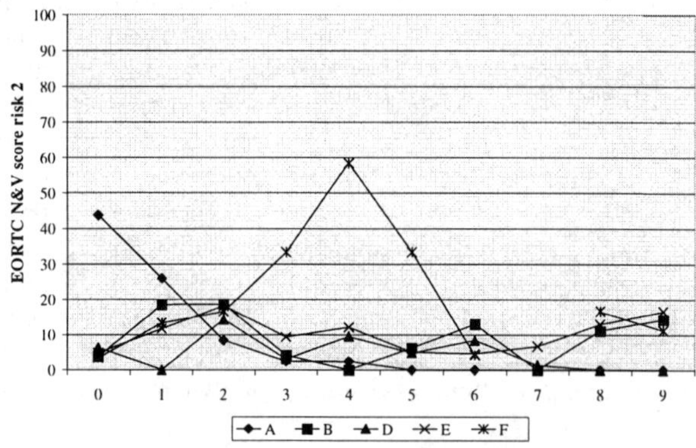

Figure 11 Nausea and Vomiting Score for Risk 2 (all Validation Sites)

Figure 12 gives the average day-to-day fatigue score during the first 10 days after a clinical event. It shows for the patient group with *risk 3* for nausea and vomiting the differences between the Validation Sites. Figure 12 shows that Site A (N=152) starts with high scores and ends up with low scores. Site B (N=78) shows a much variable status but there is less control for the first two days of the nausea and vomiting problem. Site E (N=155) seems to have problems the first two days after a clinical event. Thereafter the scores are low. At the 9th and 10th day the nausea and vomiting problem appears again. Site F (N=9) does not have many measurements, but the nausea and vomiting problem is strongly present. Site G (N=219) seems to have their nausea and vomiting problem under control. However the problem never disappears during the ten days.

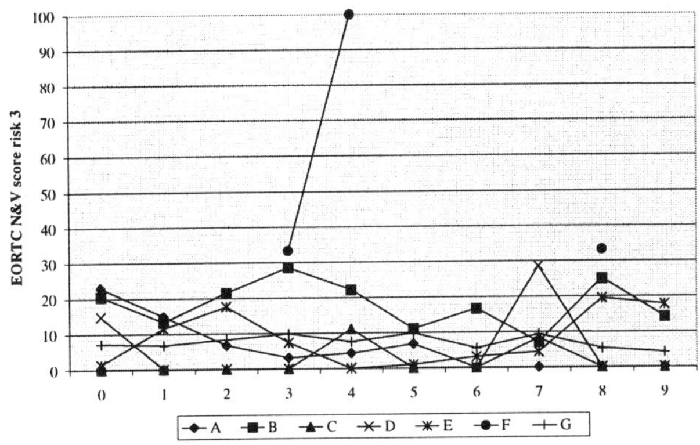

Figure 12 Nausea and Vomiting Score for Risk 3 (all Validation Sites)

4.4 Impact of Clinical Management on Patient Outcomes

During 18 months, more than 13000 patient assessments have been made for 280 patients and 590 treatment episodes. The local feedback graphs are used to discuss symptom control with patients, nurses and physicians. Two global feedback reports were generated. Table 5 shows that for every clinical indicator, there is a significant decrease in the average scores comparing the first Time Period (April 1998–December 1998) to third Time Period (April 1999–September 1999).

Table 5 Evolution in Symptom Management during the Project (N=total number of patient assessments)

Clinical indicator	First Period	Third Period	differences	
average fatigue score	44%	33%	-25%	(N=3259)
average nausea & vomiting	11,8%	5,6%,	-53%	(N=4349) (N=3276)
average pain score	23%	19%	-18%	(N=2134)
average oral problems	22,3%	18,5%.	-18%	

Table 5 to 12 confirm these findings in more detail. Table 5 and 6 show the impact of clinical management on *oral problems* using the Oral Assessment Guide (OAG).

Table 6 Number of Patients in the 4 OAG-Severity Groups

	PERIOD			
OAG_severity group	1	2	3	Total
No problems (score 8)	234 (28,5%)	107 (31,7%)	314 (32,4%)	655 (30,7%)
Mild problems (score 9-10)	239 (28,9%)	111 (32,8%)	267 (27,6%)	617 (28,9%)
Moderate problems (score 11-12)	107 (12,9%)	39 (11,5%)	120 (12,4%)	266 (12,5%)
Severe problems (score 13-24)	247 (29,9%)	81 (23,9%)	268 (27,6%)	596 (27,9%)
TOTAL	827	338	969	2134

Difference between period 3 and period 1 is significant (p=0,0123), by Wilcoxon Mann-Withney U test, Monte-Carlo exact p-interval estimates 99%CI : 0,0095-0,0151 (All 17 categories (8-24) are taken into the analysis)

Table 5 shows that in Time Period 1, 71,5% (N=593) of all patient assessments show oral problems, in Time period 2 this number is decreased to 68,3% (N=231) and further to 67,6% (N=655) in Time Period 3.

    L. Delesie / Global Feedback on Clinical Management

Table 7   Average OAG-scores (EORTC data manual algorithm) per LCRA-risk Category

LCRA-risk	Description	PERIOD 1	2	3	TOTAL
0	Average OAG (stdev): (Number)	0,149 (0,168) N=168	0,332 (0,298) N=81	0,219 (0,236) N=329	0,215 (0,235) N=578
1	Average OAG (stdev): N=	0,275 (0,270) N=324	0,149 (0,214) N=150	0,080 (0,139) N=228	0,185 (0,239) N=702
2	Average OAG (stdev): N=	0,140 (0,121) N=160	0,071 (0,060) N=65)	0,135 (0,148) N=235	0,128 (0,131) N=460
3	Average OAG (stdev): N=	0,272 (0,339) N=175	0,273 (0,275) N=42	0,321 (0,215) N=177	0,294 (0,283) N=394
Global average OAG (stdev) N=		0,223 (0,255) N=827	0,193 (0,246) N=338	0,185 (0,210) N=969	0,201 (0,235) N=2134)
Difference with period 1			P=0,069 NS	P=0,0005 Significant	

Table 6 confirms this decreasing trend over the 3 periods. The global average score starts at 0,223 in Time Period 1 (N=827), over 0,193 in Time Period 2 (N=338) to 0,185 in Time Period 3 (N=969). Table 7 and 8 give the impact of clinical management on *fatigue* using the EORTC-QLQ-C30 Fatigue subscale. In Time Period 1, 84% (N=659) of all patient assessments show a degree of fatigue, in Time period 2 this number is decreased to 78% (N=257) and further to 72,5% (N=640) in Time Period 3 (Table 8). It results in a decrease of the global average score for fatigue from 0,435 (N=1975) in Time Period 1, over 0,360 (N=1627) to 0,327 (N=4859) in Time Period 3.

Table 8   Number of Patients in 4 Fatigue Severity Groups

Number of Fatigue Fatigue	PERIOD 1	2	3	TOTAL
0	317 (16%)	360 (22,1%)	1652 (34%)	2329 (27,5%)
1	466 (23,5%)	129 (7,9%)	667 (13,7%)	1262 (14,9%)
2	1003 (50,7%)	1039 (63,8%)	2291 (47,2%)	4333 (51,2%)
3	189 (9,5%)	99 (6%)	249 (5,1%)	537 (6,3%)
TOTAL	1975	1627	4859	8461

Difference between period 3 and period 1 is highly significant (p<0,0001), by Wilcoxon Mann-Withney U test, Monte-Carlo exact p-interval estimates 99%CI: 0,0000-0,0005

Table 9   Average Fatigue-Scores (EORTC data manual algorithm) per LCRA-Risk Category

LCRA-risk	Description	PERIOD 1	2	3	TOTAL
0	Average Fatigue score (Stdev) N=	0,365 (0,226) N=317	0,368 (0,254) N=360	0,284 (0,248) N=1652	0,308 (0,249) N=2329
1	Average Fatigue score (Stdev) N=	0,459 (0,184) N=466	0,410 (0,151) N=129	0,427 (0,224) N=667	0,437 (0,204) N=1262
2	Average Fatigue score (Stdev) N=	0,429 (0,265) N=1003	0,350 (0,232) N=1039	0,321 (0,248) N=2291	0,353 (0,252) N=4333
3	Average Fatigue score (Stdev) N=	0,523 (0,233) N=189	0,369 (0,314) N=99	0,400 (0,319) N=249	0,438 (0,297) N=537
Global average Fatigue (stdev) N=		0,435 (0,242) N=1975	0,360 (0,238) N=1627	0,327 (0,253) N=4859	0,359 (0,252) N=8461
Difference with period 1			P<0,0001 Significant	P<0,0001 Significant	

Table 9 and 10 give the impact of clinical management on *nausea and vomiting* using the EORTC-QLQ-C30 nausea and vomiting subscale. In Time Period 1, 28,6% (N=270) of all patient assessments show a degree of Nausea and Vomiting, in Time period 2 this number is decreased to 27,3% (N=236) and further to 18,2% (N=461) in Time Period 3 (Table 10).

Table 10 Number of Patients in 4 Nausea and Vomiting Severity Groups

	PERIOD			
N&V_severity group	1	2	3	TOTAL
No problems (score 2)	674 (71,4%)	628 (72,7%)	2079 (81,8%)	3381 (77,7%)
Mild problems (score 3-4)	183 (19,4%)	138 (15,9%)	386 (15,2%)	707 (16,2%)
Moderate problems (score 5-6)	52 (5,5%)	77 (8,9%)	51 (2%)	180 (4,1%)
Severe problems (score 7-8)	35 (3,7%)	21 (2,4%)	25 (1%)	81 (1,8%)
TOTAL	944	864	2541	4349

Difference between period 3 and period 1 is significant (p<0,0001), by Wilcoxon Mann-Withney U test, Monte-Carlo exact p-interval estimates 99%CI: 0,0000-0,0005 (All 7 categories (2-8) are taken into the analysis)

Table 10 gives the evolution over time concerning Nausea and Vomiting scores per risk category. Time Period 1 (N= 944) and 2 (N=864) are quite similar. Time Period 3 (N=2541) shows a significant decrease in global average scores. There is a high variability over the 3 periods with a decrease of the scores of all risk groups in comparison to the first period. Table 11 and 12 give the impact of clinical management on *pain* using the EORTC-QLQ-C30 pain subscale.

Table 11 Average Nausea and Vomiting scores (EORTC data manual algorithm) per LCRA Risk Category

		TIME			
LRCA – risk	Description	1	2	3	Total
0	Average N&V-score (Stdev) N=	0,116 (0,222) N=417	0,143 (0,243) N=388	0,047 (0,119) N=1067	0,082 (0,182) N=1872
1	Average N&V-score (Stdev) N=	0,165 (0,251) N=96	0,056 (0,156) N=150	0,068 (0,178) N=555	0,077 (0,187) N=801
2	Average N&V-score (Stdev) N=	0,087 (0,201) N=243	0,177 (0,300) N=112	0,060 (0,169) N=340	0,088 (0,210) N=695
3	Average N&V-score (Stdev) N=	0,140 (0,259) N=188	0,108 (0,234) N=214	0,058 (0,146) N=579	0,085 (0,196) N=981
Global average N&V-score (stdev) N=		0,118 (0,229) N=944	0,123 (0,239) N=864	0,056 (0,147) N=2541	0,083 (0,191) N=4349
Difference with period 1		944	P=0,639 NS	P<0,0001 Significant	

In Time Period 1, 64% (N=422) of all patient assessments show a degree of pain, in Time period 2 this number is decreased to 49,2% (N=315) and there is a slight increase to 50,5% (N=997) in Time Period 3 (Table 12).

Table 13 show the evolution over time of the average pain scores for the different risk groups. Although the global average scores are decreasing slightly and there is some variability within the risk groups there is still a significant decrease over time from Time Period 1:0,231 (N=660) over 0,178 for Time Period 2 (N=641) to 0,185 for Time Period 3 (N=1975).

Table 12 Number of Patients in 4 Pain-Severity Groups

	PERIOD			
Pain_severity group	1	2	3	TOTAL
No problems (score 2)	238 (36%)	326 (50,8%)	978 (49,5%)	1542 (47%)
Mild problems (score 3-4)	306 (46,4%)	228 (35,6%)	770 (39%)	1304 (39,8%)
Moderate problems (score 5-6)	88 (13,3%)	80 (12,5%)	175 (8,9%)	343 (10,5%)
Severe problems (score 7-8)	28 (4,2%)	7 (1,1%)	52 (2,6%)	87 (2,6%)
TOTAL	660	641	1975	3276

Difference between period 3 and period 1 is significant ($p<0,0001$), by Wilcoxon Mann-Withney U test, Monte-Carlo exact p-interval estimates 99% CI: 0,0000-0,0005 (All 7 categories (2-8) are taken into the analysis)

Table 13 Average Pain-Scores (EORTC data manual algorithm) per LCRA-Risk Category

		PERIOD			
LCRA - Risk_Pain	Description	1	2	3	TOTAL
0	Average pain score (Stdev) N=	0,202 (0,229) N=304	0,140 (0,200) N=285	0,100 (0,178) N=810	0,130 (0,199) N=1399
1	Average pain score (Stdev) N=	0,223 (0,197) N=134	0,235 (0,207) N=63	0,284 (0,236) N=196	0,255 (0,220) N=393
2	Average pain score (Stdev) N=	0,259 (0,259) N=186	0,197 (0,237) N=264	0,204 (0,236) N=833	0,211 (0,240) N=1283
3	Average pain score (Stdev) N=	0,370 (0,249) N=36	0,259 (0,266) N=29	0,434 (0,237) N=136	0,397 (0,250) N=201
Global average N&V-score (stdev) N=		0,231 (0,236) N=660	0,178 (0,223) N=641	0,185 (0,233) N=1975	0,193 (0,232) N=3276
Difference with period 1			P<0,0001 Significant	P<0,0001 Significant	

References

[1]　　Fayers P. et al. EORTC QLQ-C30 Scoring Manual, 1997.

Global Nursing Resource Feedback

Luc Delesie, Kris Vanhaecht

1 Nursing Resources in WiseTool

Nursing resource data are collected on a random day once a week chosen by the project co-ordination. The nursing resource indicators are collected in WiseTool and are included to the WiseHoos database. The collected data were indicators on nursing staff as well as on patients.

The indicators on nursing staff are nurse qualification level (from 1 to 4) [1] and the amount of nursing hours during a 24 hour period. These data are needed to calculate the indicator "nursing hours per patient day".

Next to indicators on staff, indicators on patients are collected: patient classification score based on the Moffitt Classification [2], the amount of hours a patient was on the unit and if the patient was included in the WISECARE project for clinical feedback.

2 Nursing Resource Feedback Production

Graphical feedback on three resource indicators is created: nurse qualification score, nursing hours per patient day score and patient classification score. These graphs are based on data from March till September 1999. Non response was less than 5%.

2.1 Nurse Qualification Score

The nurse qualification score ranges from 4 (lowest score) to 1 (highest score): see Chapter 2, Data Collection Manual, for more extensive definitions. Feedback is given in a graphical way. A ridit score is calculated for every Site. A ridit is a valid aggregate score for ordinal data: between 0 and 1, where 0.50 is the benchmark for the total group or between -0.50 and +0.50 where 0.0 is the benchmark for the total group. Figure 1 shows Validation Site A with a nurse qualification level that varies over the 6 months period. In March, April, May and July the qualification level for this Site is higher than the qualification level for the group of Validation Sites which is standardized at the value 0.0. In June and August the qualification level for this Site is lower than the qualification level for the group of Validation Sites.

Table 1 and 2 show the distribution of the Nurse Qualification Level (NQL) between the WISECARE Validation Sites.

Most of the Validation Sites have a majority of nurses with Nurse Qualification Level 1 (NQL1) or 2.60% of the nurses of Validation Site D have a NQL 1. Validation Site F is the outlier. All the nurses have a NQL level 3 which means that they haven't recorded any Registered Nurses' level.

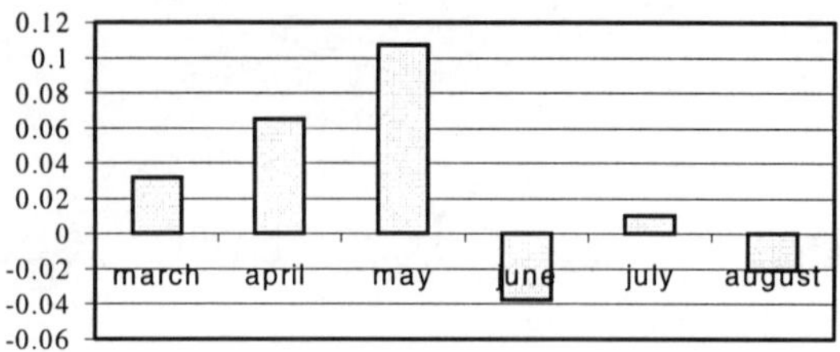

Figure 1   Nurse Qualification Score for Validation Site A between March and August 1999

Table 1   Distribution in absolute numbers of Nurse Qualification Level

NQL	NQL1	NQL2	NQL3	NQL4	Total
Site A	93	62	18	16	189
Site B	166	77	25	62	330
Site C	22	227	0	10	259
Site D	149	100	0	0	249
Site E	129	167	4	35	335
Site F	0	0	356	0	356
Site G	18	60	6	1	85
WISECARE	577	693	409	124	1803

Table 2   Distribution in Nurse Qualification Level in %

NQL %	NQL1 %	NQL2 %	NQL3 %	NQL4 %	Total
Site A	49	33	10	8	100
Site B	50	23	8	19	100
Site C	8	88	0	4	100
Site D	60	40	0	0	100
Site E	39	50	1	10	100
Site F	0	0	100	0	100
Site G	21	71	7	1	100
WISECARE	32	38	23	7	100

2.2 Number of Nursing Hours Per Patient Day (NHPPD)

The number of nursing hours per patient day gives some indication of the care that nurses give to their patients. The indicator is based on the number of hours that all patients were cared for on the unit during the previous 24 hours and the number of hours all nurses worked during the same 24 hours.

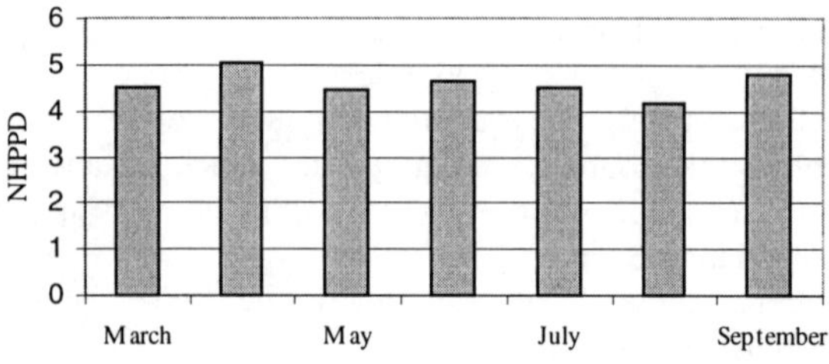

Figure 2   Nursing Hours Per Patient Day for Validation Site B during a 7 month Period

The histogram (Figure 2) shows the NHPPD for seven consecutive months for Validation Site B. It reveals that the number of NHPPD stays constantly over the whole project time. In other Validation Sites the NHPPD shows variation from month to month.

In Table 3 the average, minimum and maximum number of Nursing Hours Per Patient Day is shown for the different Validation Sites within Europe. The differences in NHPPD within Europe are obvious. Site A has the lowest NHPPD (average 3,08 hours with a minimum of 2.21 hours) and Site D the highest (average 26,39 hours with a maximum of 28,8 hours).

Table 3   Distribution of NHPPD

NHPPD	Average	Minimum	Maximum
Site A	3.08	2.21	3.53
Site B	4.58	4.19	5.02
Site C	5.76	5.19	8.71
Site D	26.39	23.11	28.80
Site E	11.04	6.66	21.55
Site F	5.87	4.86	7.81
Site G	9.61	2.63	17.24
TOTAL	9.03	2.21	28.80

2.3 Patient Classification Score on the Nursing Unit

The third resource indicator concerns the aggregation of the patient classification score with respect to the variability of nursing care, based upon the Moffitt score. The patients are divided in three groups: WISECARE patients, Non-WISECARE patients and all patients.

Figure 2 shows the Moffitt score for Validation Site B. This Validation Site has a higher patient classification score than the average WISECARE patient classification for all the months except for the WISECARE patients in September while the Ridit Score is lower than 0,5.

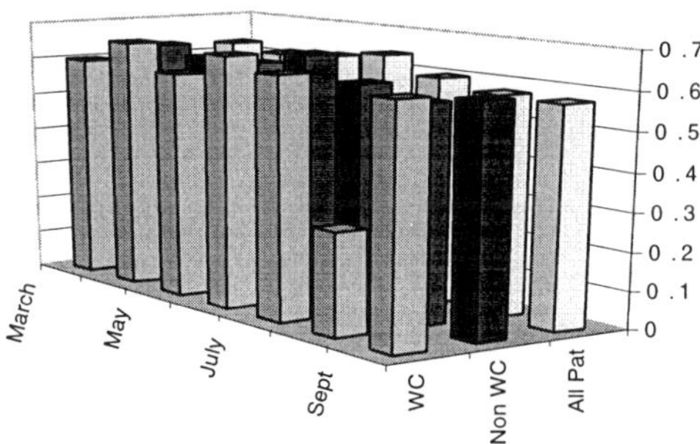

Figure 3   Patient Classification Score for Validation Site B over a 6 Month Period

Table 4 Distrubution of Moffitt Scores in absolute Numbers

MOFFIT	Wisecare					Non Wisecare				
TOTAL %	Moffitt 1 %	Moffitt 2 %	Moffitt 3 %	Moffitt 4 %	Total %	Moffitt 1 %	Moffitt 2 %	Moffitt 3 %	Moffitt 4 %	Total %
site A	64	33	3	0	100	51	33	10	6	100
site B	11	47	38	5	100	9	45	40	5	100
site C	0	50	50	0	100	5	43	42	10	100
site D	100	0	0	0	100	82	18	0	0	100
site E	0	23	73	5	100	3	30	55	12	100
site F	20	80	0	0	100	77	22	1	0	100
site G	100	0	0	0	100	15	22	57	6	100
WISECARE	24	40	32	3	100	45	29	22	4	100

Table 5 Distribution of Moffitt Scores in %

MOFFIT	Wisecare					Non Wisecare				
TOTAL	Moffitt 1	Moffitt 2	Moffitt 3	Moffitt 4	Total	Moffitt 1	Moffitt 2	Moffitt 3	Moffitt 4	Total
site A	23	12	1	0	36	261	168	49	32	510
site B	9	40	32	4	85	55	278	248	33	614
site C	0	1	1	0	2	22	180	176	43	421
site D	1	0	0	0	1	992	218	0	0	1210
site E	0	5	16	1	22	12	114	212	44	382
site F	1	4	0	0	5	327	95	3	1	426
site G	3	0	0	0	3	38	55	139	14	246
WISECARE	37	62	50	5	154	1707	1108	827	167	3809

Table 4 and 5 give the distribution of the Moffitt Scores which explains the differences between the various Validation Sites with respect to their patient classification. Only 2 Validation Sites have got WISECARE patients with a Moffitt Score 4. This is 3% of all WISECARE patients. Most of the in-patients during the WISECARE data collection had a Moffitt 1 or 2 classification.

References

[1]   Versiek K, Bouten R.(1995) Manpower problems in the nursing/midwifery profession in the EC: Country Reports Volume 1. Leuven: Katholieke Universiteit Leuven. Hoger Instituut voor de Arbeid, 268p.

[2]   Lovett RB, Reardon MB, Gordon BK, McMillan S (1994) Validity and reliability of medical and surgical patient acuity tools. Oncology Nursing Forum. Vol 21, No 10, pp1709-1717.

Experiences of the Clinical Nursing Sites

Pirkko Bellaoui, Anne Henttinen, Marja-Leena Hyvärinen, Marita Kaltea,
Tarja Seppänen-Savela, Finland
Jop Helleman, The Netherlands, Shelley Dolan, United Kingdom
Lieve Goossens, Xavier Lefever, Gert Peeters,
An Roelants, Catherine Servaes, Kris Vanhaecht, Belgium

1 Finland

1.1 Nursing Care at HUCH

Nursing care at the Helsinki University Central Hospital (HUCH) is based on nursing science and its humanistic conception of human being. It emphasizes uniqueness of each human being, integrity, individual responsibility and freedom, and self-determination. At HUCH, we have chosen primary nursing as our model of nursing care delivery. By the implementation of primary nursing, HUCH strives to guarantee objectivity and equity in the delivery of nursing care and to take into account the patients' security and individuality.

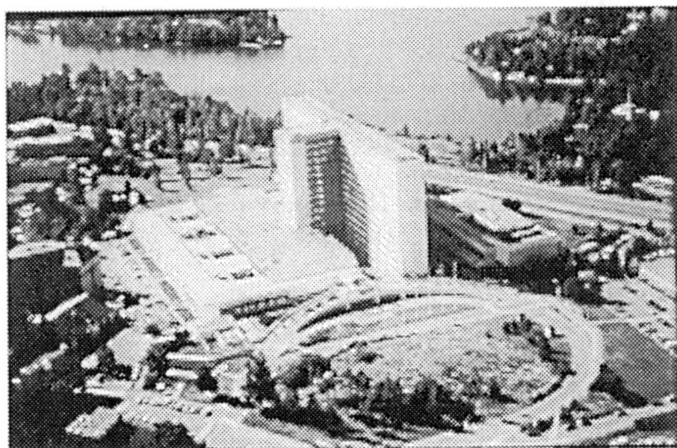

Figure 1   Helsinki University Central Hospital, Main Building

1.2 HUCH Ward 82

The ward for pulmonary diseases is one part of the Department of Internal Medicine. Patients with lung cancer are the biggest patient group. Other diseases that are treated in the unit are mesothelioma, pneumonia, asthma and sleep apnoea. There is an outpatient unit attached to the ward where patients have one-day treatments and toxic treatments e.g. cisplatin-gemcitabine/vinorelbine or paclitaxel-carboplatin. Patients stay at the ward if they are having treatments that last many days, if their physical status is poor or if they are suffering from severe side effects. In the ward we have 15 + 3 beds (3 beds are for patients with sleep apnoea), and the average length of stay is 4.6 days. In the outpatient unit there are about 60 treatments per month. Most of our WISECARE patients have been outpatients. The staff is working both in the ward and at the outpatient unit which is staffed with two RNs and one ward assistant work. At the beginning of year 2000 there were nine medical trials for the treatment of lung cancer or mesothelioma, some of them included questionnaires about patient's quality of life as we also had done at the beginning of the WISECARE project.

Table 1   Staff and Common Chemotherapeutics on Ward 82

No	Staff	Common chemotherapeutics
1	Departmental medical officer	Carboplatin
2	Physicians	Cisplatin
1	Head nurse	Docetaxel
13	Registered nurses	Etoposide
4	Licensed practical nurses (or enrolled nurses)	Gemcitabine
2	Ward assistants	Ifosfamide
3.5	Domestics staff members	Ironotecan
		Paclitaxel
		Vinorelbine

1.3   HUCH Chemotherapy OPD

The chemotherapy outpatient department at the Department of Oncology is specialized in administering chemotherapy during a few hours stay. Before and during the treatments all patients visit an oncologist. A primary nurse who is specialized in cancer nursing administers the drugs. In our unit there are five primary nurses who administer the chemotherapy protocols and two nurses who work at the oncologists reception. In general, the Department of Oncology in HUCH aims to promote the patients' optimal health in cancer care effectively and economically by emphasising the best possible patient care and nursing management, scientific research and continuous education.

Table 2   Common Patient Groups and the Principles of Nursing Care at the Chemotherapy OPD

Patients	Principles of nursing care
Breast cancer	Primary nursing
Colorectal cancer	Physical, emotional and social rehabilitation
Mb Hodgkin	Early detection of symptoms
* 60 - 70 patients/day	Prevention of health risks
* 17 000 patients/year	

Table 3   Staff and Breast Cancer Patients' most common Chemotherapy Regimens at the Chemotherapy OPD

No	Staff	Most common chemotherapy regimens
1	Departmental medical officer	Cyclophosphamide-methotrexate-5-fluorouracil
3	Physicians	Cyclophosphamide-epirubicin-5-fluorouracil
1	Head nurse	Vinorelbine
5	Registered nurses	Methotrexate
1	Licentiate practical nurses (or enrolled nurses)	Single-adriamycin
2	Ward assistants	Single-epirubicin

1.4   HUCH Ward 12

The haematological ward is a part of the Department of Internal Medicine. The capacity of the ward is 14 beds, but often there are more patients than that. As in HUCH, also on our ward the nursing care is based on nursing science and its humanistic conception of human being.

Table 4 Commonest patient groups and the principles of nursing care on ward 12

Patients	Principles of nursing care
AML	Holistic nursing
ALL	Individualized nursing
Myeloma	Nursing documentation
Lymphoma	Primary nursing
MDS	Mutual communication
CML	Security
CLL	Patient education
* 3 800 patient days	Patient's rights
* 380 hospital admissions per year	Continuous learning
* average length of stay 10.5 days	In the future: Peer evaluation
	Equality assurance

Table 5 Staff and common chemotherapeutics on ward 12

No	Staff	Common chemotherapeutics
1	Haematologist	Carmustine
1	Physician	Cisplatin
1	Head nurse	Cyclophosphamide
15	Registered nurses	Cytarabine
5	Licentiate practical nurses (or enrolled nurses)	Daunorubicin
1	Ward assistant	Doxorubicin
4.5	Domestics staff members	Etoposide
		Fludarabine
		Idarubicine
		M-Amsakrine
		Melphalan
		Metotrexate
		Mitoxantrone
		Vincristine

1.5 Pros and Cons of the WISECARE project Experienced at HUCH

Useful learning experiences	Frustrations
• Learning more English language • Learning to use a computer: e-mail, Internet • Learning to evaluate patient's care by comparing with others in order to find the best practices • Getting to know colleagues locally and internationally • Getting to know other sites and hospitals • Possibility to participate in the meetings • Receiving instant feedback from WiseTool • Receiving global feedback • Obtaining a scale to assess patient's oral health • Possibility to assess the impact of WISECARE on clinical behaviour by WiseCompass • Learning project work	• Many diagnosis and many different treatments make it difficult to compare and to draw conclusions • IT-programs are not compatible, are made for one-user system, not a part of every day work • The shortage of travelling allowance to attend the meetings • Lack of time • Moffit is not suitable for outpatient departments

Good To Remember: "WISECARE is a learning process" - W. Sermeus

2   The Netherlands

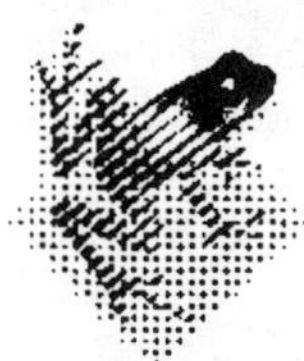

ACADEMISCH ZIEKENHUIS GRONINGEN

The Groningen University Hospital

The AZG can be described as an enormous company. Every day treatment, research, training and knowledge are passed on for the benefit of people's health. The hospital has 1056 beds. 26,000 patients are admitted annually, around 350,000 people visit the outpatient clinics and it is the workplace for 5,500 people.

2.1   The AZG and Wisecare

The AZG is a Validation Site for WISECARE. The unit for surgical oncology is involved with 20 beds. Seventy patients participated in WISECARE. All usual surgical treatments are performed, including state of the art treatments such as the sentinel lymph node procedure.

2.2   Pain Outcomes

All patients complaints about pain at a moderate level. This was of a temporary nature in all of the cases and was concurrent with the risk assessments made previously. Out of 70 assessed patients, 14 showed an increase of pain after discharge. Of notable interest is the group of patients, which received an excisional biopsy. 8 out of 14 patients reported increasing pain after discharge, although nurses consider the treatment as less severe.

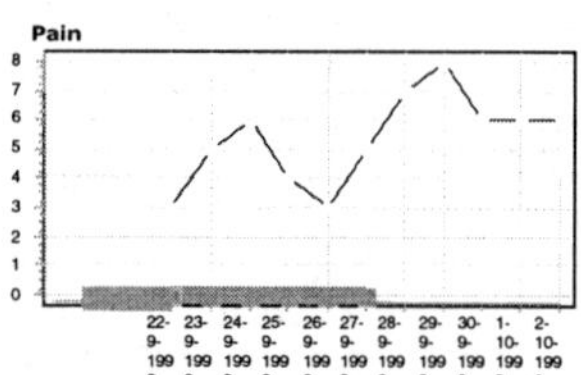

Figure 1   Pain Outcomes of a Patient after receiving an Excisional Biopsy. Discharged at 09/27/99 (taken from Wisetool).

2.3   Fatigue Outcomes

Fatigue occurred during hospitalization. Most patients experienced a moderate problem, occurring during the first days after surgical treatment. This tended to resolve to a normal or mild problem. 15 patients grew more fatigued after discharge.

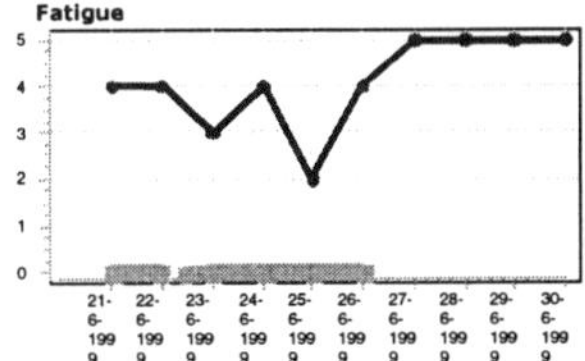

Figure 2   Fatigue Outcomes of a Patient after receiving a Modified Radical Mastectomy.
Discharge at 06/26/99 (taken from Wisetool)

2.4 Nausea & Vomiting Outcomes

Approximately 75% of the patients experienced problems with nausea or vomiting after surgical treatment. These problems ranged from mild to moderate, but always resolved during hospitalization. After discharge, nausea did not occur.

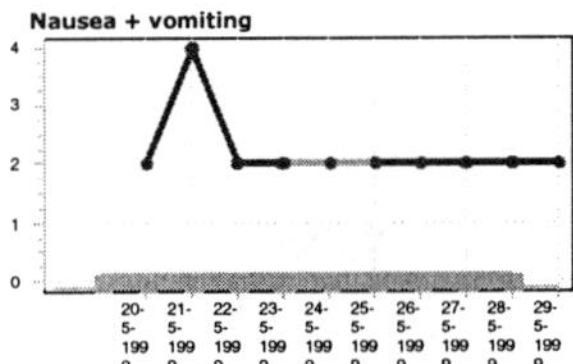

Figure 3   Nausea/Vomiting Outcomes of a Patient receiving an Ablatio.
Discharge at 06/28/99 (taken from Wisetool)

2.5 Conclusion

Patient evaluation illustrated that the patients health status incorporated in the WISECARE project have improved during hospitalisation. WISECARE has focussed the attention on these problems, initiating nursing interventions, even after discharge. Further research is necessary to continue to evaluate the nature of the problems.

3   Slovenia

History of WISECARE project in University Medical Center Ljubljana, Slovenia from June until December 1999

The Beginning:

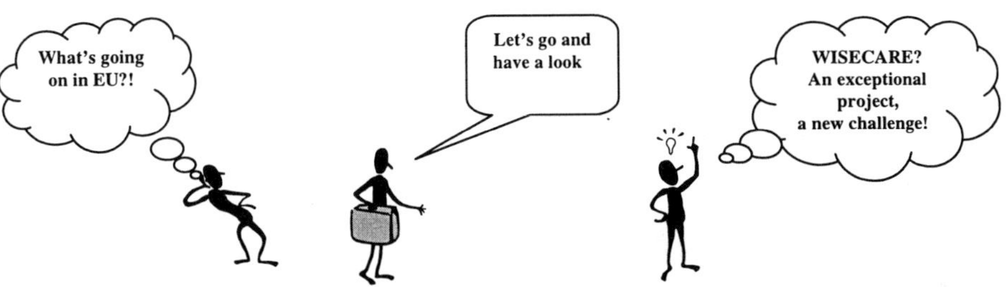

Further Steps:

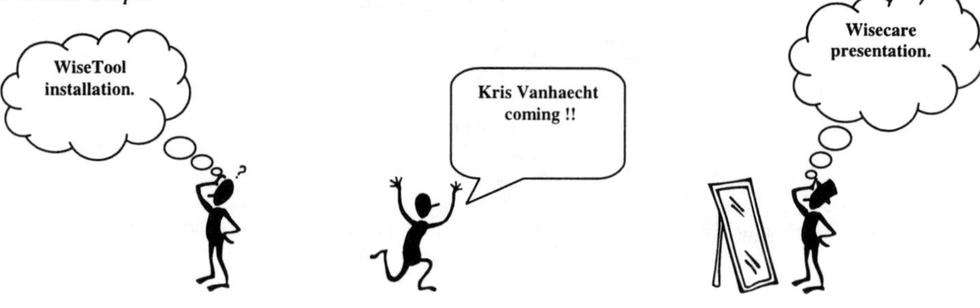

Hard Work:

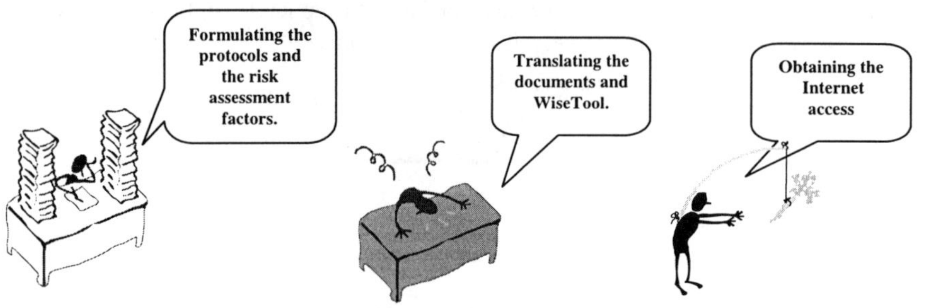

Benefits:

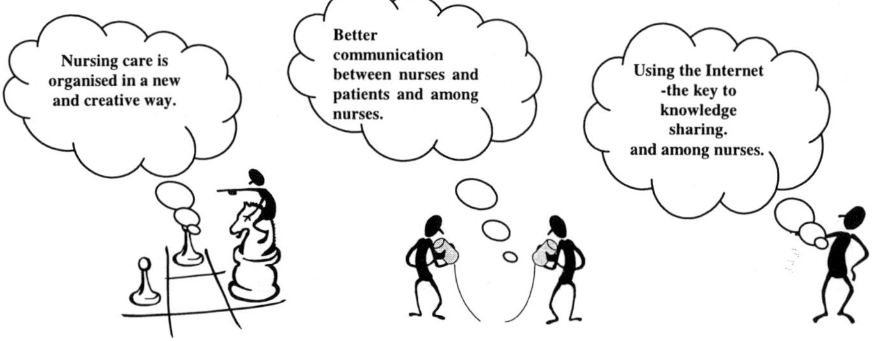

By way of Conclusion:

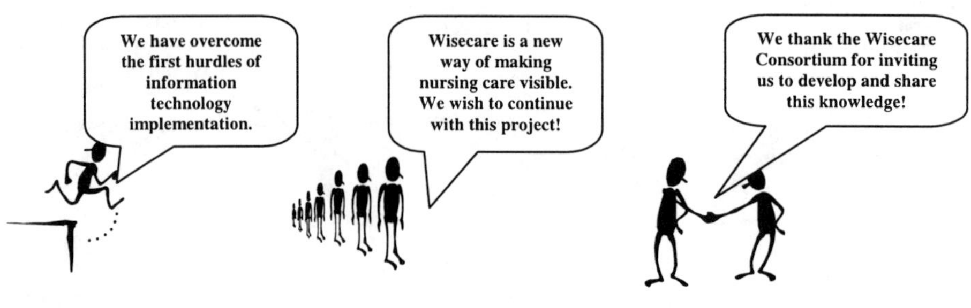

4   The Royal Marsden Experience

The nurses of the Royal Marsden Hospital joined the WISECARE project on the 13th September 1999 and since then have recruited over 20 patients. These patients have been recruited from the Breast unit, Lymphoma and Sarcoma units.

The overall experience of the project has been very positive for the following reasons:

4.1 Patient's Experience

The patients have stated that they feel safer when they know that their symptoms are being formally examined and recorded.

Many of the patients receiving chemotherapy for Breast cancer attend the hospital every 3-6 weeks for cyclical therapy — these patients are opting to complete the questionnaires on each cycle so that they can compare their symptoms.

As is often seen the women are very altruistic and are anxious to help knowledge and growth of awareness to help other women in the future.

Two patients who have completed 2 cycles felt that because of the project they felt more empowered to discuss their symptoms.

4.2 Staff Nurse's Experience

After the first 10 patients had been recruited with no problems many of the clinical staff on the wards have been directly involved either with recruiting themselves or witnessing for consent.

Following positive benefits are remarked:

- For many staff nurses this is their first chance to be involved in actual clinical nursing research in their ward area.
- The WISECARE project is a chance to narrow the practice-research gap and to make 'research' more 'user-friendly'
- There have been several 'spin-off' discussions each time I have been on the various wards - with mini spontaneous teaching sessions on: Informed consent, Questionnaire design, Research Ethics Committees.

Finally the impression is that all of those who have been involved in the project would very much like the project to continue and almost to become a part of the way working on every unit.

If it was able to continue the nurses might be able to approach the Research Ethics Committee again and widen the patient accrual to include patients from other clinical units such as Leukaemia and Lung Cancer.

5   Belgium

WISECARE was a challenge! The close cooperation between the WISECARE project staff of the Centre for Health Services and Nursing Research (who co-ordinated the project) and the staff of the Validation Site made the ward a pilot Validation Site within the project. The project staff from the University Hospitals Leuven and the research centre had a weekly meeting to keep track of the project. Suggestions and comments were made on the status of the project.

Within the University Hospitals Leuven, nurses of the ward gave several seminars. It was an opportunity to show colleagues what WISECARE was all about.

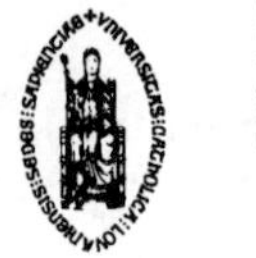

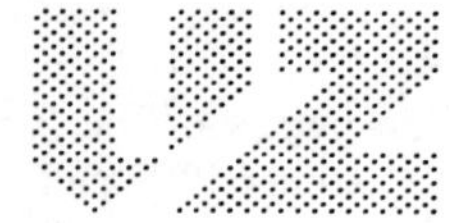

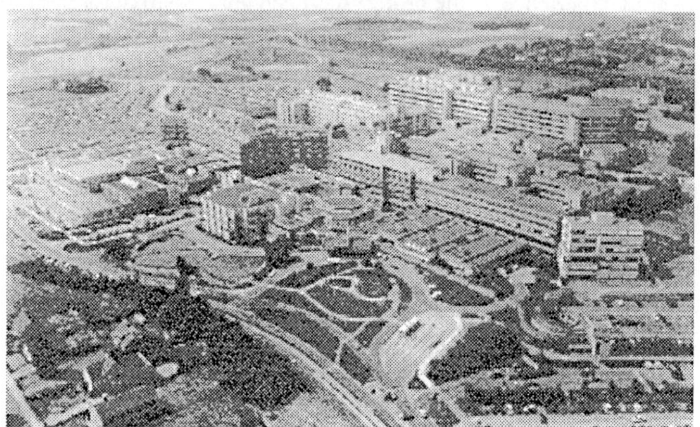

Figure 2   University Hospitals Leuven, Gasthuisberg Site

The use of WISECARE and WISETOOL has been evaluated very positive. WISECARE taught the nursing staff to work in a structured way and taught us to use structured follow-up forms for clinical indicators. Participation in the project resulted in the development of a new patient admission form wherein 15 clinical indicators are used. WISECARE gave us the chance to make by-products of the project: clinical pathways with risk assessment and clinical time, new chemotherapy follow up forms, some new procedures on specific clinical indicators, and further development of the Leuven Chemotherapy Risk Assessment Scale (LCRAS).

The Leuven Validation Site wants to go on with WISECARE because we have just started our journey towards providing better patient care.

WISECARE
W. Sermeus et al. (Eds.)
IOS Press, 2000

Modelling and Simulation of Patients Undergoing Chemotherapy

Jeff Tansley

1   Background

A small part of the WISECARE project was devoted to looking at the potential benefits that might accrue if nursing practice and the patient's self-care could be simulated on a computer. This would provide an opportunity to explore the importance of nursing care in a safe environment. It can also provide a basis for training nurses and instructing patients on the benefits of their self-care activities.

The computer simulation was based on nursing practice and the patient's self-care derived from the WISECARE patient model from the empirical investigations conducted at the Sites participating in the project.

2   Computerized Patient Model

Chemotherapy treatment gives rise to several side effects that, left unmanaged, can cause severe discomfort. In the extreme, these side effects can lead to treatment discontinuation and life threatening situations.

As described elsewhere in this report the WISECARE project studied, for each patient, four adverse affective states that arise because of the chemotherapy treatment. These were: fatigue, nausea, mucositis and pain.

These states dominate, although others may occur. Each state gives rise to similarly named side effects of varying degrees of magnitude. The severity of the side effects that a patient experiences from a given therapeutic dosage will depend on factors such as the patient's sensitivity, their self-care activities and their life-style. In the study, the side effects were measured using variants of existing psychometric scales, each with its own scoring mechanism and range of values.

In addition to the adverse affective states, the computer model also incorporates three "normal" affective states: hunger, thirst and activation.

These manifest themselves as similarly named main effects. The first two have obvious psychological/physiological analogues (eating, drinking) but the third is a modelling attempt to reflect a level of arousal, a desire to do things and live a normal life. The model codes this as the proportion of the day on three levels of patient behaviour (active, resting and sleeping).

For the purposes of the computer model [1] the affective states are the motivation for behaviour [2]. They are represented as normalized scale on an interval 0 to 25 and follow the law of initial values [3]. Thus, if a computer generated patient has a value of 0 then this represents a day on which they experience no fatigue, nausea, mucositis or pain, whereas one with a value of 25 is representing a day on which they are experiencing extreme conditions.

The resulting magnitude of the side effects is proportional to initial values of "personal characteristics". (Currently this is based on a simple model). As each day passes, so the magnitude of side effects change. The extent of change is determined by the patient's own behaviour in managing side effects and the interaction between affective states.

Indirectly this relates to the quality of instruction given to the patient and the extent to which a patient is under direct interventionist care.

In summary, Table 1 shows the compensatory care and behaviour in the patient model for each side and main effect.

Table 1   The Compensatory Care and Behaviour in the Patient Model for each Side and Main Effect

Affective states as side effects	*Compensatory care*
Fatigue	Rest
Nausea	Medication (anti-emetics)
Mucositis	Oral care
Pain	Medication (analgesics)
Affective states as main effects	*Normal behaviour*
Hunger	Eating
Thirst	Drinking
Activation	Sleeping, resting, daily activity

3   Computerized Nursing Model

Nursing care attempts to counter side effects. It does this through a complex mixture of direct interventions and patient education. Nursing practice has evolved on demand, through experience and based on perceived individual patient needs, rather than through systematic evaluation. There is a requirement for improved efficiency, efficacy and quality.

Each of the WISECARE nursing Sites has documented their nursing care protocols. These describe, in detail, the way in which a patient might respond according to the side effects they may exhibit. Five different protocols per side effect per Site have been collected and are being evaluated.

The computer model illustrates the presence/absence of a protocol for managing each of the 5 side effects.

Currently the "with-protocol" model allows a patient to receive a nominal "best care". This assumes that they remain in contact with a comprehensive interventionist nursing care programme for the whole of the period of chemotherapy treatment. This is obviously artificial in that it assumes that the patient eats/sleeps/medicates perfectly according to a prescribed programme.

The alternative "no-protocol" model is equally artificial in that it assumes that the patient does not follow any of the compensatory care, and their condition deteriorates.

4   Calibration

The computer model was calibrated using data collected in the study. Calibration was done in terms of initial conditions, which included a model of sensitivity to chemotherapy.

5　Simulation Methodology

The model as described was coded in a simulation language EpiScript [4]. The language executes according to a discrete event mechanism. In this study, it was set to be day by day. Table 2 shows the measurements made in the simulation for each category of patient behaviour.

Table 2　The Measurements made in the Simulation for each Category of Patient Behaviour

Behaviour	*Recorded activity*
Sleeping,	Hours/day
Resting	Hours/day
Active	Hours/day
Eating	Times/day
Drinking	Times/day
Medication anti emetics	Doses/day
Medication analgesics	Doses/day
Mouth care, teeth cleaning	Times/day
Mouth wash	Times/day

6　Model Dynamics

Based upon WISEDATA, the model generates virtual patients that will undergo chemotherapy.

It should be emphasized that the examples discussed here are not real patients and are not intended to imply that any real patients have been cared for in the ways discussed.

We will explain the coding using examples.

Box 1 and 2 show the side effect profiles of a virtual patient who has their first chemotherapy on day 14 of the simulation. Box 1 simulates "with-protocol" model whereas Box 2 simulates the "no-protocol" model.

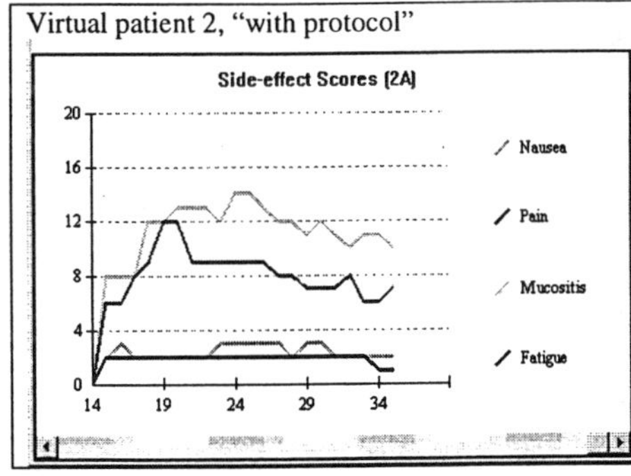

The chart shows the side effect profile from the day of the patient's first chemotherapy (day 14 of the simulation).

The virtual patient exhibits low levels of nausea (3) and pain (2). Over the next 20 days, these remain at about the same levels, with pain finally decreasing to level 1.

The patient's mucositis score rises to 12 within 5 days of chemotherapy, peaking at 14 and then gradually falling, but only to 9 or 10.

The patient also experience high levels of fatigue, rising to 12, and remaining at 6 or higher

Box 1　"With-Protocol" Model for Virtual Patient 2

Box 2 shows the side effect profile for the same virtual patient as in Box 1. However, in this scenario the care is quite different, following the "no-protocol" model, i.e. there is no systematic intervention. The patient is left to make his own responsive decisions with little help and no pre-emptive care. The patient continues with their previous daily activities influenced by the adverse effects of the treatment.

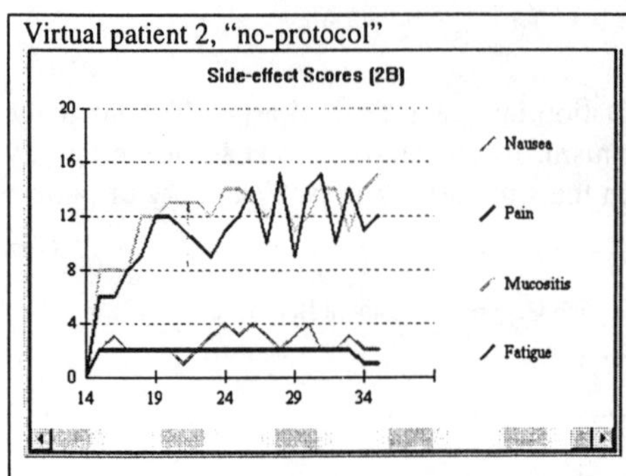

These are the simulated charts for the same virtual patient with a "no-protocol" model.
Again side effects of mucositis and fatigue dominate.
There appears to be an interesting oscillatory effect on fatigue. This arises from the nature of the simulation using a daily event interval, and thus showing a daily average.

Box 2   "No-Protocol" Model for the same Virtual Patient 2

The charts also reflect the individual nature of each of the virtual patients and situations generated in the simulation. They are different when they start the simulation and behave differently each day. This is shown in Boxes 3 and 4. These contain the side-effect profiles for two virtual patients, the one on the right being more sensitive to chemotherapy than the one on the left (whose profiles were explained in Boxes 1 and 2). Box 3 shows the "with-protocol" model and Box 4 the "no-protocol" model.

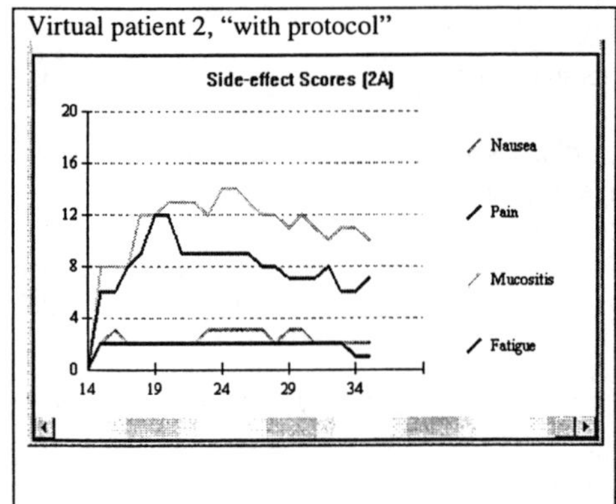

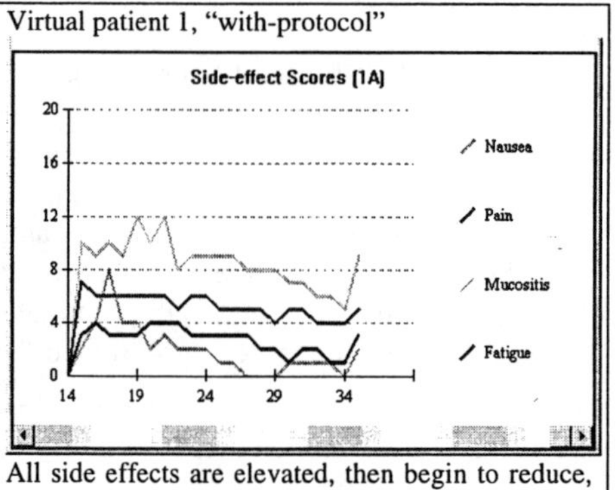

All side effects are elevated, then begin to reduce, with nausea gradually diasppearing

Box 3   Patient Individuality - the "With-Protocol Model for Virtual Patient 2 and 1

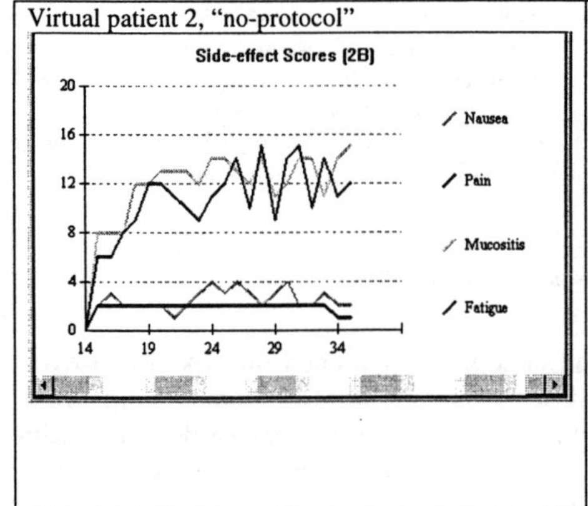

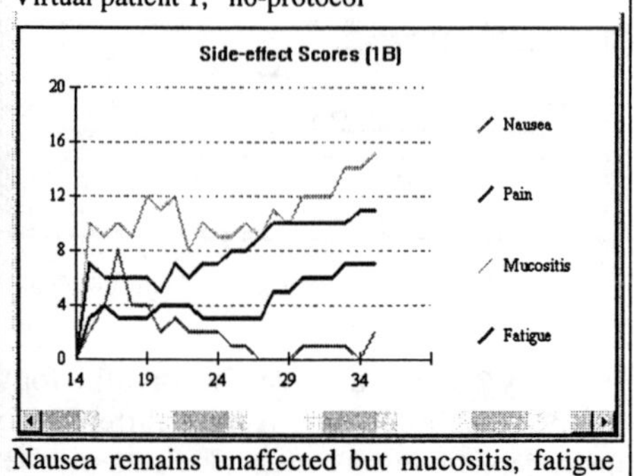

Nausea remains unaffected but mucositis, fatigue and pain increase for the whole of the monitoring period.

Box 4   "No-Protocol" Model for the two Virtual Patients

The simulation also reports how patients spend their time. We show some of the charts in Boxes 5, 6 and 7, and include the two weeks prior to the chemotherapy (administered on day 14).

Box 5 charts are for two patients (the two discussed above). They show that time is divided between sleeping, resting and waking activities. The patient on the right is the more active before chemotherapy, but less active afterwards.

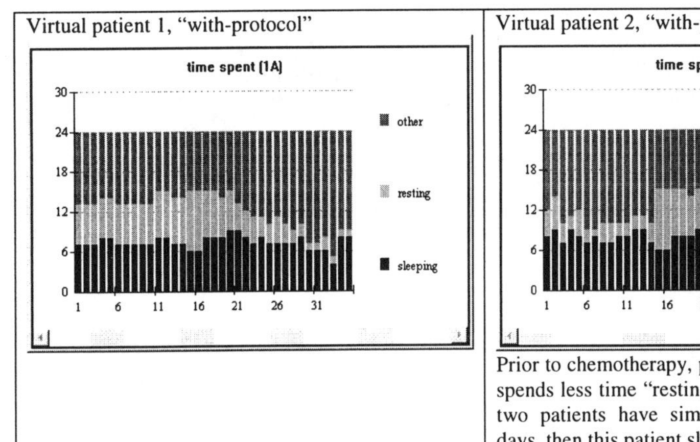

Prior to chemotherapy, patient 2 is more active and spends less time "resting". After chemotherapy the two patients have similar profiles for about 10 days, then this patient sleeps more than the other.

Box 5　Time Spent for the two Virtual Patients under the "With-Protocol" Model

In Box 6 the two charts are from the same patient in the two models, so the differences between the two graphs result from different care protocols - "with-protocol" is on the left (1A), "no-protocol" is on the right (1B).

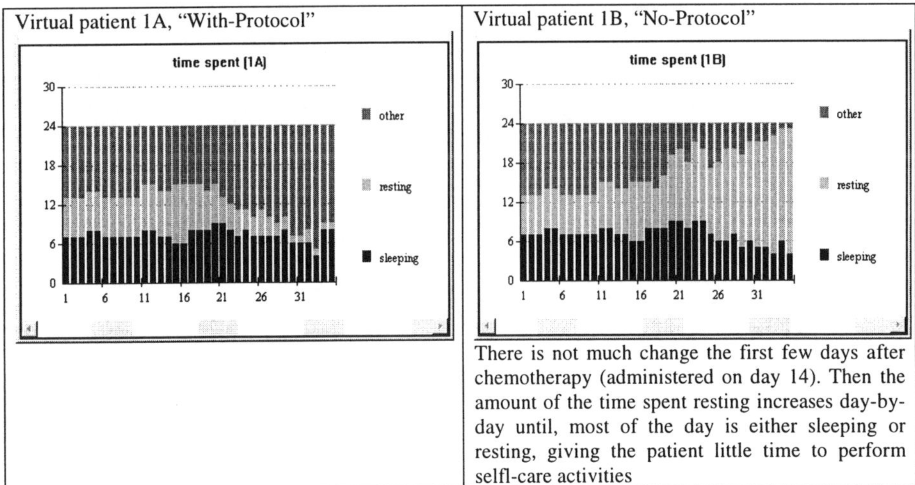

There is not much change the first few days after chemotherapy (administered on day 14). Then the amount of the time spent resting increases day-by-day until, most of the day is either sleeping or resting, giving the patient little time to perform self-care activities

Box 6　Time Spent for Virtual Patient 1 under the two Models

Box 7 shows the number of times each day the virtual patient eats and drinks under the two different care protocols

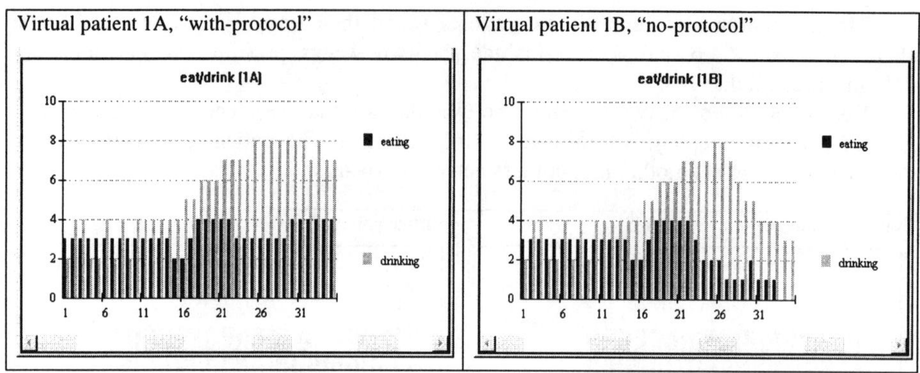

Box 7   Eat & Drinking by Virtual Patient 1 for the two Protocols

7   Simulator Output

Boxes 8 and 9 below show the form of the simulator output. Four graphic quadrants can be viewed at any one time as the simulation proceeds. Different collections of graphs can be selected and the user can structure these to meet their investigation needs.

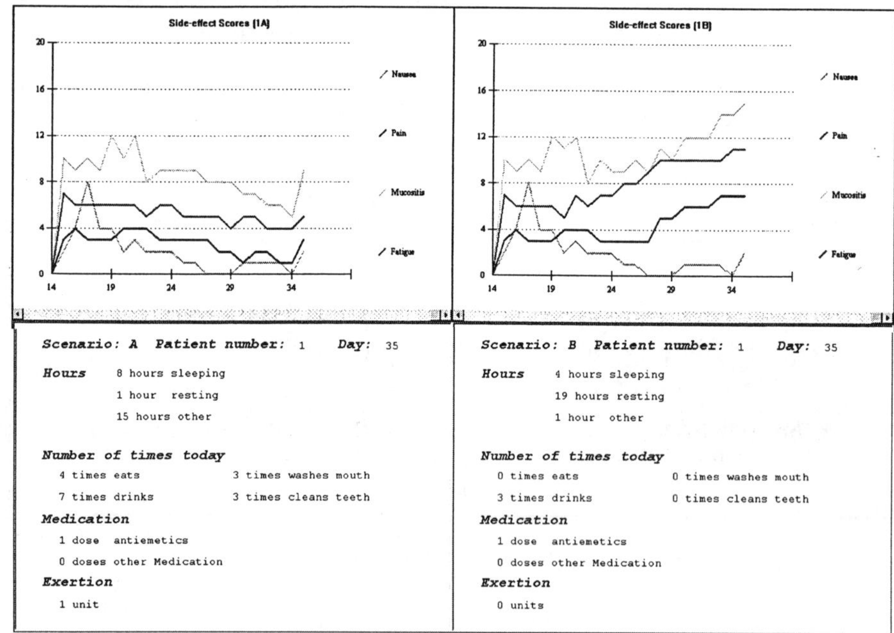

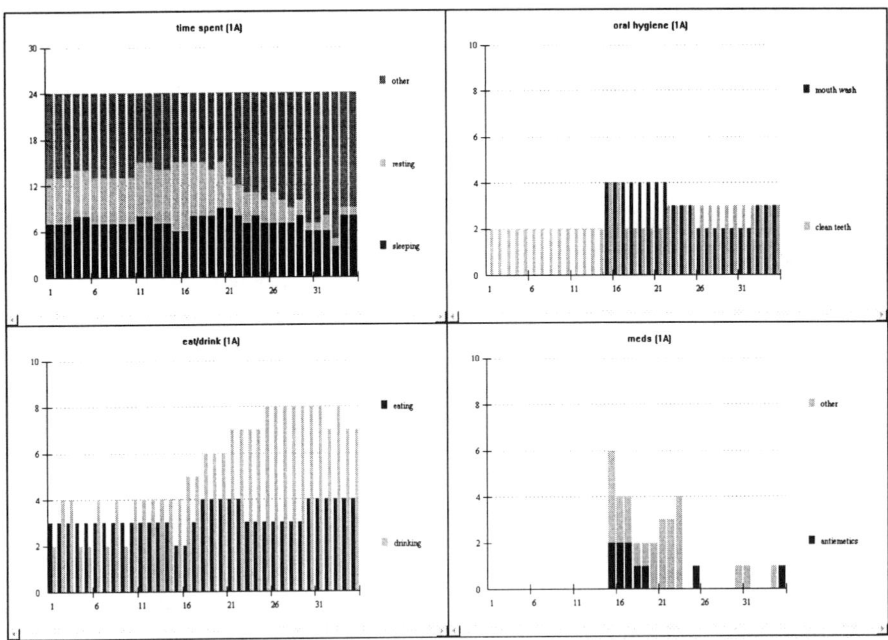

Box 8　Full Side Effect and Activity Report for "With-Protocol" Model, Virtual Patient 1

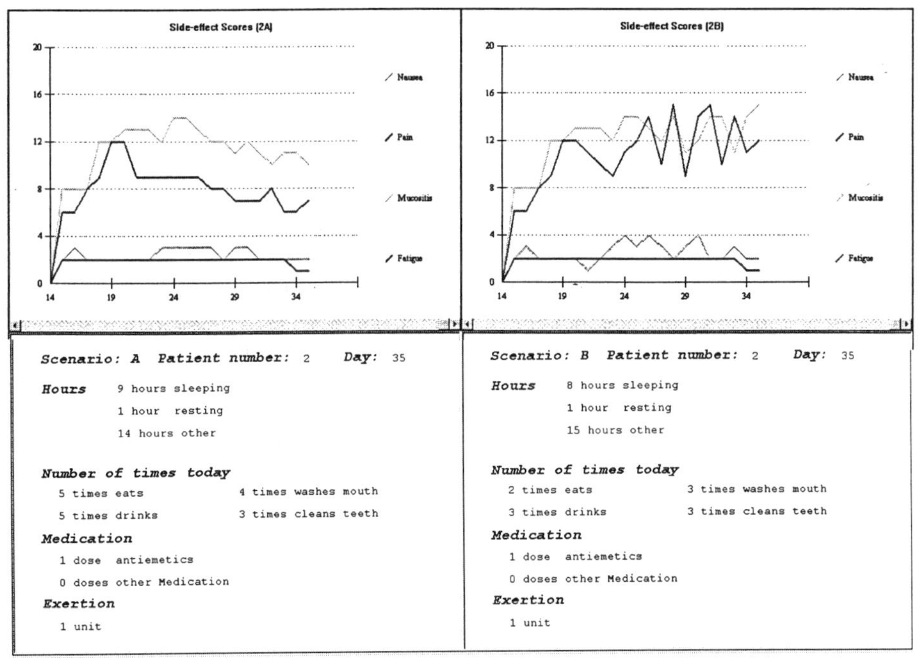

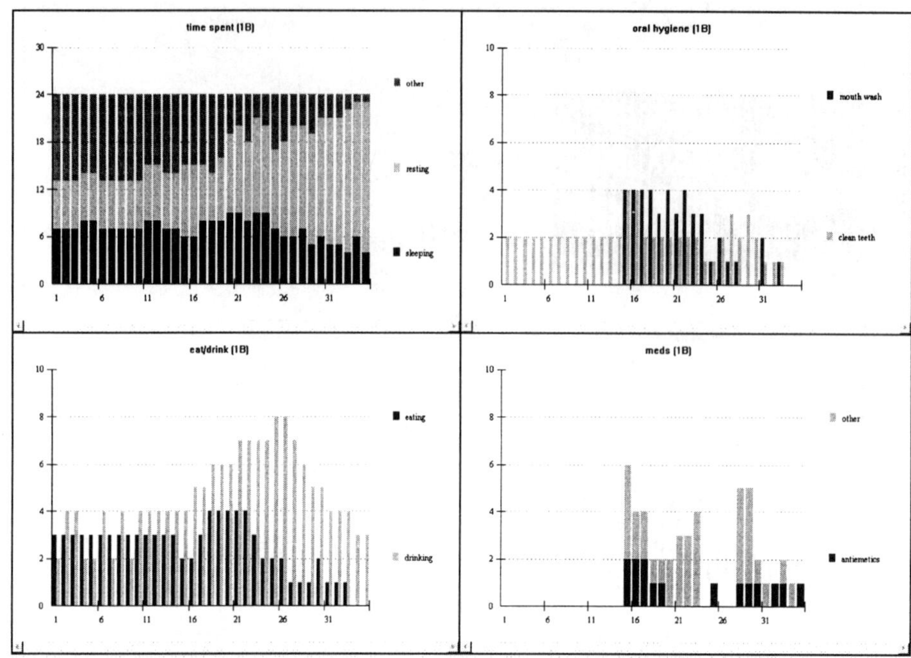

Box 9   Full Side Effect and Activity Report for "With-Protocol" Model, Virtual Patient 2

8   Conclusions

The simulation of the individual patients and care protocols is a relatively new technology, particularly in health care. The small incursion of simulation into the WISECARE project has shown the contribution this technology has yet to make.

It is still early days and much more can be achieved. As recently as the formation stages of the WISECARE project the cost of suitably powerful computing equipment seemed inhibitory. This has now changed. Powerful computers are now relatively inexpensive. Further, the simulation of this model takes only a few seconds to complete 32 days of activity. Considerable complexity can be added to the model without loss of user interactive capability but with considerable gain in utility. It is possible to explore care profiles at the level at which they are recorded and discussed by practitioners. Simulations can run the on-going workload of a busy unit up to six months ahead of current times

References

[1]   Sloman A. Prolegomena to a theory of communication and affect. In: Ortony A, Slack J & Stock O.
[2]   Communications from an artificial intelligence perspective: Theoretical and applied issues. Springer, 1992.
[3]   Picard R. Affective computing. MIT Press, 1997.
[4]   Sternbach R. Principles of psychophysiology. Academic Press, 1966.
[5]   Bryan-Jones J & Tansley J. EpiScript Users Manual. An Teallach Ltd, 1997.

Part IV

Evaluation

WISECARE
W. Sermeus et al. (Eds.)
IOS Press, 2000

Multicentre Research

Morven Miller, Nora Kearney, Walter Sermeus

1 Introduction

Collaborative research ventures are increasingly viewed as the optimal way of conducting research in nursing and health care [1]. This is mostly because of the increased likelihood of funding, increased accessibility to practice settings and increased access to resources such as research and clinical expertise [2]. As a result, collaborative research is now one of the most desirable strategies for accomplishing the goals of research. However, while glowing pictures can be painted of what can be achieved through the collaborative process, the reality of collaboration can be fraught with difficulties for the research team to overcome.

2 What is Collaborative Research

While the term 'collaboration' can have negative connotations, associated with working with the enemy, the Oxford Dictionary [3] defines 'collaboration' as 'working in partnership'. However, review of the nursing literature reveals that within research, the term 'collaboration' is understood and used in a variety of ways. The meaning of collaboration can be as diverse as individuals working on various facets of research projects fairly isolated from one another or teams of individuals working together on all facets of the project from the conceptual stage to final report writing. Additionally, collaboration can refer to work between professionals within a group, various organisations and also between various disciplines. To further complicate matters, any project could involve any or all of these levels of collaboration.

In particular, two definitions help to capture the complexity and diversity of such a collaborative research process. Firstly, Engstrom [4:78] defined collaborative research as, "a research endeavour that pools the resources of any of a variety of researchers, agencies, scientists, clinicians and representatives from various disciplines". Ten years later Henneman et al. [5:363] suggested that "Collaboration is a process by which members of various disciplines share their expertise. Accomplishing this requires that these individuals understand and appreciate what it is that they contribute to the whole".
These definitions help us to focus on the positive aspects of the collaborative research process such as sharing expertise, feeling that each member of the team is making a contribution and of understanding and therefore 'owning' whatever the research team hope to accomplish.
Although involved in collaborative research for many years, nurses have slowly changed their roles, moving from positions of data collectors and research assistants to those of project directors and principle investigators of interdisciplinary projects. This has brought about a new level of awareness of the intricacies that collaborative ventures entail [6].

This article will draw on the authors' experience of WISECARE, a European collaborative cancer nursing project to ground the discussion of the benefits and pitfalls of multicentre nursing research.

3   Setting the WISECARE Scene

Throughout Europe, the impact that nursing has on the quality of care for Europe's citizens is not evaluated. Given the changes in health care financing that are taking place across Europe, it is imperative that hospitals focus their cost-containment efforts in this area. Furthermore, it is essential that the relationship between costs of nursing and outcomes of care be established. One could argue that the vast amounts of data generated by nursing staff should be used constructively for the development and evaluation and improvement of nursing protocols and guidelines. However, the vast majority of data stored in patient records are merely used for individual and operational communication between individual caregivers, hospitals and community care.

It is within this European situation that the Workflow Information Systems for European Nursing Care (WISECARE) project has been conceived. WISECARE turns actual clinical care information into data ready for the development and evaluation of protocols and guidelines. Through dissemination and sharing of information, the WISECARE project aims to provide international guidelines and protocols and the facility to compare actual practice with benchmarks. Despite the multidisciplinary nature of the team members, the focus of the project is nursing care. Additionally, focussing the project on oncology care has allowed a wide range of clinical settings and nursing care to be incorporated.

Using clinical problems as the vehicle for the project, WISECARE aims to quantify and make visible factors vital to patient care and nursing practice. These include the diversity of patient population, the variability of patient care across Europe, patient outcomes and nursing resources. Using this information and pooling the experiences of cancer nurses across Europe will lead to the development of a knowledge base of best practices and facilitate a move away from individual knowledge to knowledge sharing and ultimately improved patient care [8].

Research must be brought closer to the practice of nursing and so consequently nearer to the practitioners in nursing [9]. In an attempt to achieve this and to ensure that the nurses involved in WISECARE have a sense of ownership of the research, clinically based nurses in five European cancer centres, Scotland, Finland, Sweden, Belgium and the Netherlands are also involved with the project. September 1999 will see them joined by nurses from Greece, Denmark, Belgium, France, England and Slovenia. These clinically based nurses have identified four priorities that allow the exploration of nursing issues within the project: oral care, fatigue, pain and nausea and vomiting.

State-of-the-art information technology (IT) systems allow these nurses to communicate and compare their current practices and patient outcomes in a way that has not hitherto been accessed by clinically based nurses on a pan-European basis. Communicating in this way has the potential to markedly alter the way that knowledge is transferred and nursing practice developed. Traditional education strategies and transfer of knowledge will be partially superseded by inductive experience-based knowledge development, driven by clinical practice and patient requirements. Additionally WISECARE aims to meet the needs of nursing management in Europe, addressing issues such as nursing workload and nurse staffing to ensure better quality care.

The ambitious nature of WISECARE makes collaboration across multiple Sites essential and the five partners involved each bring differing expertise to the project. The European Oncology Nursing Society is a pan-European cancer nursing society and brings an established network of cancer nurses to the project. Within WISECARE, the School of Nursing and Midwifery within the University of Glasgow supports the European Oncology Nursing Society. The Catholic University of Leuven, co-ordinator of the WISECARE project, is involved in the provision of statistical analysis and also simulation work. The Glasgow Caledonian University and University of Kuopio have been involved with defining user requirements, building the databases and data collection. University of Kuopio and HISCOM, an independent company concerned with hospital management systems, have been involved in the WISECARE project as evaluators of the technology employed and validation of the project. Finally, the University of Athens is responsible for networking within the project and the development of the WorldWide Website of WISECARE. Such is the diversity of the main partners, collaboration has not been without its problems. Using the WISECARE project for illustration, the advantages and disadvantages of this type of research can be illuminated.

4   Positive Aspects of Multicentre Research

4.1   Increased Productivity of Individual Studies

While common criticisms levelled at nursing research include the recruitment of small sample sizes and the use of largely descriptive research methods resulting in fairly superficial findings [10], utilising multicentre research offers a solution through increasing the productivity of individual studies and contributing substantially to the scientific knowledge base.

Multicentre research has the potential to contribute substantially to the scientific knowledge base for a variety of reasons. Firstly, it allows complex patient care problems to be addressed: such as the WISECARE project focussing on the four patient problems, i.e. nausea and vomiting, pain, oral care and fatigue, alongside addressing nursing management issues. A collaborative project also allows the generalisation of clinically relevant research through the acquisition of larger sample sizes and within the WISECARE project, this relates not only to patient sample size but also to a larger sample size of nursing staff with varying skills and abilities. This larger size of samples is also reflected in the clinical settings included in the WISECARE project that facilitates access to both surgical and medical oncology locations, incorporating in-patient, out-patient and ambulatory care settings. The pooling of both human and non-human resources in this way assists in the expansion of nursing knowledge that ultimately impacts on patient care. Utilising multicentre research in this way also prevents years of delay in replicating the studies. Furthermore, the sharing of resources prevents unnecessary duplication, which can amount to considerable cost.

4.2   Financial Support

Financial support is crucial to the successful implementation of both data collection and analysis, especially when a project involves a substantial number of collaborators and multiple Sites. While both nursing service and education have long traditions of 'investment', in many countries, investment in nursing research is at best sporadic and limited and at worst non-existent [11]. Within oncology nursing, as with many other specialities, the need for significant financial support will become increasingly more likely as cancer nurses seek to design and implement studies that have a high degree of generalisability across Europe. Securing funding for projects can involve a great deal of time in the preparation and submission of a proposal. Currently, cancer nursing is generally disadvantaged in securing such financial backing primarily because of the lack of an adequate infrastructure and interest to facilitate the submission of competitive applications. However, as a profession, we must learn to generate bids of high quality and compete on equal terms with other disciplines.

While economic restraints and cutbacks, in both educational and health care delivery settings have made sharing resources a necessity [12], collaborative nursing research is one approach that allows the provision of the scientific basis for nursing practice whilst observing the economic realities. Although the need for financial support is dependent on the research project, the quality and generalisability of multicentre research often make it more likely to receive financial backing. Indeed, the WISECARE project is fortunate to have received financial backing from the European Commission. However, while financial support is essential for the initiation and sustenance of such a project, support for the personnel involved in the project is also essential. Such support comes from the network of fellow professionals involved with the project and the importance of this supportive network in maintaining the impetus of the project should not be underestimated.

4.3 Mutual Learning and Support

While not every nurse can or should be a researcher, all nurses should be involved in some aspect of the research process [13] and involvement in the WISECARE project offers not only individual nurses the opportunity to learn but also the nursing profession the chance to develop. As team members differ in terms of their experience and educational backgrounds, mutual learning and sharing is often an outcome of collaborative research. WISECARE offers all levels of nursing the opportunity to participate in collaborative nursing research that will foster growth and understanding of the importance of nursing research. At the same time it also has the advantage of fostering critical inquiry for all nurses involved and allows nurses of varying levels of education and experience to participate.

Furthermore, as is so often the case in research, and lengthy research in particular, enthusiasm for a project wanes over a period of time. Unforeseen events in the clinical setting and other clinical priorities can often result in the research project lagging behind time with personnel becoming stale and loosing interest. The WISECARE project overcomes this potential problem through the use of a supportive network that allows all research team members involved to support each other, discuss their clinical concerns and pressures and overcome the feelings of isolation that are often felt by researchers. Consequently this maintains the impetus of the project so ensuring the successful realisation of the research agenda.

WISECARE has created this supportive network primarily through the use of electronic mail, which can be used by both clinical and non-clinical research team members either between individual team members or via a general WISECARE mailing list. It allows clinically based nurses to communicate and discuss any concerns they have with, for example, patient recruitment or the process of data collection. However, more recent communication has been directed towards discussions regarding patient outcomes between individual Sites and differences in the nursing resources available to each of the Sites/countries. The flexibility of this communication medium appears well suited to both clinical and non-clinical areas. It affords nurses the opportunity to communicate at a time convenient for them, be that during a quiet spell in the day or during night shift. Other forms of communication have been discussed, such as video or telephone conferencing. However, it is problematic for clinically based staff to negotiate an appropriate time for these and the preferred method of communication continues to be e-mail; an appropriate choice for a project that aims to promote the use of IT within cancer nursing. Building such flexibility into a multicentre research project is essential and makes for the successful completion of the project. While such supportive links allow problems to be shared and solutions found, they also foster understanding and the building of strong working relationships. Such understanding allows complementary viewpoints to be shared in an unthreatening environment and these complementary viewpoints are also an advantage of multicentre research projects.

4.4 *Complementary Viewpoints*

All nurses have a responsibility to strive to develop the scientific body of knowledge required to guide nursing practice. This includes nurses involved in clinical practice, education, research and management. The combined skills of the research team allow complementary viewpoints to be explored within the multicentre research project. Team members from the academic setting can be particularly valuable in the development of the research proposal and instrument development as a result of their experience in these areas, while clinical personnel ensure that the project has value for clinical practice. Tierney and Taylor [14] illustrated that problems can arise as practising nurses are inevitably suspicious and sometimes apprehensive of academically qualified nurses who work in 'ivory towers'. However, they also highlighted that nurse researchers can often feel overawed by the aura of competence exuded by experienced nurses. Ultimately, as the aims of the research findings are first and foremost meaningful to nurses, there is great value in having the more objective and theoretical approach of academics tempered by the clinically orientated and down-to-earth observations of clinically based nurses. These complementary viewpoints are evident in the WISECARE project as clinically-based nurses were involved from the outset and have established the patient indicators they believe would be most beneficial, while support for these nurses comes from the academic setting.

Reflecting on these positive aspects, it would seem that collaboration and multicentre research offer a solution to many of the problems that have plagued nursing research in the past. However, the pitfalls must be explored before one can make an informed choice regarding the overall power of this form of research.

5   Problems of Multicentre Research

5.1 *Organisational Aspects*

Research must be organised and methodical in its approach. For WISECARE, such organisation is complicated as the project not only involves co-ordinating a variety of research Sites but also must constantly consider the diverse backgrounds of the partners. Furthermore, this co-ordination takes place in various research Sites, all of which except one speak English as a second or third language. From crucial requirements such as ethical approval to more basic requirements such as access to facilities such as a computer, co-ordination has been essential. As the WISECARE project, by its very nature, is keen to implement IT within health care, much of the co-ordination has been communicated via electronic mail which has had positive results as it offers flexibility across a variety of settings and gives individuals the time to consider issues for discussion.

Standardised data collection is essential within multicentre research to ensure that the results of the research are comparable. The geographical distance between Clinical Sites makes frequent meetings for all those involved impossible with the result that most information is communicated via e-mail. Standardisation of data collection has been achieved through the use of a comprehensive staff manual for data collection, and in some cases this has been translated. In addition, regardless of the language, this manual is subject to interpretation by each of the Clinical Sites and despite all attempts to avoid variations in interpretation, small, local variations in data collection are evident.

5.2 Differing Expectations

Organisational issues aside, a number of individuals working together can be further complicated because each member of the research team may have different expectations regarding the research project's aims, methods, purpose and process. The differing expectations of individual researchers within a multicentre research project can be problematic, with the result that one could surmise that there appears to be an inherent conflict of interest between practice and research. Hinshaw et al. [15] identified differing goals for research held by clinicians, administrators and researchers. While practitioners can be seen to place value on relevance, realism and immediately applicable information, researchers put a premium on accurate, precise data informed from theory and a clearly stated research problem. However, negotiating and resolving such conflicts through recognising individual's concerns and expectations allows all parties to reach a mutually acceptable position.

Such differing expectations have become evident during the WISECARE project in the shape of tensions between the practical, clinical reality of data collection and textbook research practices. This has resulted in a change to the data collection process more than halfway through the project. Original data collection involved the completion of a quality of life questionnaire (the EORTC QLQ-C30 [16]) and the Piper Fatigue Scale [15] once weekly with the Oral Assessment Guide [16] completed daily during patients' stay in hospital. A major drive for the change to data collection came from the data managers who believed that a large amount of data was being collected from which only a small amount was being extrapolated for use in this particular research project. This feeling regarding the large amount of data being collected was mirrored by the clinically based nurses who felt that the questionnaires selected for use within the project were too lengthy for patients to complete, and they questioned whether modifications in the data collection process were possible. Despite concerns expressed by academic team members regarding the reliability and validity of the subsequent data collected, compromise was essential. Data collection is now completed for ten consecutive days during each treatment cycle (day 1 being the start of treatment). It involves the completion by the patient of the Oral Assessment Guide and seven additional questions that reflect the patients' experiences of nausea and vomiting, fatigue and pain. Considering the multiple perspectives of the team members, one should not be unduly surprised at the need for compromise. Optimistically, since data collection has been modified there has been a resultant increase in patient compliance, improvements in nursing enthusiasm and positive feedback from data managers.

Differing expectations were also evident with regards to the timeframe of the WISECARE project, with the clinically based nurses demanding feedback quicker than data managers were able to give it. Disillusionment and loss of enthusiasm in the project were evident among the clinically based nurses regarding this lack of feedback. Through discussion and negotiation, the research team was able to reach a consensus regarding the production of meaningful and possible feedback. The outcomes of these discussions were the production of two types of feedback. Firstly, local feedback which is instantly produced for each clinical problem for each patient, allowing nursing staff to identify patterns of patient problems, establish when nursing interventions should be implemented and evaluate the effectiveness of these nursing interventions. Secondly, global feedback allows the comparison of patient outcomes across each Clinical Site. Determining such timeframes and feedback and ensuring they are adhered to has resulted in increased enthusiasm among the clinically based members of the research team.

Differing expectations also includes those of the supporting organisations. As a European Commission funded project, funding for each supporting organisation arrives in the form of the Euro. However, fluctuating financial markets can and do impact on this, with the result that supporting organisations may receive less funding depending on the strength of the Euro against their particular currency. Understandably, this is a bone of contention for supporting organisations but is outwith the power of the research project to resolve.

5.3 Communication and Language Problems

Problems in communication can occur at both individual and group levels [12]. Individuals may fail to communicate their own needs, desires and expectations, leading to frustration, or on a larger scale, the physical separation of individual institutions and group members may be problematic. Recommendations for promoting good communication within collaborative ventures advocate flexible methods of communication [12]. The variety of communication methods available to the WISECARE team, primarily, electronic mail, telephone, facsimile and post, appear to have ensured adequate communication. The use of the general WISECARE e-mail list has kept all team members involved in the project and has allowed the momentum of the project to be maintained. This frequent communication throughout the project has been essential, not only because not all members have been involved in all facets of the project, but also because it has provided all members of the research team with a sense of progress. Communication within the WISECARE project has been further facilitated, as all members of the team have been aware of each other's personal objectives from the outset, while issues such as individual roles have been clearly delineated through the regular distribution of 'to do' lists.

Understandably a multicentre research project such as WISECARE requires vast amounts of communication for both co-ordination and feedback purposes. Considering this level of communication, one can appreciate that misunderstandings have occurred innocently as individuals' interpretations of discussions have varied tremendously. Again, the multinational nature of WISECARE further complicates communication as the majority of team members speak English as a second or third language. A perfectly reasonable request in one language can sound abrupt in another. Indeed, considering the potential for communication problems, it is surprising that more problems have not occurred.

The question of translation has significant implications for multicentre and multinational research projects such as WISECARE. It is not uncommon in the absence of a common European language to default to English for historical reasons. Nevertheless, for such collaborative endeavours, it is essential that we remember that many European citizens neither can nor want to speak English and that we ensure accurate translation. The tool for data collection, patient information sheets and consent forms and the staff manual for standardised data collection are just some examples of the documentation that have required translation in this project. Members of the WISECARE team have accepted responsibility for translating the tools because it was felt that this required interpretation and contextual understanding to ensure that the meaning was reconstructed appropriately.

5.4 Culture

However, while language is an obvious consideration when one is working alongside many countries, it is essential that culture is given equal consideration. We are often told that the world is getting smaller, thanks to television, advances in telecommunications and transportation. While it may be true that on the surface we appear to converge, differences in culture exist beneath the surface [19]. The same myth holds true for management. It is often thought that management consists of a set of principles and techniques that can be universally applied and therefore transcend national boundaries. However, the fact that management deals with human beings, means that the application of the rules must differ extensively. In collaborative research, both types of differences are met.

One particular example from the WISECARE project highlights the potential impact of culture. Data collection within the project relies heavily on the participation of patients through the completion of standard questionnaires. However, it came to the notice of the researchers that Belgian responses to the questionnaires were poorer than other Sites. Closer discussions with clinical staff identified that within Belgium questionnaires have a notoriously poor response rate. It seemed that 'culturally' Belgians did not comply well with questionnaire completion. Additionally, the lengthy nature of the questionnaires being used also contributed to the poor response rates. This illustrates that what appears on the surface to be a reasonable request in one country is quite inappropriate in another. This poor response rate was one factor that led to alterations in the data collection process, with a subsequent improvement in response rate.

An example of cultural difference in management is the different understanding of managing in various countries [18]. In Latin countries, organisations are characterised by high formalisation, hierarchy and input control, with overall control held by one person. Examples include France, Italy, Greece, Belgium and Latin American countries. These countries place high value on relationships, colleagues and friends. An alternative to this is the management style of the Anglo-Saxon culture. This culture is characterised by low formalisation, decentralisation and low hierarchical structure. The leader has considerably less control as hierarchy, power and status are downplayed and the emphasis is put on tasks, merits and business. Examples of this type of culture are found in Sweden, Denmark, United Kingdom, The United States and the Netherlands. Time is viewed differently and this has implications for conducting a meeting. Anglo-Saxon cultures perceive time as a finite resource whereas managers from Latin-European cultures believe that time expands to accommodate necessary activities. Such difference are very real and have a great impact on conducting a project such as WISECARE as they have the potential to lead to mutual frustrations as a result of not understanding differences in culture.

If the nature of the collaborative relationship is not supportive for individual group members to express their fears and uncertainties, both the project and the individual suffer. It is essential that team members reflect on why they feel the way they do and discuss these feelings with the team. Within the WISECARE project, demonstrating mutual respect and value through open discussion and acknowledgement of cultural differences has often helped to ameliorate tensions and anxieties. Discussions with members of the research team from all Sites have allowed both anxieties to be aired and frustrations expressed and so managed sensitively and appropriately.

In any multicentre research project, culture should be given adequate consideration as it can differ greatly, even across small geographical areas. However, the multinational nature of the WISECARE project heightens the importance of culture.

5.5 Availability of Facilities

Whether each individual Site has the appropriate facilities to be involved in a multicentre research project is a crucial consideration. Strict guidelines regarding requirements that potential members of the research team must fulfil are essential if the project is to run smoothly following its conception. While facilities are required to initiate, implement and evaluate valid research, one can argue that nursing must remain realistic about the desirability and possibility of nursing becoming involved in research activities. The availability of facilities such as access to computers and the ability and knowledge to operate advanced IT equipment was a requirement for involvement in the WISECARE project. However, nursing remains in its infancy in some countries with little or no support for the basics of nursing practice let alone research or research-based practice. Ultimately some interested parties were unable to participate as a result of not having access to or understanding of technological facilities. However, as advocates for our less fortunate European fellow professionals, we must question whether the countries excluded from participation are those that would ultimately have benefited most from the increased communication, knowledge sharing and supportive network that underpins the WISECARE project. The frustration that this exclusion leads to must drive us to develop research projects that are as straightforward to participate in as possible whilst ensuring nurses receive appropriate education in the skills required for nursing research.

6   Conclusion

The improvement of health care is dependent on a strong scientific foundation and collaborative research across Europe provides one method to facilitate the rapid development of such a scientific knowledge base. Disbrow believes that rewards seldom accrue without payment of a certain price, noting that frustrations frequently occur when persons from several disciplines collaborate [6]. The literature highlights the positive and negative aspects of collaborative research and generally concludes that the advantages outweigh the disadvantages. From the WISECARE perspective, we agree. At times the respective contributions of the research team seem so naturally complementary, rather than in conflict, that the problems we have worked so hard to overcome are forgotten. We believe recognising the potential obstacles in the collaborative process and determining methods to overcome these obstacles will assist nurses to continue to develop and participate successfully in collaborative nursing research.

Better patient care and outcomes are the raison d'être of research in nursing. They are the common ground that researchers and clinicians share, regardless of different interests and priorities. Ideally, research should be focussed on relevant and practical problems with clinical decision based on logical and valid data [21]. We believe that transforming such ideals into reality is more likely if clinical research is based on a collaborative model in which both researchers and clinicians are decision-makers. Despite the difficulties encountered along the way of the WISECARE project, we can echo the observations of Hinshaw et al. [13] who stated that the challenges faced when conducting research in a practice setting are only partially predictable and only partly resolvable but always exciting.

References

[1]   Beattie J, Cheek J & Gibson T. The politics of collaboration as viewed through the lens of a collaborative nursing research project. *Journal of Advanced Nursing* 1996; **24**: 682-687.

[2]   Hanson SM. Collaborative research and authorship credit: Beginning guidelines. *Nursing Research* 1988; **37**: 49-52.

[3]   *The Oxford Popular Dictionary*. Oxford University Press, 1995.

[4]   Engstrom J. University, agency and collaborative models for nursing research: an overview. *Image: Journal of Nursing Scholarship* (1984): 16: 76-80

[5]   Henneman EA. Nurse-Physician collaboration: a post-structuralist view. *Journal of Advanced Nursing* 1995; **22**: 359-363.

[6]   Disbrow M. Conducting interdisciplinary research: gratifications and frustrations. In Chaska N (ed.). The Nursing Profession: A Time to Speak. McGraw-Hill, New York, 1983.

[7]   Kearney N, Campbell S & Sermeus W. Practising for the future: utilising information technology in cancer nursing practice. *European Journal of Oncology Nursing* 1998; **2**: 169-175.

[8]   Auld M. Some problems in nursing. *Health Bulletin* 1981; **39**: 117-124.

[9]   Smith M & Stullenberger E. An integrative review and meta-analysis of oncology nursing research 1981-1991. *Cancer Nursing* 1995; **18**: 167-179.

[10] European Health Committee. Nursing Research - Report and Recommendations. Council of Europe, Strasborg, 1996.

[11] Chenger PL. Collaborative nursing research: advantages and obstacles. *International Journal of Nursing Studies* 1988; **25**: 295-300.

[12] Haller KB. Research in clinical settings. *Maternal-Child Nursing* (1986): 11: 290

[13] Tierney AJ & Taylor J. Research in practice: an 'experiment' in research-practitioner collaboration. *Journal of Advanced Nursing* 1991; **16**: 506-510.

[14] Hinshaw AS, Chance HC & Atwood J. Research in practice: a process of collaboration and negotiation. *The Journal of Nursing Administration* 1981; **11**: 33-38.

[15] Aaronson NK, Ahmedzai S, Bergman B, Bullinger M, Cull A, Duez NJ, Filiberti A, Flechtner H, Fleishman SB, de Haes JCJM, Kaasa S, Klee M, Osoba D, Razavi D, Rofe PB, Schraub S, Sneeuw K, Sullivan M & Takeda F. The European Organisation for the Research and Treatment of Cancer QLQ-C30: A quality of life instrument for use in international clinical trials in oncology. *Journal of the National Cancer Institute* 1993; **85**: 365-376.

[16] Piper BF, Lindsey AM, Dodd MJ, Ferkeitch S, Paul SM & Weller S. The development of an instrument to measure the subjective dimension of fatigue. In Funk SG, Tornquist EM, Champagne MT, Copp LA & Wiese RA (eds.). Management of Pain, Nausea and Fatigue. Springer Publishing Company, New York, 1989.

[17] Eilers J, Berger AM, Petersen MC. Development, testing and application of the Oral Assessment Guide. *Oncology Nursing Forum* 1988; **15**: 325-330.

[18] Schneider SC & Barsoux JL. Managing across Cultures. Prentice Hall, London, 1997.

[19] Hofstede G. Cultures and Organisations: Software of the mind. 1995 McGraw-Hill, London, 1991.

Patient Outcome Measures for Oncology Care

Nora Kearney, Morven Miller

1 Introduction

Considerable time, energy and resources are being directed towards the pursuit of quality and have been invested in developing and implementing a range of systems to evaluate the quality of nursing care. This is not surprising given the current drive towards cost-containment, which puts nurses under increasing pressure to evaluate the effects of their care. It is concerning therefore, its impact is rarely formally scrutinised [1]. This situation is becoming untenable given the ever changing context of quality - with the current drive towards clinical effectiveness, outcomes measurement and developing collaborative, multiprofessional approaches to quality.

Expanding and enhancing education to ensure more competent and effective nursing has become increasingly complex. Consequently, the task of assessing the quality of nursing care as well as maintaining and raising standards presents a wide-ranging challenge. Without evidence to prove the complex nature and value of nursing there is little nursing can do to stop the tide of increasing numbers of nursing assistants who perform tasks under nursing supervision. It has been shown that investment in qualified staff, ensuring post-registration education and developing effective methods of organising nursing care have a positive impact on the delivery of quality patient care [2]. Add to this the fact that oncology nursing is a speciality that is continuously evolving and so creating a demand for excellence in nursing care provision and it would appear essential for oncology nurses to evaluate the impact of their interventions on patient outcomes.
This report will

- present a historical background of measures developed to evaluate quality nursing care;
- explain the drive towards the evaluation of patient outcomes;
- highlight the benefits of patient outcome measures within the WISECARE project and
- make suggestions for the future use of patient outcome measures.

2 The Concepts and Techniques of Measurement in Nursing Care

In recent years there has been a surge of interest and activity in the field of measuring nursing care and the quality of that care. It can be argued that such measurement and evaluation stems from an ever-increasing need for cost-containment within the health service. However, viewed in a more positive light, measuring and evaluating patient care gives nursing the opportunity to evaluate care, define and develop standards of care and alter professional nursing practice with the aim of continuously improving patient care and consequently patient outcomes.

Two objectives of the WISECARE project were to describe the variability of the patient population and evaluate the outcomes of care. Both these objectives were archived using patient measurement techniques. While the priority of this section is to concentrate on the later of these objectives, it is important to briefly describe the options and method selected to measure the variability of the patient population.

2.1 Evaluating Patient Acuity in Oncology Nursing

A review of the literature identified a number of patient acuity classification systems designed specifically for use in the oncological setting.

2.1.1 Oncology Patient Classification System (OPCS)

The Oncology Patient Classification System (OPCS) [3] was primarily based on the special nursing needs of patients receiving treatment for haemopoietic disorders and categorised patients according to the acuity of their illness into 5 levels of care. According to this system, patients were categorised using therapeutic indicators for which a predictable sequence of nursing interventions had been developed. Based on this categorisation, the number of nursing hours per patient day can be calculated. After careful evaluation, the OPCS was considered inappropriate for use in the WISECARE project primarily because of its medical focus and its relation to specific patient groups.

2.1.2 The Critical Care Oncology Tool

The Critical Care Oncology Tool [4] was developed from the OPCS and involved modification of the tool making it appropriate for the services of an intensive care unit. However, as intensive care units and patients requiring intensive care were not included in the WISECARE project, this tool was considered unsuitable.

2.1.3 Moffitt Tool

A more appropriate tool was developed, again from the OPCS, called the Moffitt tool [5]. This tool was developed for use both in medical and surgical oncology areas. Following a number of modifications to the OPCS which included: removal of the highest acuity bracket; replacement of medical diagnoses with nursing diagnoses and the incorporation of additional nursing diagnoses, the Moffitt tools were developed. These tools have been used in a number of surgical and medical oncological settings and have established reliability and validity. Based on the advantages of the focus being on nursing diagnoses, their simplicity and speed of use, no calculations required and the provision of reliable quantification of nursing based on medical and surgical oncological patients' needs of care, they were selected for use within the WISECARE project.

2.2 Evaluating Quality in Nursing Care

Quality assessment instruments commonly used within the UK include Monitor [6], QualPacs [7] and The Dynamic Standard Setting System (DySSSy) [8]. All are derived from externally generated criteria and claim to provide a valid index of the quality of nursing care delivered in a ward [8]. A marked increase in the use of pre-formulated generic quality assessment instruments has been seen, with Monitor and its versions for different client groups being the most popular and QualPacs used primarily in acute medical and care within elderly units [8]. Although such generic tools have benefits in their standardisation unfortunately they are not without their problems.

Generic instruments are apt to give a broad evaluation of care as opposed to specific aspects of nursing care. Redfern and Norman [8] highlight some of the problems associated with the use of generic instruments as difficulties of administration, problems of accessing information, interpretation of items, disruption of ward staff, unwieldiness, obscurity, and poor inter-rather reliability.

Furthermore, it may be argued that the development of a generic instrument to evaluate the outcomes of nursing care is impossible because the outcomes of care should be compared with the individual objectives for care, which are both patient and problem specific. Monitor has been shown to be the most centrally controlled of these generic tools and external assessors are known to provoke anxiety in nursing staff [10]. Although QualPacs is a pre-formulated system, it is less rigid than Monitor and less threatening, however, there would seem to be less follow up of the results when compared with Monitor [10]. DySSSy has been shown to be the most flexible of these standard assessment instruments and improvements in quality can take place prior to completion of the implementation process [10].

However, the pitfalls of these measures mean that they have limited impact in terms of driving changes in practice to improve patient care. Despite this, nurses are being constantly encouraged to demonstrate the value of their nursing practice in terms of its effects on patient outcomes. This attention can be seen to complement the established process orientated methods of using instruments like Monitor or QualPacs by including an assessment of what care actually achieves in terms of patient outcomes. If nurses' traditional concern with measuring quality is to be conserved, they must become familiar with the complexities of patient outcome measures. This is in line with other healthcare professionals, such as the medical profession, where patient outcomes are increasingly being used as a yardstick against which to evaluate the efficacy and efficiency of medical care [11].

3   Patient Outcomes

As the patient should be the focus of care, one could argue that health care professionals should evaluate the impact of their care and services on patient outcomes. Outcome usage and measurement have moved from a focus on death, disease, disability, discomfort and dissatisfaction to a broader focus that includes areas such as quality of life and satisfaction with care [12]. Such evaluation and quality assurance may be regarded as a positive step in professional self-monitoring as Donabedian stated that professionalism is perhaps the most fundamental safeguard of quality [13]. Indeed, as nursing continues to strive for recognition as an autonomous profession with a collegial as opposed to subservient relationship to medicine, identifying outcomes that are responsive to nursing care supports nursing's claims for greater independence, recognition and professionalism. Furthermore, this professionalisation theory will support the argument for nursing care to be delivered only by those qualified to do so, as opposed to unqualified nursing aides. However, while cost-effectiveness can be quantified, patient outcomes are less easily measured and, in many cases, have still to be adequately documented. The term 'outcomes' is used in a variety of contexts, with little assessment of whether or not the word is conceptualised in the same way or not. Before pursuing the argument of the importance of outcome measurement, it is crucial to consider what exactly we mean by the term 'patient outcome' in this report.

3.1 Definitions of Patient Outcomes

Donabedian defined an outcome as [13]
"not simply a measure of health, well-being or any other state. Rather it is a change in status confidently attributable to antecedent care".
This importance of linking the outcome to antecedent care is also evident in Redfern and Norman's [3] definition that explains that
"outcome refers to the expected changes in predetermined factors such as the patient's behaviour, health status or knowledge following the completion of nursing care".
It has also been argued that unintended or unexpected consequences of nursing interventions are also valid as outcomes as well as maintaining a steady functional status, especially if patients are very frail or have chronic health problems [14]. Based on this theory, Maas et al. [15] define nurse sensitive client outcomes as:
"variable client or caregiver states, behaviours or perceptions at a low level of abstraction that are responsive to nursing intervention".

3.2 Problems of Patient Outcome Measurement

While such definitions are useful, attributing one single patient outcome solely to nursing care as opposed to the multidisciplinary team can also be problematic. This makes it essential for one to be clear about the specific outcomes being measured. Furthermore, the choice of outcome measure must be tailored to the purpose of the study and the questions being addressed. Consequently certain challenges must be overcome regarding the measurement of outcomes.

Firstly, Bond and Thomas [14] identify that it is important to consider that patients are exposed to a number of health professionals and informal carers during any illness experience. This poses the problem of identifying whether nursing alone can be responsible for a specific patient outcome. Although a number of authors have argued that identifiable outcomes exist that can be primarily attributable to nursing care [16, 17], it is disappointing that they fail to give examples of such outcomes. Secondly, patient outcomes are influenced by factors such as individual restorative procedures, environmental and social influences [18], further complicating the process of identifying the impact of specific nursing interventions. The nebulous nature of the concept of 'quality' is the third problem to complicate the measurement of patient outcomes. Assessing the worth of an outcome is impossible if there is lack of specificity regarding what constitutes a positive or negative outcome. In an effort to overcome this Bond and Thomas [14] suggest that nurses should avoid global questions regarding quality of care and concentrate on specific effects of nursing on specific patient outcomes. In this way it would be possible to ascertain which nursing interventions under which circumstances and with which patients result in optimal patient outcomes, as defined by both health professionals and patients. Finally, limitations in the body of nursing knowledge mean that it is often not possible to predict the consequences in relation to patient outcomes of even the most standard nursing practices [18].

3.3 Patient Outcomes in the WISECARE Project

'Top-down' approaches to quality measurement may fail because of factors such as resentment, lack of initiative or personal responsibility, buck-passing and scapegoating [17]. Outcome measures themselves are perhaps of less importance than the context in, and the process by which, they are derived and applied. Clinically based nurses were responsible for the selection of the specific problems included in the WISECARE project based on their knowledge of the problems their patients experience. Such a 'bottom up' approach means that the nurses involved viewed these particular outcomes as valuable for informing their clinical practice, improving patient care and structuring their delivery of care. The integration of the WISECARE project into clinical nursing practice has turned the measurement of specific patient outcomes from an alien concept into an integral part of nurses' daily clinical practice. As a consequence this has encouraged clinically based nurses to perform their own quality assessments of the care delivered based on these individual patient outcomes. As the nurses themselves chose the particular patient outcomes to be evaluated, a sense of ownership exists regarding the collected data and its relevance for the formulation, implementation and evaluation of nursing care. Again, as a result of the 'bottom-up' approach implemented here, nurses have made the emotional and moral commitment necessary to assess and improve the quality of their nursing practice. Through the supportive environment of the WISECARE project, an organisational culture has developed that has motivated the nurses involved to incorporate such an innovative process for care delivery into clinical practice. The specific patient outcomes evaluated in the project are: pain, fatigue, oral problems and nausea and vomiting.

4　The Use of Patient Outcomes in the WISECARE Project

These four patient outcome measures are used in a variety of ways in the project and these will now be discussed in relation to their importance in influencing nursing care delivery.

4.1　Instant Feedback

It can be argued that how patients rate their care depends on what they want from treatment and the only way to find out is to ask them. Indeed, an outcome perceived positive by nurses may not be perceived as such by patients and may not accord with their wishes. Consequently, it is important to acknowledge that what constitutes a desirable outcome should not be left to the professionals alone but instead should be viewed in light of individual patients' needs and wishes [14]. Instant feedback takes this argument into consideration. Through the instant feedback facility, patients are able to articulate their own outcomes as they perceive them.

Instant feedback is designed to impact on daily clinical practice on an individual patient level. It is received immediately patient data is entered to the WiseTool, which is the integrated patient data input/feedback interface used in the project [20]. This feedback involves all four patient outcomes measured within the project (pain, fatigue, oral problems and nausea and vomiting) for each individual patient and is presented in both numerical and graphical forms.

Patients are asked to complete a questionnaire daily for the first ten days of their treatment cycle documenting their perception of specific symptoms of pain, nausea and vomiting, fatigue and oral problems over the past 24 hours (see annex 7). This 'ownership' of their outcomes, gained through patients' articulation, gives them not only the opportunity to describe their symptoms as they experience them but also a common language to facilitate in-depth meaningful discussions with health care professionals regarding the importance of these symptoms for them as individuals. Through the WiseTool patients can be presented with a graph of their outcome scores for each specific problem over a period of time either for one treatment cycle or to compare outcomes between a number of treatment cycles. Presenting outcomes in this way has been shown to have implications for both nursing staff and patients, which will now be discussed.

There are a number of ways in which instant feedback based on specific patient outcomes can impact on nursing care delivery (Figure 1). Based on the specific patient outcomes measured, appropriate nursing interventions can not only be planned, but their impact on specific patient outcomes can be evaluated. Through such cyclical evaluative process, specific positive interventions can be identified for individual patients and nursing care tailored appropriately to ensure positive patient outcomes. This process provides a powerful motivating factor for nurses to constantly evaluate their care in relation to patient outcomes. It also identifies ineffective nursing interventions and ensures their perpetuation is not encouraged.

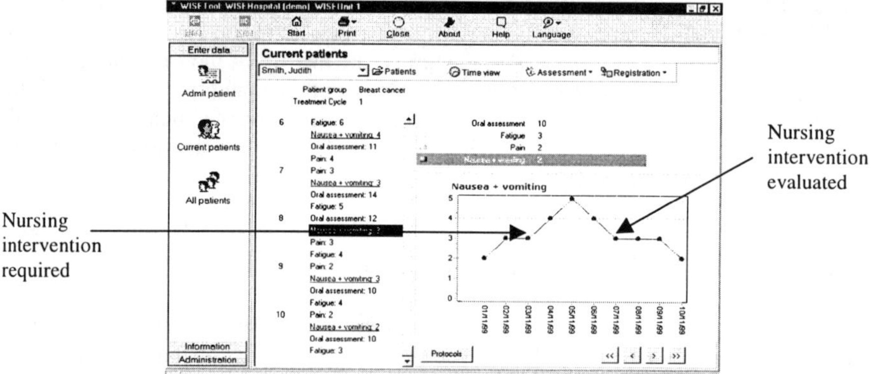

Figure 1   WiseTool Graph of Patient's Problem regarding Nausea and Vomiting

However, it is not solely nursing staff who benefits from using patient outcome measures in this way. Informal feedback from patients involved in the project indicates that they find the instant feedback, based on their personal outcomes, a valuable tool for them to visualise their problems and participate in meaningful, appropriate and individualised nursing interventions. Patients have explained that they feel more in control of their care and involved in the planning and evaluation of interventions. They also develop an understanding of the pattern of their symptoms, which helps them to initiate appropriate interventions to improve their outcomes even following discharge.

Overall, using patient outcome measures to produce instant feedback has been a simple and straightforward process for nurses to follow and has encouraged the development of a culture that promotes structured patient assessment, appropriate individualised nursing interventions and evaluation of nursing care. Furthermore, there has been increased patient partnership in care leading to an altered way of working in which the patient drives care according to their individual outcomes.

4.2 Global Feedback

Global feedback consists of all patient outcomes from all participating Sites and facilitates comparison of patient outcomes between Clinical Sites. It is designed to result in the evaluation and improvement of clinical nursing practice and planned to occur on a regular basis. Global feedback is designed to be delivered by the data managers through the WISECARE Website.

Nursing should not study outcomes because they happen to be easily measured or outcomes in isolation, but outcomes as the anticipated and theoretically meaningful effects of particular practices [14]. Taking such advice into consideration, global feedback in the WISECARE project compares the patient outcomes between Clinical Sites for each diagnosis and is stratified for each clinical indicator according to the known risk factors associated with each specific cancer treatment. In this way, only treatments with similar risks are compared across the Clinical Sites, making comparisons increasingly meaningful.

A 'benchmark' derived from the collective patient outcomes from all the Clinical Sites involved has been developed for each clinical indicator and risk factor. This allows individual Clinical Sites to compare their clinical performance in terms of patient outcomes not only across specific Clinical Sites but also with the 'WISECARE average' (Figure 2).

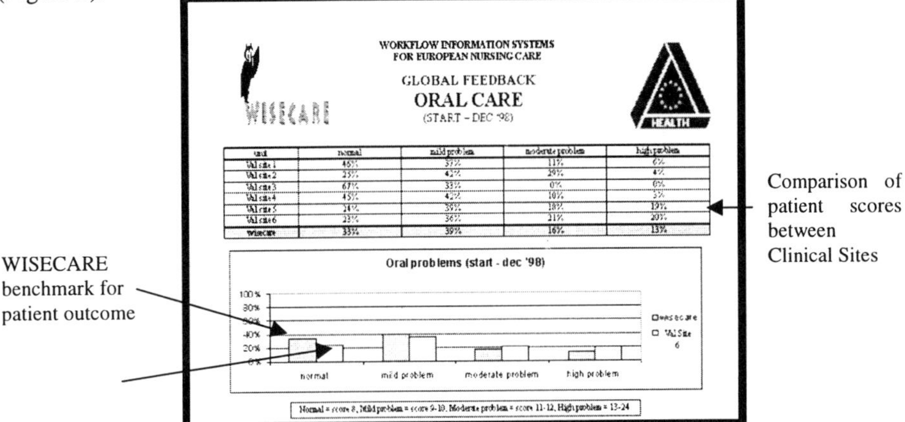

unit	normal	mild problem	moderate problem	high problem
Val site 1	45%	37%	11%	6%
Val site 2	25%	42%	29%	4%
Val site 3	67%	33%	0%	0%
Val site 4	45%	42%	10%	3%
Val site 5	24%	39%	18%	19%
Val site 6	23%	36%	21%	20%
wisecare	33%	39%	16%	13%

Figure 2   The Possibilities for Benchmarking offered by the Global Feedback

This process provides the nurses involved with a 'quality cycle', represented in figure 3 below. For example, firstly comparing patient outcomes between Clinical Sites and with the benchmark gives a 'definition' of the level of quality to be aimed for and developed. Secondly, Clinical Sites are able to 'measure' their practice against the current 'benchmark' and identify the level of care they are presently delivering. Finally, they are encouraged to take appropriate 'action' to improve or maintain their level of care through the sharing of protocols, standards and guidelines.

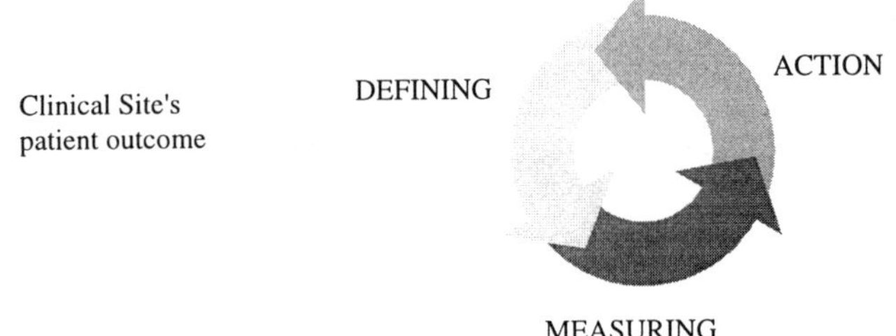

Figure 3   Quality Cycle

Participating in this 'quality cycle' and using the global feedback information to gauge the difference between patient outcomes across various Clinical Sites, encourages the clinically based nurses to compare their clinical practice and emulate the nursing interventions of the Clinical Sites that achieve the most positive patient outcomes. Such knowledge sharing and collaboration can be viewed as a dynamic concept within the project, located in the general context of organisational development and change. Some of the most recent global feedback results can be used to illustrate the benefits of this process of knowledge sharing and the 'quality cycle' when comparing the patient outcomes recorded for the highest risk factor of nausea and vomiting over the duration of data collection. It can be shown that patient outcomes have improved over the total period of data collection and are at their lowest recorded value during the third period of data collection, see figure 4 below.

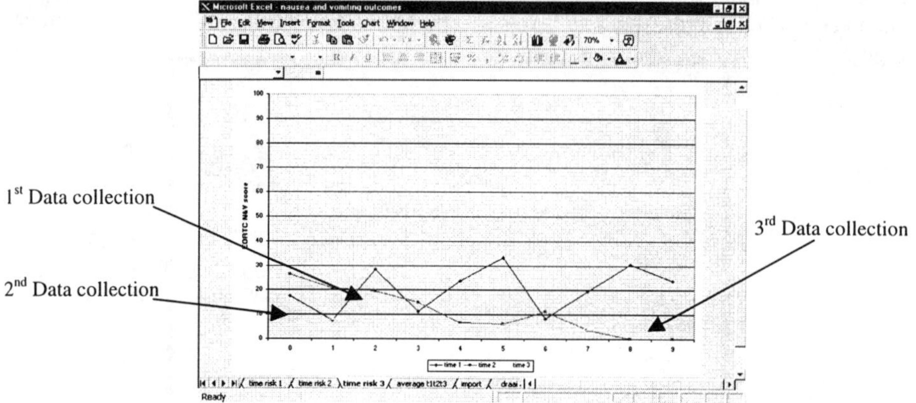

Figure 4   Patient Outcomes related to Nausea and Vomiting (highest risk chemotherapy)

4.3 Patient Modelling using Patient Outcome Measures

Patient outcome measurements have also been used to develop computerised 'patient models' within the WISECARE project. Based on 'real' patient data and the known risks of specific cancer treatments on the clinical indicators, the pattern of symptoms that would be experienced by patients receiving specific treatments can be predicted. From this information the impact of different types of nursing care on these patient outcomes can be illustrated for teaching and learning purposes. Through the development of patient scenarios, based on the knowledge of experienced cancer nurses, and the patient data gained in the WISECARE project, models have been created that compare the effects of nursing care on patient outcomes, see Figure 5. This illustrates the positive impact that appropriate nursing interventions (the left hand side of the screen) have on patient outcomes and activities of daily living, whereas inappropriate nursing interventions have no impact on patient outcomes, allowing them to grow worse and impact negatively on patients' acitivities of daily living resulting in one patient being unable to perform self-care (the right hand side of the screen). Using scenarios in this way illustrates the importance of appropriate and timely nursing interventions on patient outcomes and the ways in which evaluating patient outcomes can be used to visualise the impact of nursing care and so establish its value.

4.4 Overall Impact of Patient Outcome Measures within the WISECARE Project

Patient outcomes are the end result of treatments [21], be they medical or nursing and linking nursing interventions to patient outcomes is critical [22]. The experiences gained through the WISECARE project endorse this statement. In the project, clinically based nursing staff have used patient outcome measures in a meaningful manner to support changes and better nursing practice, resulting in improved patient outcomes in the four clinical indicators selected.

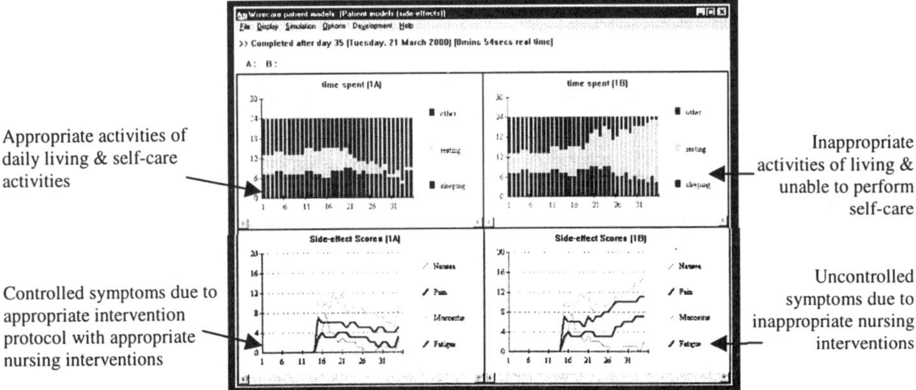

Figure 5   Patient Modelling

Instant feedback for individual patients has provided nursing staff with a powerful motivating factor to evaluate and initiate timely, appropriate nursing interventions. The selected patient outcomes measured are highly relevant to the practice of nursing staff and the structured approach to care provision that has been driven by the WISECARE project is being integrated into mainstream clinical practice in all participating Sites. The bottom-up approach to the project which was adopted at the start of the project, and which persisted throughout, has promoted a sense of ownership in the results. Indeed, although the project is drawing to an official close, nursing staff has been motivated to ensure the WISECARE system of care continues. Global feedback has encouraged nursing staff in the project to become involved in an entire quality improvement cycle and comparing patient outcomes across Clinical Sites and against benchmarks has ensured nurses' commitment to the quality cycle. This quality cycle is a dynamic concept that drives nursing staff to constantly evaluate the impact of their care on patient outcomes and strive to improve this.

The patients' perspective is also valuable to consider. Although nursing staff decided the specific outcomes for the project, the increased patient participation in outcome measurement has resulted in care being patient driven according to their individual outcomes. It has encouraged a meaningful partnership in care delivery between patients and health care professionals and has given patients the sense of control over the direction of their care. This has encouraged a culture of care in which the patient is valued, respected and trusted and in which change and improvements to ensure positive patient outcomes are promoted.

5   Conclusions

Despite the number of quality systems to evaluate nursing care, the experiences gained from the WISECARE project suggest that evaluation of patient outcomes provides one solution to illustrate the value of nursing care.

The project ensured clarity in the patient outcomes and measures chosen and the process of evaluation was straightforward with clear ideas of both positive and negative outcomes. The choice of measurement was tailored to the purpose of the study and the specific aims of the project. Patient outcome measures were also relevant to the nursing speciality under evaluation. Knowledge regarding the specific risks associated with specific cancer treatments meant that the comparisons made between Clinical Sites and patients were meaningful. The bottom-up approach fostered throughout the project encouraged a sense of personal responsibility in the nursing staff while ensuring that the information gained was valuable for informing their clinical practice.

Through both instant and global feedback based on patient outcome measurements, nursing care in the WISECARE project has been evaluated. Informal communication with patients has highlighted the value they place on the opportunities that participating in the project has given them. From the nursing perspective, instant feedback is invaluable in identifying problems promptly and initiating and evaluating nursing care. Using this patient information to build patient models that can be used to illustrate the positive impact of best nursing practices on patient outcomes also strengthens the case for proving the value of nursing. Furthermore, the evidence to support the benefits of knowledge sharing and European collaboration is now more concrete than ever. Illustrating that patient outcomes are now better than at the start of data collection is extremely encouraging and suggests that a network of cancer nurses across Europe is not only possible but also has positive implications for improving patient outcomes.

References

[1]   Kearney N, Campbell S, Sermeus W Practising for the future: utilising information technology in cancer nursing practice. European Journal of Oncology Nursing (1998): 2: 169-175

[2]   Carr-Hill R, Dixon R & Gibbs I. Skill mix and the effectiveness of nursing care. Centre for Health Economics, University of York, York, 1992.

[3]   Arenth LM. The development and validation of an oncology patient classification system. *Oncology Nursing Forum* 1985; **12** (6): 17-22.

[4]   Lovett RB, Reardon MB, Gordon BK & McMillan S. Validity and reliability of medical and surgical oncology patient acuity tools. *Oncology Nursing Forum* 1994; **21**(10): 1709-1717.

[5]   Marsee VD, Lovett RB & McMillan SC. Validity and reliability of an oncology critical care patient acuity tool. *Oncology Nursing Forum* 1995; **22** (6): 967-971.Redfern SJ & Norman IJ. Quality assessment instruments in nursing: towards validation. *International Journal of Nursing Studies* 1995; **32**: 115-125.

[6]   Goldstone LA, Ball JA & Collier MM. Monitor: an index of the quality nursing care for acute medical and surgical wards. Newcastle upon Tyne Ploytechnic Products, Newcastle upon Tyne, 1983.

[7]   Wandelt MA & Ager JW. Quality patient care scale. Appleton-Century-Crofts, New York, 1974.

[8]   Royal College of Nursing. Quality patient care: the Dynamic Standard Setting System. Scutari, Harrow, Middlesex, 1990.

[9]   Redfern SJ & Norman IJ. Quality assessment instruments in nursing: towards validation. International Journal of Nursing Studies **32**:115-125.

[10] Harvey G & Kitson A. Achieving improvements through quality: an evaluation of key factors in the implementation process. *Journal of Advanced Nursing* 1996; **24**: 185-195.

[11] Hopkis A & Costain D. Measuring the outcomes of medical care. The Royal College of Physicians, London, 1990.

[12] Nies MA, Cook T, Bach CA, Bushnell K, Salisbury M, Sinclair V & Ingersoll GL. Concept analysis of outcomes for advanced nursing practice *Outcomes Management for Nursing Practice* 1999; **3**: 83-86.

[13] Donabedian A. Quality assessment and assurance: unity of purpose, diversity of means. *Inquiry* 1988; **25**: 172-192.

[14] Bond S & Thomas LH. Issues in measuring outcomes of nursing. *Journal of Advanced Nursing* 1991; **16**: 1492-1502.

[15] Maas ML, Johnson M & Morehead S. Classifying nurse-sensitive patient outcomes. *IMAGE: Journal of Nursing Scholarship* 1996; **28**: 295-301.

[16] Haussman RKD & Hagyvary ST. Monitoring quality of nursing care, Part III Professional review for nursing: an empirical investigation. US Department of Health, Education and Welfare, Hyattsville, Maryland, 1977.

[17] van Maanen HMT. Evaluation of nursing care: quality of nursing evaluated within the context of health care and examined from a multinational perspective. In Willis LD & Linwood ME (eds.). Measuring the Quality of Care Churchill Livingston, Edinburgh, 1984.

[18] Horn BJ & Swain MA. Criterion measures of nursing care quality (final report). National Centre for Health Services Research, US Department of Health, Education and Welfare, Hyattsville, Maryland, 1978.

[19] Lower MS & Burton S. Measuring the impact of nursing interventions on patient outcomes - the challenge of the 1990s. *Journal of Nursing Quality Assurance* 1989; **4** (1): 27-34.

[20] Redfern SJ & Norman IJ. Measuring the quality of nursing care: a consideration of different approaches. *Journal of Advanced Nursing* 1990; **15**: 1260-1271.

[21] Hoy D. Data Input Programme. Deliverable 3.4: Workflow Information Systems for European Nursing Care, 1998.

[22] Moritz P. Innovative nursing practice models and patient outcomes. *Nursing Outlook* 1991; **39** (3): 111-114.

[23] Fitch M & Thompson L. Fostering the growth of research-based oncology nursing practice. *Oncology Nursing Forum* 1996; **4**: 631-637.

Impact of WISECARE on Clinical Behaviour of Oncology Nurses and on Patient Outcomes

Tiina Nyberg, Juha Kinnunen

1 Introduction

In Europe, nursing services represent approximately half of the national health care budgets. Nurses and midwives also comprise the largest single group of health professionals in Europe [1]. Yet the impact of nursing care on the total quality of care for the patients has not been evaluated sufficiently [e.g. 2-4]. Nor is there any national database that would continuously follow up the impact of nursing on patient outcomes [5].

As nursing has become more grounded in science due to improved academic education and research and the costs of care have increased, the central question has shifted from whether nursing care helps to make the patient better to whether the approach to care or the actual intervention is the most effective and efficient [6]. By identifying the "best practices" for particular situations, it is believed that the costs of care can be reduced without compromising the quality of patient outcomes [4].

The aim of this report was to provide insight into the added value of the WISECARE project on the clinical behaviour of oncology nurses and on patient outcomes.

1.1 The WISECARE Project

The WISECARE project was a pan-European project, which aims to develop cancer nursing practice in several cancer centres in Europe through the utilisation of information technology. Five European nursing Sites specialising in oncology participated in the verification and validation phases of the project. These clinical settings included medical and surgical locations and in-patient, outpatient and ambulatory care settings. The project was demonstrated at another seven Sites.

The ultimate goal of the WISECARE project was to exploit clinical nursing data stored in electronic patient records systematically. Instead of using this data for individual patient care, in the WISECARE project the data were exploited for clinical and resource management. This would enable a shift from individual knowledge to knowledge sharing, allowing the nurses to learn from their past patients and from their own ways of practising nursing care [7]. The method of the project is simplified in Figure 1. See more detailed description about the project in the Overview of WISECARE.

1.2 Oncology Nursing

Sitzia and Wood refer to Gullatte (1994) who has pointed out that cancer is the second common cause of death in the western world. They continue that according to Parkin et al. (1993) and Otto (1994) many common cancers are treated with cytotoxic chemotherapy.

More than one half of all patients diagnosed with cancer receive chemotherapy treatment, and the volume of treatment is seen to increase as cytotoxic agents become more powerful. These drugs are also known to have a vast range of adverse reactions like nausea, fatigue, alopecia, and stomatitis just to mention a few. Effective management of side effects is critical as poor management can lead to further complications [8].

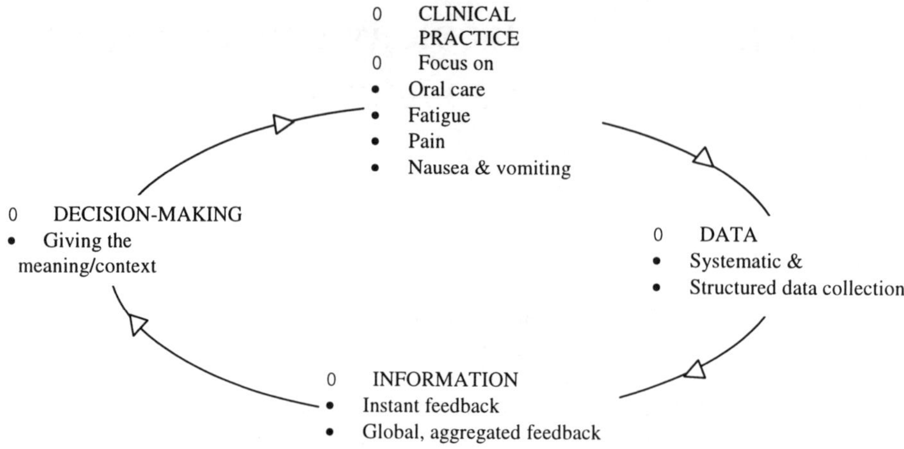

Figure 1   The Working Method of the WISECARE Project

When Margaret Fintch in her study identified a Canadian research agenda with relevance to cancer nursing practice, she found out that the main areas of interest should be: home care, patient education, symptom management, evaluating care delivery and research instrument development. Among the most frequently cited symptoms by nursing staff as troublesome to patients were pain, nausea and vomiting, and fatigue [9].

Oncology nurses who administer chemotherapy play important roles in managing the side effects and working as part of a multidisciplinary team to alleviate symptom distress. Although it has been stated that research directed only toward the management of symptoms and not at their underlying causes would be inadequate and incomplete, Hegyvary has indicated two reasons, why the research into management of symptoms is an essential adjunct to research about disease and treatment. First, symptoms usually are manifestations of disease processes. People have to live with the symptoms before and during successful treatment. Management of symptoms during that time is important to individuals, families, and practitioners. Second, naming and treating the disease may not cure the symptoms, as some become chronic even when the disease process is under control [10].

Consistent with these views from the literature, nurses in the Validation Sites were asked to identify common topical issues and specific areas of care, which WISECARE should tackle. The WISECARE nurses (i.e. WiseNurses) decided to focus on particular problems. The WiseNurses identified *oral health, fatigue, pain*, and *nausea and vomiting* as the most specific problems for patients in their care [11]. As shown, these issues are also in line with the results of previous oncology nursing research.

The lack of a systematic approach to *oral care* for patients receiving chemotherapy was identified as an important nursing issue for the nurses involved in the project. Maintaining good oral health has found to be necessary to prevent infection, for eating, and communicating either through speech or non-verbal expression such as smiling [12]. There is a prevalence of oral complications in oncology, and mouth care for these patients is particularly significant. In the management of cancer, oral dysfunction is a potential hazard for the majority of patients and is therefore a major oncology nursing concern. The impact of oral problems on patients' quality of life is a significant dose-limiting factor potentially affecting prognosis, and can result in prolonged hospital admission for treatment of infections and nutritional support [13].

However, it has been found that this area of care engenders negative attitudes in nurses who find it unrewarding and unpleasant, making it a low priority and often delegating the role to unqualified care assistants [12, 14]. According to Kearney, Date, Daeffler (1980) and Moore (1995) mouth care has become a ritualistic and banal activity, a topic of conflicting advice and subjective conclusions from sporadic research [13].

Fatigue is perceived by more than 90% of patients with cancer [15] and is the most frequently reported symptom of cancer and cancer treatment [16]. The nurses involved in the WISECARE project identified fatigue as one of the most significant problems for the patients in their care and being a problem, which is not always dealt with adequately, either in terms of assessment and effective intervention strategies [13].

Chang refers to the World Health Organization Cancer Pain Relief Programme and states that world wide about 5 million people experience *cancer pain* on daily basis. This pain is known to be often inadequately treated. Unrelieved cancer pain has been shown to lessen patients' activity, function, appetite, and sleep and induce fear, and increase suffering. Comprehensive management of cancer patients with pain is regarded as being accomplished best through multidisciplinary collaboration [17-19].

Grant, Goodman and Richardson have pointed out that chemotherapy-induced *nausea and vomiting* have remained a nursing research priority since Oberst first identified it in 1978 as the most urgent problem for oncology patients and nurses. According to them, nausea and vomiting are two of the commonest symptoms associated with chemotherapy. Some of the very common cytotoxic agents, like carmustine, cisplatin, cyclophosphamide, doxorubicin and ifosfamide, have been shown to have high emetic potential. The level of distress associated with these symptoms is profound, and the resulting interference with normal daily activities has made it essential that these symptoms be well managed. A nurse plays a pivotal role in assessing, teaching, intervening, and evaluating drug and non-drug approaches to chemotherapy-induced nausea and vomiting [20-22].

1.3 Patient Outcomes

Donabedian [4] defined outcomes as "those changes, either favourable or adverse, in the actual or potential health status of persons, groups, or communities, that can be attributed to prior or concurrent care". Patient outcomes are the end results of treatments or interventions performed by health care professionals.

Outcomes are being used to describe the impact of care on patients' health and well-being, to establish a basis for clinical decision-making, to evaluate the effectiveness of care, and to identify areas for improvement in care. Therefore, choosing outcome measures that are meaningful to the patient is essential [23]. Fundamental to outcome selection is also that they are associated with antecedent processes and establishing these relationships is a key to progress. This means making explicit the intended outcomes of nursing actions, while permitting opportunities for unintended or unanticipated outcomes to emerge [24].

Outcomes are time-dependent and temporary or permanent by nature. Thus, the selection of an appropriate time frame to determine the selected patient outcomes must be established [23, 25]. It is generally acknowledged that longer-range outcomes are less specific to a period of treatment because of the probability of numerous intervening factors. Even so, it is desirable that evaluation of care and treatment include more than one time, as in a repeated measures approach. Ultimately, the designation of end-results or outcomes is arbitrary and reflects a modern, Western view of both the meaning of time and the causation of events and is more or less based on mutual agreement among those who use the information [26, see also 23, 27].

The work by Johnson and Maas [28, 29] to classify nursing-specific patient outcomes (i.e. Nursing Outcomes Classification NOC) is one of the most extensive in nursing. In addition, Marek [30, 31-32] has synthesised the patient outcome categories described in literature into fifteen categories. Kleinpell uses slightly similar conceptualisation as Marek but has been able to aggregate the descriptive categories into three: patient, provider and payer-specific outcomes. Patient-specific outcome measures include broad categorical measures such as functional status, health status, patient satisfaction, and quality of life and individual measures such as symptom control, medication and treatment side effects, and knowledge [23].

In nursing the aim of outcomes research is to ascertain which nursing interventions under what circumstances and to which patients result in optimal patient outcomes. Nurses and their managers need to know whether what amount, and what kind of nursing makes a difference to patient outcomes [24]. In the WISECARE project one of the leading ideas has been that establishing the effectiveness of nursing care in the "real world" is an important aspect of outcomes research and evidence-based practice. This is so because establishing the efficacy of a procedure or intervention under well-controlled conditions suggests only that it is likely to work in real-life situation [e.g. 33].

1.4 Evidence-Based Practice

Information drives the practice of health services ever more. It has been seen as one of the essential antecedents to power, i.e. to the actual or potential ability or capacity to achieve objectives through an interpersonal process [34]. Information represents a key source to those managers or clinicians who feel that change is needed to improve the services [35]. In the acute care hospitals of England, doctors and nurses have been found to spend a quarter of their time finding, sorting and using information [36], which probably is the case in other European countries as well.

There has been no uniform agreement as to the definition of evidence-based health care (services). Christine Tanner [37] suggests that the McMaster University, Evidence Based Medicine Group (1996) offers a definition that is comprehensive in its view of what counts as evidence and what should figure into decisions regarding patient care:
"The collection, interpretation, and integration of valid, important and applicable patient-reported, clinician-observed, and research-derived evidence. The best available evidence, moderated by patient circumstances and preferences, is applied to improve the quality of clinical judgements and facilitate cost-effective health care."

The aim of evidence-based practice is to reduce wide variations in individual clinicians' practices, eliminating the worst practices and enhancing the best practices, thereby improving quality and reducing costs [37]. In other words, to do right things, in a right manner, to right patients, at right time [38].

Thus evidence, characterised as something that furnishes proof for decision-making, encompasses the findings of formal research as well as the consensus of recognised experts. Within an organisational setting it is realistic also to include data related to operations and improvement activities as evidence [37, 39-40]. However, quite often the concept of evidence-based practice has been viewed as synonymous with research-based practice. Thus, during the 1990's there has been a strong evidence-based movement in medicine, e.g. the International Cochrane Collaboration, the institutionalisation of health technology assessment (national offices for health technology assessment, OHTA), and the activities of the AHCPR (Agency for Health Care Policy and Research, U.S.A.). During this development, critical quantitative meta-analysis of existing research reports has partially replaced 'expert opinion' reviews as a basis for guidelines and health care decisions. Inevitably, this has an impact on the criteria used to evaluate medical research, overall research and development activities, and also the clinical practice of medicine.

When it comes to evidence-based nursing, there is a thrust towards research-oriented activities similar to those that have taken place in medicine. At the same time, nursing research has been heavily criticised for not producing the necessary information needed in clinical settings [41-43]. As an alternative, Rolfe suggested that clinical research, if it is to make a difference to practice, should be practitioner-based. He argued this by explaining that, in addition to scientific knowledge about the general effects of treatment X on an average patient, nurses also require personal knowledge about patient P and experiential knowledge about situation S [42]. Also some of the phenomena in nursing have a nature that cannot be quantified and thus not reached through quantitative meta-analyses.

The WISECARE project seeks to provide evidence for clinical decision-making. Instead of engaging itself in an international effort to find and summarise research from any one area of interest, it has taken a bottom-up approach to the issue by exploiting large, shared databases and by creating information networks for sharing knowledge. Although this method has the disadvantage of offering less scientifically sound evidence, it has the advantage of laying more emphasis on practice and clinical effectiveness [44].

1.5 Information Technology in Nursing

Gorn [45-46] defined the term "informatics" as computer science plus information science. Used in conjunction with the name of a discipline, it denotes an application of computer science and information science to the management and processing of data, information and knowledge in the named discipline. Thus nursing informatics is a combination of computer science, information science and nursing science designed to assist in the management and processing of nursing data, information and knowledge to support the practice of nursing and the delivery of nursing care.

According to Saranto and Ensio [46] Saba and McCormick have defined a nursing information system as a

"computer system that collects, stores, processes, retrieves, displays, and communicates timely information needed to do the following: administer the nursing services and resources in a health care facility; manage standardised patient care information for the delivery of nursing care; link the research resources and educational applications to nursing practice".

In addition to the above-mentioned definitions, information technology in nursing can be seen to refer to all manners of data and information management, manual and automated systems, and communication devices used by nurses in the performance of their work [47].

Sermeus et al. [48] have pointed out that the real impact of information technology in nursing is not in the automation of existing processes but on the discovery of new ways to organise and practice nursing. This requires certain shifts in the patterns of knowing: knowledge sharing instead of traditional dissemination, a shift from individual to organisational (aggregated) knowledge, and a shift from deductive prescriptive knowledge towards inductive experience-based knowledge. Explicitly sharing the experiences gained through everyday decision-making at work allows them to become learning experiences beyond mere individual insight. Information technology can help to extend these experiences across boundaries of nursing units, hospitals and even countries. Furthermore, as knowledge has become a key resource in the health care sector, it has become more obvious that the professionals' knowledge must be managed as a strategic resource and not just left to the individual initiative of health practitioners. In the WISECARE project the main goal is to go beyond the interactive level and exploit the formalised experience and knowledge found in the databases. When databases are linked up in a network, the body of knowledge that was earlier intangible for practitioners, will be available in a completely different way [48].

Information technology is being used daily by nurses working in diverse roles and settings. Nurse managers use information technology to capture and measure nursing workload, to support the management of human and fiscal resources, and for the purposes of quality assurance monitoring. Information technology has been incorporated into the provision of patient care through the automation of clinical activities: order entry, nursing care planning, and documentation. Although available, a very small percentage of health care organisations have implemented a clinical information system. The spread and application of proven, well-tested models has been slow. It seems difficult to create acceptable European standards, even to find unanimity concerning the information content of the so-called "minimum data sets" [47, 49].

Nurses have indicated that they want to see system developments which: increase the focus on clinical practice, increase the meaningfulness of clinical data and support clinical decision-making. According to Nagle et al. [47] fully exploiting the possibilities of information technology for nursing necessitates moving beyond the traditional conceptualisations of nursing information system to that of an integrated clinical information system. The principle of integration here means that each patient data element is entered into the system with minimal replication and is accessible to all health care providers as necessary [50].

According to Suzanne Bakken [51-52] databases that support informed clinical decision-making are still largely non-existent. However, it is known that information technology could provide an infrastructure for evidence-based practice in nursing in a number of ways that maximise the utility of a continuum of evidence. First, standardised terminologies represented in computer-processable ways facilitate the capture of what it is that the nurses do. Second, information technology could support the collection of nursing-sensitive patient outcomes during the routine course of care. Third, and most important, information technology can support the processing of these types of data in ways that enable evidence-based practice, e.g. risk-adjustment of patient outcomes, triggering of decision support rules, benchmarking, tailoring of interventions based on patient data, and incorporating patient beliefs or preferences into the health care decision-making process. Bakken [51-52] sees also that it is essential that as a practice discipline nursing embraces informatics as a way of both building the body of practice-based knowledge and applying that knowledge towards the improvement of the nursing practice.

To develop oncological nursing, the WISECARE project seeks to apply information technology in form of structured data collection, following up patient outcomes and processing data to enable evidence-based practice.

1.6 Nursing Process

In this evaluation, the clinical behaviour of oncology nurses was interpreted through the concepts of nursing process. During the last decade, nurse authors have vigorously discussed and criticised the nursing process. The criticism has been wide-ranging and varied, and has questioned the philosophical underpinnings, stage of development, components, uses, effects and focus of the nursing process. The theoretical critiques have pitted the nursing process against the art of nursing, intuition, patient-centred care and holism. The argument that the nursing process is philosophically committed to science, rationality, empiricism and positivism has been challenged by the many different views of what the nursing process is and the fact that different authors have viewed the nursing process from various philosophical positions [53-56]. But as Colleen Varcoe [57] has pointed out, this merely suggests that the nursing process is compatible with various philosophical positions, and that the theoretical criticism of the nursing process is really criticism of a positivist-philosophical orientation, which has been illogically identified with the process itself.

In contrast to the criticism of the philosophical orientation and theoretical characteristic of the nursing process, other criticism has concerned the role of the nursing process within the nursing profession. It has been seen as a professional strategy to 'carve a niche' for nursing and promote the independent practice of nursing, thereby serving the interests of the nurses over the interests of the patients. It has also been criticised because of the negative consequences in practice, e.g. it is said to require burdensome documentation, which is time-consuming, jargon-laden and static [58-61]. Varcoe [57] emphasised that these concerns have confused the actual use of the nursing process with criticism of the administrative implementation of the nursing process. Extensive documentation is not required by the nursing process, but is rather a consequence of specific implementation decisions.

The criticism seems to have attributed tremendous power to the nursing process, far beyond the basic premise that *nurses should think systematically* and *know what is going on before they take action*. In spite of all the doubts, practitioners continue to use the nursing process. The language of everyday clinical practice is filled with reference to doing assessments, knowing problems and plans, and finding out how the patients 'are doing'.

In this evaluation, the nursing process is seen, in particular, as a mental process related to clinical judgement in order to help patients. Furthermore, it is not regarded as being linear, although it might look like that from the written nursing care plans' point of view. Thus we have wanted to emphasise the value of the judgements on which the actions are based, in contrast to the beliefs that nurses are 'doers' rather than 'thinkers'. This is congruent with the underlying principles of the WISECARE project, which emphasise experiential learning as a basic method of development in practice – learning 'in-action' and more specifically learning 'on-action', which both require reflective thinking before one is able really to learn from experience.

2   Methods

2.1 Project Evaluation

Øvretveit [62] has defined that evaluation is the attributing of value to an intervention by gathering reliable and valid information about it in a systematic way and making comparisons against standards for the purpose of making more informed decisions or understanding causal mechanisms or general principles.

Evaluation is a practice almost always requiring revision and modification of the initial evaluation plan, making compromises in the types, quantity, and sometimes quality of data collected, and responding to shifts that occur in the conduct of a process and in the composition and interests of the stakeholders involved. The design and implementation of evaluations depend upon the specific purposes they are to serve. Evaluations differ according to the type of question being asked, the stage the process is in, and the type of decision the evaluation is intended to inform. The three major classes of evaluations are: analyses related to the conceptualisation and design of interventions, monitoring of implementation and assessment of impact and efficiency [63-64].

Project evaluation provides information to improve the project as it develops and progresses. Project evaluation may also include examination of specific components, like in this case the impact of the WISECARE project on clinical behaviour of oncology nurses and on patient outcomes. Information is collected to help determine whether the project is proceeding as planned; whether it is meeting its stated project objectives according to the proposed timeline [65-66].

Project evaluation can focus on (a) planning evaluation (i.e. assessing the understanding of project's objectives, strategies and timelines), (b) formative evaluation (i.e. assessing ongoing project activities) or (c) summative evaluation (i.e. assessing the project's success). Formative evaluation is a continuous process, which quite often provides data also for the summative evaluation. Formative evaluation may consist of two parts, namely implementation evaluation (i.e. assessing whether the project is being conducted as planned) and progress evaluation (i.e. assessing the progress in meeting the goals of the project). On the other hand, summative evaluation takes place after ultimate modifications and changes have been made, after the project is stabilised and after the impact of the project has had a chance to realise [66].

The current evaluation of the impacts of the WISECARE project on clinical behaviour of oncology nurses and on patient outcomes took place after the verification and validation phases of the project, when the original project participants had completed the product development and were ready to step to the demonstration phase. Thus this evaluation represents *progress evaluation* where data were collected to determine what impact the activities and strategies have had on the participants before the final phase of the project. This progress evaluation seeks to answer the following questions:

- *Does the WISECARE method make a difference in the clinical practice of the oncology nurses and in patient outcomes?*
- *Which of the activities and strategies are aiding the nurses to move toward the set objectives?*

This evaluation is an internal evaluation, where the evaluators come from one of the project partners. The target of the evaluation consists of measuring the changes brought about by the WISECARE project in the core processes of clinical oncology nursing in the Validation Sites. The evaluation approach consists of the application of objective-based and theory-based measures. The objectives of the project act as one set of criteria and the previous research findings as the theory basis. As the main purpose of this evaluation is to shed light on the added value of the verification and validation phases of the WISECARE project on clinical behaviour of oncology nurses and on patient outcomes a combination of qualitative and quantitative approaches were chosen to develop the evaluation design.

2.2 Sampling

At least five nurses from each of the WISECARE Validation Sites were asked to participate in the evaluation during each data collection period. Out of these five, three should be WiseNurses who had worked closely in the WISECARE project collecting data and using the feedback. From each Site two nurses should have been non-WiseNurses, i.e. nurses who had not been involved in the project but working on one of the units, in a participating unit. Thus, during each data collection period the best possible responses possible were 5 x 5 = 25 responses.

The sampling technique used was nonprobability sampling, which makes it difficult to know how well the oncology nurses population on these wards were represented. At the same time the sampling was purposive. We wanted to include also those nurses in the sample who had not been involved in the project. Though, in some of the nursing units most of the nurses had been, at least, a bit involved with the project.

2.3 Measurement

The majority of the data for the evaluation was collected through a survey. The participants completed the WiseCompass questionnaire, which had 59 questions concerning the impact of the WISECARE project on clinical oncology nursing practice and on patient outcomes, use of the different project products, and general project management. The evaluators had developed the questionnaire in collaboration with the other members from Workpackage 5 Mr. J. Hofdijk and Mr. M. Steegh from HISCOM, the Netherlands. The major categories were identified from nursing literature, national nursing standards and literature related to the evaluation of information technology, e.g. the work of the MEGATAQ and VATAM projects. The level of measurement was mainly ordinal; some background variables were nominal. The project participants (partners and users) were able to view the questionnaire during its development stage and were able to identify questions which were difficult to understand. The questionnaire was in English and it was not translated into the different national languages.

The data collection took place three times during the verification and validation of the project. The first data collection was in March 1999 before the first global feedback, the second in May 1999 after the global feedback, and the third in September 1999 in the end of the validation phase. Two Demonstration Sites were able to join the 3rd, WiseCompass data collection.

In addition to the survey, qualitative methods were also used to enrich the data. For the evaluation four members of the local clinical WISECARE teams were interviewed. All written project documents (i.e. the contract, periodic reports, minutes from the meetings, deliverables, articles written about the project, presentations in the meetings and the global feedback sheets) were also checked together with the peer reviewers' statements for any additional information.

2.4 Data Analysis

During the first data collection with the WiseCompass questionnaire 20 papers were returned, 16 from the second and 30 from the third, giving a total of 66 questionnaires. They were checked visually and two of them were so poorly completed that they were excluded; otherwise the accuracy of responses appeared good: responses were readable and important questions were mostly answered. The following step was the data reduction, which included the design of the file format, codes and coding of the data as well as data entry to the SPSS 8.0 programme. Data cleaning consisted of final check on the data file for accuracy, completeness and consistency.

The way of deleting missing data while calculating a correlation matrix was to exclude all cases that had missing data in at least one of the selected variables, i.e. by casewise deletion of missing data.

As the samples were not independent, and the sample size was relatively small, the possibility that the variables were not normally distributed was high. Thus nonparametric tests were used for statistical analysis of the data. These included the use of Kendall Tau$_b$, Chi-square test or the Fisher exact test when the expected frequencies were too small.

3 Results

3.1 Nursing Assessment

Nearly one third of the nurses (28%, n = 32) indicated that WISECARE had improved the nursing assessment in their units. There was no statistically significant difference between the WiseNurses or non-WiseNurses in their views on this matter (Fisher's exact test sig. = .69). The perceived improvement in nursing assessment due to the WISECARE project related modestly positively (Kendall's tau$_b$ correlation coefficient varying from .54 to .60, p = .01, n = 32) to the use of WISECARE products (i.e. the WiseTool, WiseWeb and WiseMailingList). These correlations were statistically significant (p = .01) and in expected direction.

More than one third of the respondents (38%, n = 32) stated that the WiseTool programme would be used in their units after the closure of the WISECARE project. These nurses unevenly represented the different Sites, which had participated in the project. Especially some of the nurses from Validation Site B felt strongly that they would use the instrument in the future. Surprising also three quarters of the non-WiseNurses thought that the use of the programme would be likely to continue in their units after the end of the project.

About one fifth of the nurses (19%, n = 32) stated that the use of WiseWeb had had a positive impact on the nursing assessment in their units; all of them were WiseNurses. Half of these nurses were from a Demonstration Site.

A few WiseNurses (14%, n = 28) regarded the use of the WiseMailingList as having improved the nursing assessment in their units. Three quarters of these nurses were from a Demonstration Site and one quarter from Validation Site B.

Altogether 16% of the respondents (n = 32) evaluated that the WISECARE-patients' needs were assessed better than those of the other patients. This did not seem to be related to whether the respondent was a so-called WiseNurse or not (Fisher's exact test sig. = .49). Especially the nurses from Validation Site C-D-E and Validation Site B indicated this improvement as shown in Figure 2.

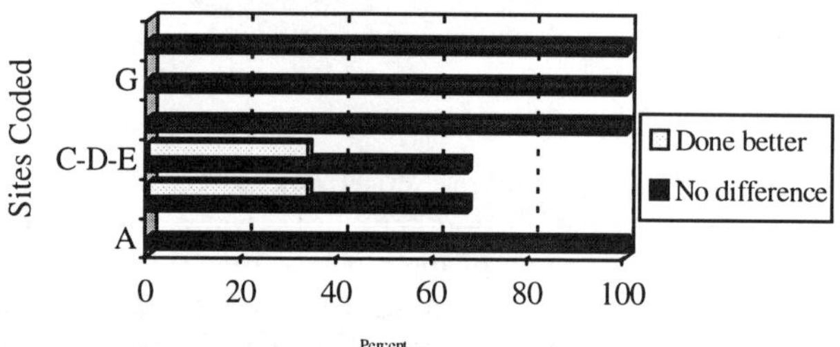

Figure 2   As per Site, Nurses' Opinions of whether the WISECARE-Patients' Needs were assessed better than those of the other Patients (n = 32);.Site C,D,E are belonging to the same Hospital.

3.2 Planning the Nursing Care

About one fifth of the nurses (19%, n = 64) indicated that the WISECARE project had improved the planning of nursing care, i.e. the setting of nursing objectives for the care and deciding the interventions. There was a statistically significant difference in this matter between WiseNurses and non-WiseNurses (Pearson chi-square value 8.150, df = 1, asymp. sig. (2-sided) .004; n = 64). One third of the WiseNurses considered that the project had improved a bit the planning of the nursing care. Half of these nurses were from Validation Site C-D-E, a quarter from Validation Site B and the remainder from Demonstration Site H (n = 64).

As can be seen in Table 1 the perceived improvement in planning the nursing care due to the WISECARE project related modestly positively to the WiseFeedback, team building initiatives and the increased use of research. These correlations were statistically significant (p = .01) and in the expected direction.

Table 1   Correlations between the perceived Improvement in Planning the Nursing Care and the WiseFeedback, Team Building and Use of Research Results (n = 64)

	Planning nursing care
WiseFeedback	.732**
Team building (e.g. multi-professional teams, QI-teams)	.729**
Use of research results	.651**
Kendall's tau_b , ** p = .01 (2-tailed)	

Altogether 17% (n = 4) of the nurses indicated that the WiseFeedback had improved the planning of nursing care either a bit or a lot. With one exception, all of them were WiseNurses, half from Validation Site C-D-E and the other half from Validation Site B.

About one tenth of the respondents (11%, n = 64) indicated that the project had promoted the team building (e.g. multi-professional teams or quality improvement teams) in their units. The answers of the WiseNurses and non-WiseNurses differed statistically significantly from each other regarding this(Fisher's exact test sig. = .01).

The answers showed that WISECARE project had enhanced the use of research results as criteria for clinical judgement among one third of the respondents either a bit (25%) or a lot (6%). This was also dependent whether nurses belonged to the group of WiseNurses or not (Pearson chi-square value 7.342, df = 1, p < .01, N=64). However, as can be seen from Figure 3, the use of research results in nursing practice promoted by the WISECARE project was more evenly distributed among the Sites than some other items in the study.

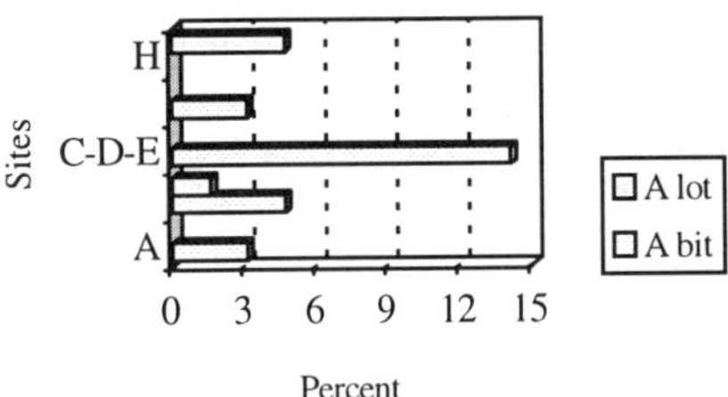

Figure 3   Percentage of Nurses (N=64) of a total from different Sites who stated that the WISECARE Project had promoted the Use of Research Results in their Nursing Practice

3.3 Nursing Interventions

Nearly half of the nurses (42%, N=64) indicated that the WISECARE project had encouraged discussions about the best nursing practices in their units. There was a statistically significant difference in this matter between WiseNurses and non-WiseNurses (Figure 4). Two thirds of WiseNurses (66%, N=64) considered that the project had promoted either a bit or a lot discussion about the best nursing practices. WiseNurses from all Sites reported this positive impact.

One quarter of the respondents (25%, N=64) indicated also that the WISECARE project had a positive impact on patient education. There was no statistical difference in this matter between Wise- and non-WiseNurses. The perceived improvement in patient education showed modest positive correlation with the improvement in written nursing procedures and the impact of the information concerning the nursing interventions included in the WiseTool (Kendall's tau_b correlation coefficient varying from .66 to .69, p = .01, N=64).

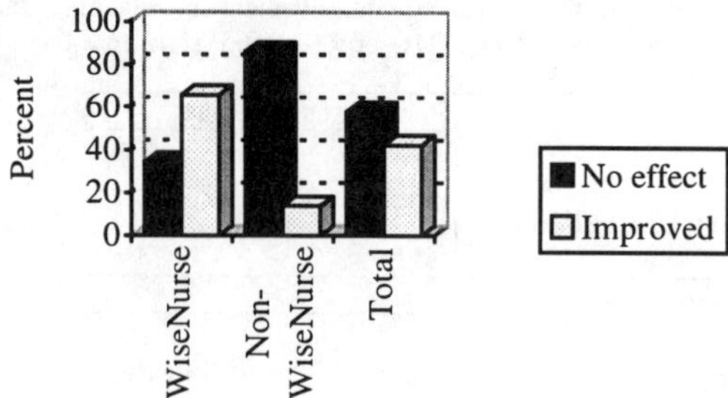

Figure 4   Difference between the WiseNurses and non-WiseNurses evaluating the perceived Impact of the WISECARE Project on encouraging Discussions about the best Nursing Practices (Pearson chi-square value 17.530, df = 1, asymp. sig. (2-sided) .000; N=64)

During the verification and validation phases of the project the different Sites shared their written nursing procedures related to oral care, alleviation of fatigue, nausea and vomiting and pain, to initiate comparison between the Sites. A quarter of the respondents (27%, N=64) stated that they had improved their written nursing procedures during the project. There was no statistical difference between the Wise- and non-WiseNurses in this issue with perceived improvement unevenly distributed among the Sites. Nearly half of the nurses from Validation Site C-D-E (44%, N=23), 60% of the nurses from Demonstration Site G (N=5) and all the nurses from Validation Site B (N=4) indicated this improvement. The perceived improvement in written nursing procedures correlated modestly positively with the use of WiseTool and WiseFeedback. The intercorrelations between the different WISECARE products in respect to the development of nursing interventions were also modestly positive.

Nearly half of the WiseNurses (49%, N=35) indicated that they had slightly altered the nursing interventions in their units due to the information obtained from the WiseTool. This was especially the case in Validation Sites B and C-D-E and in Demonstration Site H. The same applied to the perceived development in nursing interventions due to the information nurses had obtained through the WiseWeb. Just one fifth of the WiseNurses (23%, N=35) had found the use of WiseMailingList helpful in this matter.

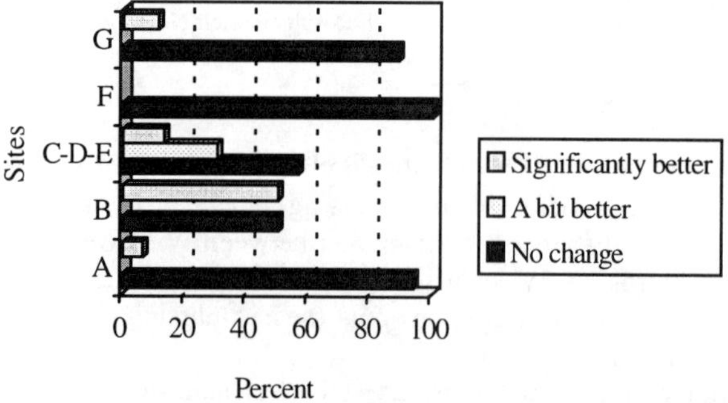

Figure 5   As per Site, Nurses' Opinions of the Degree to which they had changed evaluating Patient's Progress during the WISECARE Project (N=64)

In response to whether the information obtained from the WiseFeedback had altered nursing interventions, one fifth of the nurses (21%, N=64) answered positive. Most of them were WiseNurses (92%). The nurses that had felt the WiseFeedback useful in altering their nursing interventions were from Validation Sites B and C-D-E, Demonstration Site H.

3.4 Evaluating Patient's Progress

About one fifth of the nurses (22%, N=64) stated that they changed their way of evaluating patient's progress during the WISECARE project so that it was now done either a bit (11%) or significantly better (11%). There was no statistically significant difference between the WiseNurses and non-WiseNurses (Pearson chi-square value 1.012, df = 1, asym. sig. (2-sided) .31; N=64). The nurses who stated that they had changed their way of evaluating patient's progress unevenly represented the different Validation Sites (Figure 5).

3.5 The Impact of the WISECARE Project on Symptom Management

Oral health as an indicator and its measurement tool had been part of the project since the start of data collection. According to the respondents (42%, N=64) the project had been most successful during the verification and validation phases in promoting the patients' *oral health*. More than half of the WiseNurses (57%, N= 35) and nearly a quarter of the non-WiseNurses (24%, N=29) were of this opinion. The difference between the two groups was statistically significant (Pearson chi-square value 7.083, df = 1, asym. sig. (2-sided) .008; N=64). All Validation Sites, except F, reported at least some degree of perceived improvement in their patients' oral health (Figure 6).

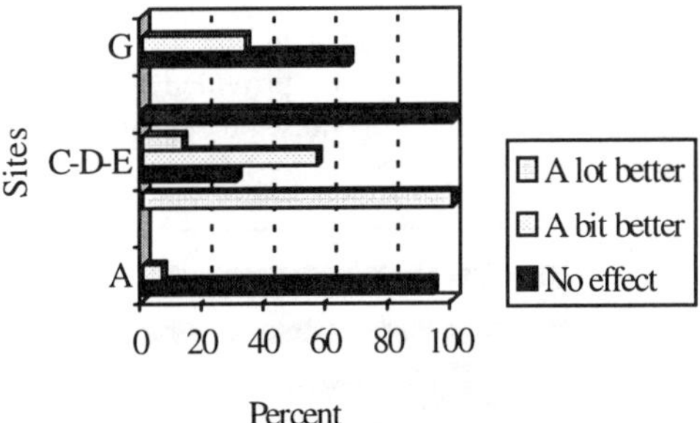

Figure 6   As per Site, Nurses' Opinions of the Impact of the WISECARE Project on Patients' Oral Health (N=64)

The perceived impact on patients' oral health correlated modestly positively with the experienced additional value of the WISECARE project on nursing practice (Kendall's tau_b correlation coefficient .66, p = .01, N=64) and the use of structured language (Kendall's tau_b correlation coefficient .64, p = .01, N=64). Oral health had slight positive correlation with patient education (Kendall's tau_b correlation coefficient .60, p = .01, N=64), written procedures (Kendall's tau_b correlation coefficient .57, p = .01, N=64), the use of instant and global feedback, and the overall exchange of information (Kendall's tau_b correlation coefficient .54, p = .01, N=64) that had been perceived to lead to the evaluation of own practice. If looking only at the results from the final data collection period (September 1999), the correlation between oral health and the use of the instant and global feedback had improved (Kendall's tau_b correlation coefficient .67, p = .01, N=64) than when viewing all the three data collection periods collectively (.55).

In relation to the other patient outcome indicators of fatigue, pain and nausea and vomiting had been part of data collection since February 1999. Eleven percent of the nurses (11%, N=64) indicated that the project had had a positive impact on patients' fatigue and pain alleviation during the verification and validation period. Just three percent (3%, N=64) of the respondents indicated this about nausea and vomiting. During the third data collection period in September 1999 pain alleviation correlated slightly positively with the use of feedback as evidence basis (Kendall's tau_b correlation coefficient = .47, p = .05). In that data collection 24% of the respondents (N=29) were of the opinion that the WISECARE project had had positively impacted a bit or a lot patients' pain alleviation. Pain alleviation had modest positive correlations with some variables describing nursing assessment, planning of the nursing care, and use of WiseFeedback to improve nursing interventions (Table 2).

Table 1   Correlations between perceived Improvement in Pain alleviation and some other Variables (N=64)

	Pain alleviation
Impact of the WiseWeb on nursing assessment	.68**
Nursing assessment	.61**
WiseFeedback and nursing interventions	.59**
Use of research results	.58**
WiseFeedback and setting patient objectives	.53**
Kendall's tau_b, ** p = .01 (2-tailed)	

3.6 Impact on Services

Nearly one fifth of the nurses (19%, N=64) stated that the WISECARE project had had an impact on the quantity or quality of services provided by their unit. This opinion was unevenly distributed among the Validation Sites; nurses from Validation Site B indicated this more than the others (Figure 7).

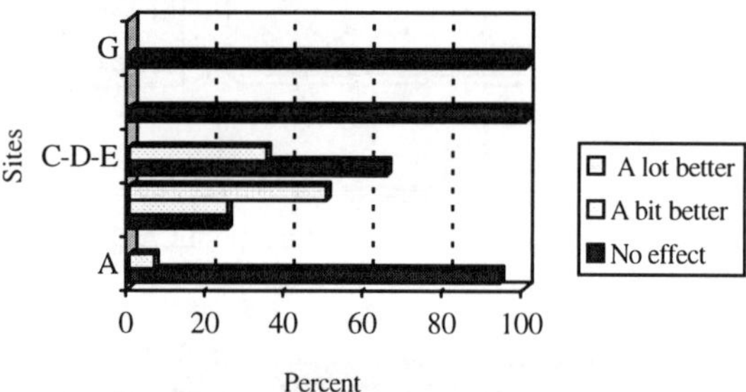

Figure 7   As per Site, nurses' opinions of the impact of the WISECARE project on the quantity or quality of services in their unit (N=64)

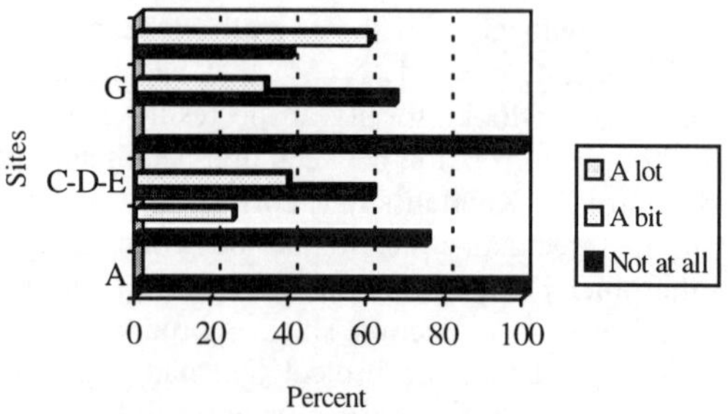

Figure 8   As per Site, Nurses' Opinions of their Ability to Use various Forms of Feedback produced in the Project as Evidence Basis in Nursing (N=64)

3.7 Feedback as Evidence Basis

One fourth of the nurse (N=64) indicated that they had been able to use the instant (WiseTool) and global feedback (WiseFeedback) as evidence basis in their work. There was a statistically significant difference regarding this between the WiseNurses and non-WiseNurses.

The use of various forms of instant and global feedback as evidence basis for clinical judgement related modestly positively to the impact WISECARE had had on patients' oral health (Kendall's tau_b correlation coefficient .60, p = .01, N=64).

The nurses who stated that they had been able to use the feedback as evidence basis represented unevenly the different Sites as can be seen from Figure 8.

4 Discussion

4.1 Clinical Behaviour of Oncology Nurses

The findings about the *nursing assessment* suggested that to some degree the WISECARE concept directed the nurses' observations and patient interviews in a meaningful and systematic way. At the same time the data collection tools gave the nurses an organised and structured language to describe and discuss their observations about important areas in their everyday patient care. The interviews revealed that one Validation Site had renewed their patient admission form to follow the WISECARE method, i.e. use focused and structured data collection on issues known to be important to patients with a particular medical problem. This supports Bakken's [40] statement that standardised terminologies facilitate the capture of what it is that patients need and nurses do.

The instant feedback from the WiseTool (e.g. the graphics showing the patterns of oral health, pain, fatigue and nausea & vomiting) gave some of the nurses, according to the interviews, additional day-to-day monitoring results, which they were able to use in the continuous nursing assessment. Some nurses explained also that as the patients themselves filled in the data collection forms it allowed the patients' "voice" better to be heard, which had encouraged the patients to discuss more freely about their various needs and concerns. One potential explanation for this could be that the four clinical indicators initially selected by the nurses reflect patients' primary concerns and from this patients perceived that nurses are particularly 'in tune' with their needs and felt able to discuss their problems with them. Another reason might be that the nurses just spent more time with the WisePatients, which enhanced the nurse-patient relationship. The fact that the patients found better means to express themselves is important because many nursing research reports have shown that when just judging from the nurse's point of view the nurses tend to under- or over-estimate the patients' problems [18, 67-69].

Bleich [70] has emphasised that nursing assessment, as a noun, is a function beyond gathering of clinical information. It includes the ordering and patterning of information to declare a professional judgement, e.g. an expression of a patient's problem. This is accurately determined only through the nurse's ability to collect, analyse, and synthesise clinical patterns in the patient. The WISECARE project helped some of the clinical nurses to deepen this true meaning of the nursing assessment by providing them tools for focused, systematic and structured data collection, assistance in data analysis and feedback and shared knowledge concerning the nursing interventions thus enhancing their experiential learning process.

The findings about the impact of the WISECARE project on the *planning of nursing care* suggested that there was not as much effort put in this aspect of the nursing process than in assessment and developing the interventions. However, as Bleich [70] has pointed out, in the planning phase of the nursing process nurses determine what can be realistically achieved for their patients. This includes priority setting.

The results suggested also that the benefits of WiseFeedback on setting the nursing care objectives were related to some other activities, which had taken place in various Validation Sites. The Sites, which reported most change, had among others established separate WISECARE-teams to guide the project, discuss the various issues emerging throughout the project and study the received feedback in relation to their knowledge of their own unit and the shared information concerning all the different Validation Sites (cf. benchmarking). Unfortunately, the team building seemed to have taken place mainly among the WiseNurses themselves, although high quality health care has been shown to depend crucially on different health care professionals working well together [71].

In addition to the use of WiseFeedback, it is encouraging that the WISECARE project promoted the use of research results among one third of the respondents as one basis for clinical judgement. During the WISECARE project the partners from Work Package 2 (User group co-ordination) conducted several high quality literature reviews for the nurses concerning the current state of knowledge related to the WISECARE clinical indicators, which may have helped the nurses to implement the latest research results into their clinical practice.

The results concerning the *nursing interventions* suggested that the WISECARE project initiated quite vivid discussions about the best nursing practices and evidence-based nursing among the WiseNurses. They found some information from the WISECARE products, which had helped them to modify their nursing interventions, even change the written nursing procedures. Interestingly, both Wise- and non-WiseNurses had perceived improvement in patient education and in written nursing procedures during the verification and validation phases of the project. The interviews revealed that one Validation Site had updated their guidelines and protocols related to the four clinical indicators, which were followed up in the project, in a multidisciplinary team. This is in tune with the principles of evidence-based practice, which emphasise the necessity to reduce wide variations in individual clinicians' practices, eliminating the worst practices and enhancing the best practices, thereby improving quality [26].

The relation between the patient education, written nursing procedures and the use of WiseTool and WiseFeedback was explained during interviews where the nurses told that they used the instant feedback from the WiseTool for patient education. It was also possible for the nurses to follow the effects of their interventions on daily basis from the WiseTool graphics when it comes to the four chosen indicators in the WISECARE project. Also the WiseFeedback helped them to describe some of the side effects better to the patients. The shared information about the nursing procedures together with the information obtained through the WISECARE products initiated the clinical discussions that in some situations led to the change of written nursing procedures.

During the interviews it became clear that as a result of the project one Validation Site created a hospital-wide chemotherapy risk assessment form. For the patient education they developed a chemotherapy follow-up form. The perceived improvement in patient education becomes even more interesting, when we remember that information and education have repeatedly been identified as primary areas of cancer patients' dissatisfaction with their care. At the same time many researchers (McHugh et al. 1982; Dodd 1983, 1988; Richardson 1995; Winningham et al. 1994) have shown that patient information is a central component of both prevention and effective management of chemotherapy side effects. The value of specific information on adverse reactions in helping patients to cope and enhance self-care has been repeatedly emphasized [8].

4.2 Patient Outcomes

The findings about the *instant and global feedback as evidence basis* suggested that, to some degree, the WISECARE concept gave the nurses that kind of feedback, which they were able to use in clinical judgement on individual patient and on patient group level. This may have depended on the use of the WiseTool and the WiseFeedback. If the data input to WiseTool was regular, preferably daily, the nurses were able to receive the instant feedback in graphics of the patient's situation and compare this to the previous data inputs and compare thus seeing the difference in outcomes. This finding is supported by the other result, which revealed that some nurses had changed their way of *evaluating patient progress*.

Global feedback was received twice during the verification and validation phases of the project. It not only gave the Validation Sites aggregated information about their own unit, but also more importantly, about the others too so that a real comparison (benchmarking) was able to begin. But as the use of aggregated clinical and management information is new for nurses, it has taken them some time to understand the various ways that the WiseFeedback can be used.

According to Haukkapää-Haara [72], Nadler (1977) pointed out the importance of feedback by explaining that feedback aims at change. It can provoke the change in the performance of individuals, groups and organisations either by motivating or steering the performance. The use of feedback is a sign of self-regulation. Thus the availability of meaningful feedback is as essential as the will to change.

Previously, the effectiveness of nursing interventions has been primarily determined through judgement rather than careful and systematic measurement. However, WISECARE has provided nurses with a tool - through the instant and global feedback - to document whether patient outcomes improve because of the care provided and which of the interventions are more effective to alleviate a symptom [cf. 6].

Guadagnoli and McNeil [61] have pointed out that in many situations the available information may not be specific enough to be applied to a given clinical situation. They have argued that the ability to provide this type of information to patients/nurses requires data collection on a large scale, in terms of both patients assessed and clinical data elements collected. Flatley Brennan [73] has said that informatics includes the processes by which information becomes accessible, interpretable, and meaningful. She correctly has stated that the WISECARE project implemented a 'wise plan' when it decided to use shared databases of patient experiences to generate the evidence needed to effectively guide practice. As of October 1999 the WISECARE database contained more than 2.000 observations in comparison to a hypothetical situation where the same data would have been collected e.g. just from one Validation Site it would have taken 5-10 years to end up with the same size of a database.

Taking into account that the WiseNurses received the first instant feedback in graphics together with the risk assessment during spring 1999, and the first global feedback nearly simultaneously, they had little time to compare their practices with others and modify their nursing practice toward 'best practices'. Working within this time frame, most of the Validation Sites put their developmental efforts in oral care. The results suggested that WISECARE approach was successful in promoting patients' *oral health*. This improved patient outcome could be due to the overall development around oral care, which consisted of a structured data collection tool, systematic data collection, availability of instant feedback with risk assessment, shared practice guidelines, global feedback results and motivated discussion through the WiseMailingList.

The inclusion of the chemotherapy risk assessment (related to the four clinical indicators i.e. oral health, fatigue, pain, nausea and vomiting) to the feedback seems to have brought additional value to the nursing practice. This supports the findings of Sitzia et al. [74] who in their study of patients' experiences of side effects associated with chemotherapy suggested that regimen-specific data is important both in formulating clinical practice and in the provision of patient education.

It might be that the management of nausea and vomiting did not receive a lot attention although it is a well-known side effect of chemotherapy. Many interventions, for example new drugs, has been developed during the recent years to control the problem. The complexity of fatigue as a phenomenon could have hindered some of the nurses to tackle this problem as their first focus of interest. To develop effective nursing interventions to alleviate this symptom with clear patient outcomes would probably take more time than has been available between the reformulation of the project and this evaluation.

5   Conclusions

During the verification and validation phases, the WISECARE project was able to develop a methodology to enable the Validation Sites to achieve the set project goals. The degree of goal attainment is dependent on the effort the respective Sites are able to put in the transition process. In other words, through the sharing of clinical information, it seems to be possible to encourage European cancer nurses to compare their actual clinical practice with other Clinical Sites and benchmarks and develop guidelines and protocols. The WISECARE method allows the nurses to learn from their past patients and their own ways clinical practise.

When viewing the impact of the WISECARE project on clinical nursing a few things must be considered: first, the opportunity to discuss and compare nursing interventions and consequent patient outcomes using the latest IT facilities on a pan-European basis has been an entirely novel concept for nurses. The nurses' skills to use computers and those available for them were less than had been anticipated during the planning phase of the project. It took some time to supply each Validation Site with a computer, not to mention the Internet connection and in some Sites training was arranged for the nurses on the use of electronic mail, World Wide Web and browsers, and the WiseTool. Second, the use and comparison of aggregated information and peer reviewing has meant a major change in professional culture. WISECARE has required a new way of thinking and developing nursing in the spirit of evidence-based nursing with a close connection to everyday nursing reality. Use of research findings or utilisation of feedback, which is received from outside one's own organisation, is not common in clinical nursing. Inevitably the WISECARE project has managed to create a method and set of tools to facilitate this through information technology.

Based on the evaluation, we as evaluators are convinced that the basic concept/procedure of the WISECARE project is relevant and useful. However, the impact of the project on patient outcomes is so far limited. This might be due to the difficulty of changing nurses' working culture so rapidly and deeply. It might have something to do with the WiseNurses position at the wards as most of them were staff nurses, and thus probably not so able to introduce new practices at ward level. The total number of patients involved in the project has so far remained relatively small in comparison to the number of units working in the project. The lower the number of patients the more limited the feedback from which the nurses can learn. The outcome results might also depend on the nurses' ability to interpret the various forms of feedback. The graphic presentation can contain so much information in a figure that it can be difficult to understand it in a practical manner. Despite these obstacles there is evidence showing remarkable progress at most of the Sites.

References

[1]   Salvage J. Introduction. In Salvage J & Heijnen S (ed.). Nursing in Europe. A resource for better health. WHO Regional Publications European Series 1997; **74**: 1-11.

[2]   French B. British studies which measure patient outcome 1990-1994. *Journal of Advanced Nursing* 1997; **26**: 320-328.

[3]   Griffiths P. Progress in measuring nursing outcomes. *Journal of Advanced Nursing* 1995; **21**: 1092-1100.

[4]   Jones K, Jennings B, Moritz P & Taylor Moss M. Policy issues associated with analyzing outcomes of care. *Image: Journal of Nursing Scholarship* 1997; **29** (3): 261-267.

[5]   Turtiainen A-M. Methods to describe nursing with uniform language: The cross-cultural adaptation process of the Belgium Nursing Minimum Data Set in Finland. Kuopio University Publications E. Social Sciences 71. Doctoral dissertation, 1999.

[6]   Strickland O. Challenges in measuring patient outcomes. *Nursing Clinics of North America* 1997; **32** (3): 495-512.

[7]   Contract between EU DG XIII and the WISECARE partners, 1997.

[8]   Sitzia J & Wood N. Patient satisfaction with cancer chemotherapy nursing: a review of the literature. *International Journal of Nursing Studies* 1998; **35**: 1-12.

[9]   Fitch M. Creating a research agenda with relevance to cancer nursing practice. *Cancer Nursing* 1996; **19** (5): 335-342.

[10] Hegyvary S. Patient care outcomes related to management of symptoms. *Annual Review of Nursing Research* 1993; **11**: 145-167.

[11] Sermeus W. Annual project review: Workflow Information Systems for European Nursing Care. Belgium: Katholieke Universiteit Leuven Centre for Health Services Research, 1998.

[12] Boyle S. Assessing mouth care. *Nursing Times* 1992; **88** (15): 44-46.

[13] Kearney N. (previously Jodrell). Report on information needs of oncology nurses. WISECARE/WP2/D2_1, 1997.

[14] Wallance K, Senko A & Thomas C. Effect of attitudes and subjective norms on intention to provide oral care to patients receiving antineoplastic chemotherapy. *Cancer Nursing* 1997; **20** (1): 34-41.

[15] Richardson A & Ream E. The experience of fatigue and other symptoms in patients receiving chemotherapy. *European Journal of Cancer Care* 1996; **5**, Suppl. 2: 24-30.

[16] Winningham M, Nail L, Barton Burke M, Brophy L, Cimprich B, Jones L, Pickard-Holley S, Rhodes V, Pierre B, Beck S, Glass E, Mock V, Mooney K & Piper B. Fatigue and the cancer experience: the state of the knowledge. *Oncology Nursing Forum* 1994; **21** (1): 23-36.

[17] Chang HM. Cancer pain management. *Medical Clinics of North America* 1999; **83** (3): 711-

[18] Berry D, Wilkie D, Huang H-Y & Blumenstein B. Cancer pain and common pain: A comparison of patient-reported intensities. *Oncology Nursing Forum* 1999; **26** (4): 721-726.

[19] Strang P. Cancer pain – a provoker of emotional social and existential distress. *Acta Oncologica* 1998; **37** (7/8): 641-644.

[20] Goodman M. Risk factor and antiemetic management of chemotherapy-induced nausea and vomiting. *Oncology Nursing Forum* 1997; **24** (7) supplement: 20-32.

[21] Grant M. Introduction: Nausea and vomiting quality of life and oncology nurse. *Oncology Nursing Forum* 1997; **24** (7) supplement: 5-7.

[22] Richardson A. Theories of self-care: their relevance to chemotherapy-induced nausea and vomiting. *Journal of Advanced Nursing* 1991; **16**: 671-676.

[23] Kleinpell R. Whose outcomes. Patients providers or payers? *Nursing Clinics of North America* 1997; **32** (3) 513-520.

[24] Bond S & Thomas L. Issues in measuring outcomes of nursing. *Journal of Advanced Nursing* 1991; **17**: 1492-1502.

[25] Burns N & Grove S. The practice of nursing research. Conduct critique and utilization. 3rd ed. W. B. Saunders Company, Philadelphia, 1997.

[26] Hegyvary S. Issues in outcomes research. *Journal of Nursing Quality Assurance* 1991; **5** (2): 1-6.

[27] Jennings B. Patient outcomes research: Seizing the opportunity. *Advances in Nursing Science* 1991; **14** (2): 59-72.

[28] Johnson M & Maas M. Nurisng outcomes classification. Iowa outcomes project. Mosby, St. Louis, 1997.

[29] Maas M, Johnson M & Moorhead S. Classifying nursing-sensitive patient outcomes. *Image: Journal of Nursing Scholarship* 1996; **28** (4): 295-301.

[30] Marek K. Outcome measurement in nursing. *Journal of Nursing Quality Assurance* 1989; **4** (1): 1-9.

[31] Lang N & Marek K. The classification of patient outcomes. *Journal of Professional Nursing* 1990; **6** (3): 158-163.

[32] Lang N & Marek K. Clinical conditions and interventions: their relationship to outcomes that reflect clinical practice. In Patient outcomes research: Examining the effectiveness of nursing practice conference. NINR. U.S.A. Maryland, 1991.

[33] Guadagnoli E & McNeil B. Outcomes research: Hope for the future or the latest rage. *Inquiry* 1994; **31**: 14-24.

[34] Hokanson Hawks J. Power: a concept analysis. *Journal of Advanced Nursing* 1991; **16**: 754-762.

[35] Scott T. Management for doctors: using information for managing clinical service effectively. *British Medical Journal* 1995; **310**: 848-850.

[36] Tonks A & Smith R. Information in practice. *British Medical Journal* 1996; **313**: 438.

[37] Tanner C. Evidence-based practice: research and critical thinking. *Journal of Nursing Education* 1999; **38** (3): 99.

[38] Perälä M-L. Towards evidence-based nursing. In Simoila R, Kangas R & Ranta J (eds.). Management in nursing. Kirjayhtymä Oy, Helsinki, 1999. [in Finnish]

[39] Sackett D, Rosenberg W, Gray JAM, Haynes RB & Richardson W S. Evidence based medicine: what it is and what it isn't. *British Medical Journal* 1996; **312**: 71-72.

[40] Stetler C, Brunell M, Giuliano K, Morsi D, Prince L & Newell-Stokes V. Evidence-based practice and the role of nursing leadership. *Journal of Nursing Administration* 1998; **28** (7/8): 45-53.

[41] Clarke C & Procter S. Practice development: ambiguity in research and practice. *Journal of Advanced Nursing* 1999; **30** (4): 975-982.

[42] Rolfe G. The theory-practice gap in nursing: from research-besed practice to practitioner-based research. *Journal of Advanced Nursing* 1998; **28** (3): 672-679.

[43] Tolley K. Theory from practice for practice: is this a reality? *Journal of Advanced Nursing* 1995; **21**: 184-190.

[44] Sermeus W & Vanhaecht K. WISECARE to support evidence in practice. An article manuscript, 1999.

[45] Graves J & Corcoran S. The study of nursing informatics. *Image: Journal of Nursing Scholarship* 1989; **21**: 227-231.

[46] Saranto K & Ensio A. Information systems in nursing. In Saranto K & Korpela M (eds.). Infromatics in social and health care. WSOY, Porvoo, 1999. [in Finnish]

[47] Nagle L, Shamian J & Catford P. Information technology developments: Issues for nursing. In Saba V, Pocklington D & Miller K (eds.). Nursing and computers. An anthology 1987-1996. Springer, New York, 1998.

[48] Sermeus W, Hoy D, Jodrell N, Hyslop A, Gypen T, Kinnunen J, Mantas J, Delesie L, Tansley J & Hofdijk J. The WISECARE project and the impact of information technology on nursing knowledge. In Gerdin U et al. (eds.). Nursing Informatics. IOS Press, Amsterdam, 1997.

[49] Kajander A & Konttinen M (eds.). Information and communication technologies in health care. A report prepared for the STOA unit of the European Parliament. STAKES National research and Development Centre for Welfare and Health, Helsinki, 1996.

[50] Ball M & Douglas J. Integration of systems for patient care. Proceedings of Fourth International Conference on Nursing Use of Computers and Information Science. Springer-Verlag, New York, 1991; 110-114.

[51] Bakken S (previously Henry). Informatics: Essential infrastructure for quality assessment and improvement in nursing. In Henry SB, Holzemer W, Tallberg M & Grobe S (ed.). Informatics – The infrastructure for quality assessment & improvement in nursing. UC Nursing Press, California, 1995; 8-19.

[52] Bakken S (previously Henry)B. A comment to an unpublished article "WISECARE to support evidence in practice" by Sermeus W & Vanhaecht K, 1999.

[53] Hagey R & McDonough P. The problem of professional labelling. *Nursing Outlook* 1984; **32** (3): 151-157.

[54] Henderson V. The nursing process: is the title right? *Journal of Advanced Nursing* 1982; **7**: 103-109.

[55] Kiikkala I & Munnukka T. Nursing research: on what basis? *Journal of Advanced Nursing* 1994; **19**: 365-371.

[56] McHugh M. Does the nursing process reflect quality care? *Holistic Nursing Practice* 1991; **5** (3): 22-28.

[57] Varcoe C. Disparagement of the nursing process: the new dogma? *Journal of Advanced Nursing* 1996; **23**: 120-125.

[58] de la Cuesta C. The nursing process: from development to implementation. *Journal of Advanced Nursing* 1983; **8**: 365-371.

[59] Donelly G. The promise of the nursing process: an evaluation. *Holistic Nursing Practice* 1987; **1** (3): 1-6.

[60] Henderson V. Nursing process: a critique. *Holistic Nursing Practice* 1987; **1** (3): 7-18.

[61] White A. The nursing process: a constraint of expert practice. *Journal of Nursing Management* 1993; **1**: 245-252.

[62] Øvretveit J. Evaluating health interventions: An introduction to evaluation of health treatments services policies and organisational interventions. Open University Press, Buckingham; 1997.

[63] Rossi P & Freeman H. Evaluation: a systematic approach. 5th ed. Sage, California Newbury Park, 1993.

[64] Sinkkonen S & Kinnunen J. Evaluation and monitoring at the public sector. Kuopio University Publications E. Social Sciences 22, Kuopio, 1994. [in Finnish]

[65] Kinnunen J & Nykänen P. Evaluation of health informatics. In Saranto K & Korpela M (eds.). Infromatics in social and health care. WSOY, Porvoo, 1999. [in Finnish]

[66] Stevens F, Lawrenz F & Sharp L. User-friendly handbook for project evaluation: Science mathematics engineering and technology education. Government Accounting Office. Program Evaluation Issues. GAO/OCG-93-6TR, 1992.

[67] Hovi S-L & Lauri S. Cancer patient's pain. University of Turku. Deparment of Nursing Science. Research and reports series A17, 1997.

[68] Lepistö M, Lauri S & Käppeli S. Patients' nursing problems: Nurses' and patients' views. University of Turku. Deparment of Nursing Science. Research and reports series A8, 1995.

[69] Suominen T. The nursing care of breast cancer patients: perceived information support and participation. Doctoral dissertation. University of Turku. Department of Nursing Science, 1994.

[70] Bleich M. Clinical judgements: Essential elements of nursing process. *Journal of Nursing Quality Assurance* 1990; **4** (4): 1-6.

[71] Casey N & Smith R. Bringing nurses and doctors closer together. Greater cooperation will benefit patients. *British Medical Journal* 1997; **314**: 617.

[72] Haukkapää-Haara P. The production of the feedback system of adverse events. Unpublished master's thesis. University of Kuopio. Department of Health Policyand Management, 1998. [in Finnish]

[73] Flatley Brennan P. A comment to an unpublished article "WISECARE to support evidence in practice" by Sermeus W & Vanhaecht K, 1999.

[74] Sitzia J, Hughes J & Sobrido L. A study of patients' experiences of side-effects associated with chemotherapy: pilot stage report. *International Journal of Nursing Studies* 1995; **32** (6) 580-600.

Oncology Nurses' Change with Respect to Clinical Management

Juha Kinnunen, Tiina Nyberg

1   Introduction

There can be little doubt that within the last decade, nursing has undergone major and significant changes. Ideally, changes in nursing should be viewed as necessary rather than inevitable and exciting rather than stressful. Unfortunately, factors such as low morale, a drop in productivity, narrow outlook and reluctance to take risks may impede the process of change [1]. Nurses' feelings regarding their lack of control and the profession's dependence on medical staff have been shown to result in the development of defensive actions against change by nurses [2]. However, as change has been our only constant in nursing and is now faster and more complex than ever before [3], nurses must develop a new mindset more in tune with a constantly changing world [4] and learn to manage change appropriately [5]. Indeed, although change can create uncertainty and discomfort, it often leads to real innovation, providing abundant opportunities for creating a better way forward [6]. This report will consider the impact of the WISECARE project on changes to oncology nurses' clinical management. In doing so, it will consider 5 aspects:
The concept and process of change in nursing:

- The instigation of the change process within the WISECARE project
- A retrospective view of the experiences of nurses from Validation Sites regarding changes to clinical management as a result of WISECARE
- The prospective expectations of nurses from Demonstration Sites regarding changes to their clinical management
- A look to the future regarding the impact of the WISECARE project on overall changes to clinical management in nursing.

2   The Concept and Process of Change in Nursing

Many synonyms exist for the word change, e.g. modification, transformation, growth or evolvement. These all imply the process of movement. Nurses often feel uncomfortable and resistant to change [1], with the common reaction being to nurture the false hope that by not addressing the change taking place, the situation will 'calm down' and everything will 'return to normal' [7]. This attitude to change must be confronted to ensure an appropriate response to the changes taking place. Change is a burden when it is done to us and rewarding when we do it [6]. However, how we, as nurses, view the change taking place, shapes our ability to respond to it. It is concerning to note then, the findings of Lima-Basto who found that nurses felt they had a limited degree of control over nursing care and change because of nurse-physician group relations, characterised by their conflicting dominating/domineered nature [2].

Considering the current climate of change, nurses must begin to view change differently. Zukowski [5] questions whether nurses resist change because they believe it to be inappropriate or because they are currently undertaking more than their share of the wrong jobs, making change more difficult to manage. She suggests that nurses must be challenged, not to take on more, but to take on what is appropriate, as well as give up what is inappropriate, advocating that change is difficult when one is doing more than ones share of the wrong jobs. [5] However, there is little doubt that some changes are accomplished easier than others. In essence, change is likely to be perceived as necessary, rather than inevitable, if it is not too large, if there is a degree of control over the change and if it appears to have benefit of some sort [6]. Five factors have been identified as crucial to the successful accomplishment of change within all aspects of nursing. First, the practicalities and realistic nature of the change must be considered, taking into account the magnitude of the change and acknowledging that big changes are more easily accomplished if broken down to smaller steps. Secondly, the environment where the change will take place should be considered, as the change has to be specific to the context. Thirdly, one has to consider those on the receiving end of the change and fourthly, those responsible for implementing the change. Finally, the change strategy itself needs to be evaluated, for example, whether the change is to be imposed from 'top to down' or from 'bottom to up', implemented as a whole or as a series of smaller changes [9].

Cartor [7] highlights some of the general assumptions about change, including the belief that change will mysteriously vanish if ignored, that changes are unnecessary or bad for individuals' careers, that becoming upset will result in resorting to the status quo and that problems during a time of transition indicate that the proposed change is unnecessary. These assumptions indicate that workers often feel threatened by change. Changing attitudes is a major part of implementing change and overcoming threatened feelings [6]. A variety of methods have been suggested to positively influence attitudes to change [3, 6, 8]. Firstly, additional communication must be instigated. One must accept that where an information vacuum exists, rumours will usually fill it. Secondly, the use of approval or disapproval through rewarding or providing incentives contingent on a particular type, magnitude or direction of attitude change may be helpful in developing positive attitudes towards a particular change. Thirdly, attitudes can be altered as a result of group influences and finally, individuals can be induced to engage in discrepant behaviour, whereby their behaviour is contrary to the attitudes they hold.

Lewin [10] was one of the original theorists to study the process of change and its impact on individuals. He believed that individuals progress through three distinct phases when confronted by change. He defines the first as 'unfreezing', a process which occurs when change is first introduced and leaves the individual involved feeling very threatened, uncomfortable and anxious. 'Moving to a new level' is the second phase and begins when the change is incorporated into the normal processes for a department, organisation or individual. During this stage the individual feels more comfortable and more in control of the situation. The final stage of Lewin's change process, termed 'refreezing', occurs when the change is permanently incorporated into normal daily operations. At this stage in the process, if the change was taken away, individuals would resist, as it has become part of their identity. While utilising Lewin's theory could explain the process of change in the WISECARE project, Post [11] proposed a five phase process of change that has been applied to the management of nurse innovation and so may be more appropriate for adequately describing the process of change within the WISECARE project.

3   The Instigation of the Change Process Within the WISECARE Project

Muller [4] has proposed that approaching change with a level of excitement and enthusiasm allows us to perceive it as an adventure and challenge that gives us the opportunity to improve both our lives and those of our patients. Indeed, it is these opportunities that underpin the WISECARE project. Viewing the WISECARE project from this perspective allows the changes to be considered more as innovation. Innovation provides a new way of doing something that, more often than not, has positive connotations or a benefit of some sort [8]. Furthermore, applying a logical and systematic process to managing change helps to reduce chaos and increase effectiveness [3]. The changes required for the instigation of the WISECARE project can be examined using the five stages of change, identified by Post [11] namely preparation, movement, synergy, the new reality and integration.

3.1 Preparation

The positive effects of preparation in the early stages of change are tremendous [3]. During this first phase, the purpose of the change must be clarified, explaining why change is appropriate at this time and why it is important for the people involved. Furthermore, it is important to relate the change to the mission of the organisation. Clarifying the purpose of the WISECARE project and relating it to the mission of nursing was not difficult. That the unique contribution of nursing is rarely formally evaluated [12], provided nursing with more than enough reason to participate in a project with the potential to change clinical management and rectify this invisibility. Health care's finite resources mean that nurses must be able to demonstrate the relationship between patient outcomes and nursing care. The fact that the project aimed to highlight the real value of nursing provided a sense of direction for those clinically based nurses within the project, on whom the change depended for its implementation. The potential for empowerment of nursing and improvements in nursing care that the project offered resulted in a number of countries being keen to participate.

The second issue of the first phase involves evaluation of the required resources for successful implementation of the change. This was an important consideration for the WISECARE project, as interested parties were required to have Internet links and information technology facilities and knowledge. Participation in the WISECARE project has led to some members of staff developing new skills to ensure the successful implementation of the change.

3.1.1 Movement

This phase considers the structural elements required for supporting the change such as the development of a committee and a vision for the future. Indeed, Manion [3] advocates that a vision for the future is essential if a cultural change is required, e.g. asking people to behave or relate to one another differently in the future. This was most definitely the case in the WISECARE project, which involved the development of a virtual organisation of cancer nurses to enhance communication and knowledge sharing. Explaining this vision to the nurses involved was essential to ensure that they internalised the concept and benefits to be gained from this virtual organisation.

Planning is the second issue to be considered during this phase of change. Manion [3] suggests that if one can see the desired end, then establishing the steps required to reach it becomes possible. For the WISECARE project, regular meetings and communication facilitated the setting of plans, targets and goals which maintained the impetus of the project, allowed all team members to feel involved and kept the project in time as far as possible.

3.1.2   Synergy

The process of synergy is smoothest if the first two phases have been successfully accomplished. Key issues during this phase are communication, co-ordination and co-operation [3]. Personnel within the WISECARE project are fortunate to have a myriad of communication facilities, for example, telephone, facsimile, electronic mail (e-mail), video conferencing and post. Prior to the commencement of the project, none of the Clinical Sites were using e-mail within their daily clinical practice and the clinically based nurses were initially dubious about the appropriateness and usefulness of this novel and unfamiliar communication channel. However, the change in their practice and attitude towards e-mail has been outstanding. There has been an overwhelming shift towards the use of e-mail in the project as the major communication channel. The flexibility it offers facilitates free flowing communication between both clinical and non-clinical team members. The problems encountered with negotiating a suitable and appropriate time for telephone calls or conferencing has been resolved by using e-mail. This flexible mean of communication has been essential for successfully accomplishing the project's goal of encouraging knowledge sharing and communication across Europe to enhance nursing care and patient outcomes. Keeping these lines of communication open through the use of both individual e-mails and the general WISECARE e-mailing list received by all members of the research team has fostered co-operation and team spirit. Such co-operative spirit has kept a tight focus on the project through re-evaluation of goals and aims and re-stating of priorities. Regular e-mail communication has allowed the additional stresses and strains of clinical practice in individual Sites to be appreciated and has allowed appropriate support to be instigated so decreasing the sense of isolation of individual Sites participating in the project. Encouraging all team members to share information with each other through the general WISECARE e-mailing list, rather than information constantly coming from the project's leaders has also helped to foster enthusiasm and motivation for change.

3.1.3   The New Reality

This phase is where the change begins to penetrate practice. Stabilisation of the change during this phase is essential, anchoring the change in reality. Within the WISECARE project, the anchoring of change in reality can be seen in the increasing volume of questions from Clinical Sites regarding their future as the end of the project draws closer.

In addition to the anchoring the change in reality, productivity is another key issue during this stage. Although productivity may drop initially during times of change, improvements are known to come later. This pattern has been evident within the WISECARE project as clinically based nurses have become increasingly comfortable and confident in the integration and value of IT in their clinical practice for improving patient outcomes.

3.1.4   Integration

This is the final phase of change and involves evaluating the impact of the change. As the WISECARE project draws to an end, report writing and evaluation of the project's effectiveness and value in clinical practice and impact on patient outcomes must be assessed. Such evaluation is essential as it provides us with logical direction for future innovations.

4   Retrospective Views of Nurses' Change to Clinical Management

While important to understand the crucial phases of change experienced by the team members to instigate the project and ensure its incorporation in clinical management, it is important to also evaluate clinically based nurses' perceptions of changes in clinical management as a consequence of participation in the project.

While the WiseCompass evaluates nurses' perceptions of the project, additional information was sought in the form of an informal questionnaire, e-mailed to all Validation Sites. This was completed by the nurse manager of each Site and at least one other nurse involved in the project. As a result of participation in the WISECARE project a third of nurses believe that further research activities have been undertaken in their unit. The remainder, however, do not believe that their involvement in the WISECARE project has encouraged further research activities. One could suggest that this could be because nurses are focussing solely on WISECARE at present, making additional research activities difficult and that following the successful completion of the project, enthusiasm for additional research activities may flourish. Indeed, the majority of nurses perceive that their participation in the project has the potential to stimulate initiation of further activities involving information technology in the future within their clinical areas.

As regards the impact of the WISECARE project on changes to *oral care*, about one third of nurses reported a change in their clinical management. Nurses explained that they are more likely to discuss oral problems with patients as a result of structured assessments and consequently oral care has a higher profile. It is reported that oral care has received increased amounts of attention during the course of, and as a result of nurses' participation in, the project. Furthermore, increased communication between nurses and other units regarding appropriate nursing interventions for oral problems has been enhanced. The nurses involved in the project report that such sharing of information has led to the development of educational activities regarding best oral care practice in their individual units. Those who reported no change in practice did so because they felt they were already performing adequate oral care with positive patient outcomes despite the fact that they were 'lacking an evidence base'.

No nurses involved in the project perceive a change to their clinical management as regards the problem of patients' pain believing that pain is always adequately managed and positive patient outcomes persistently achieved. However it is important to consider this perceived satisfaction with pain management in conjunction with patients' perceptions of their pain management. Despite the arsenal of pharmacological and non-pharmacological interventions available with which to manage pain, many patients continue to endure unnecessary suffering [13]. Pain assessments made by health care professionals are often inaccurate and sometimes biased [14]. Time constraints, lack of appropriate facilities and poor staff mix cause problems for appropriate pain assessment [15]. Indeed, concerning results were highlighted by Grossman et al. [16] who established that health care providers' perceptions of patients' pain are often quite different from that of the patient and that such discrepancies become more prominent for patients experiencing significant pain. This is in keeping with, and may go some way to explaining, the perceptions of the nurses involved in the WISECARE project. However, it is also important that we consider this perceived lack of change in pain management alongside the information gathered from each of the Clinical Sites regarding current nursing practices at the start of the project. This indicated that none of the Sites were currently using a pain measurement tool. However, merely participating in the project involves objectively assessing patients' pain regularly and consequently indicates a change in pain management. Furthermore as the project has spanned two and a half years, a change in the nursing staff responding to these questions may explain why nurses fail to perceive a change in their practice.

The majority of nurses participating in the project believe that their involvement in the project has resulted in a change to their clinical management of patients' *fatigue*. Objective assessment of the problem of fatigue for patients has resulted in increased nursing attention being directed towards this particular issue. Additionally, patients have been observed as becoming more aware of the problem. Increased communication and discussion between patients and nursing staff regarding fatigue's aetiology and management, as a consequence of this increased attention, has resulted in patients and nurses working together to develop methods of ameliorating or alleviating patients' fatigue.

The majority of nurses reported using effective, established medical and nursing protocols to successfully manage the associated problems of *nausea and vomiting* with positive patient outcomes. However, there is the general perception by participating nurses that there has been some improvement in the management of these symptoms as a result of sharing knowledge and information. Although positive, this improvement is noted to be variable across all Sites and dependent on individual patients.

Reflecting on the results regarding the specific changes in clinical management, one could conclude that the integration of the project has resulted in changes in clinical management for the patient problems of oral care and fatigue as they have not enjoyed the high profile often given to cancer-related pain and nausea and vomiting. These high profile symptoms and side effects have revelled in the attention that they have received in the past and are subsequently better managed, with successful patient outcomes. One could argue that this would result in less change to their management being required. However, this leads us to question why, at the outset of the project, clinically based nurses chose to focus on these specific patient problems, if they were already managed appropriately? This raises several questions. Should the project have focussed on less obvious patient problems? Are nurses conditioned to believe that the main problems for patients are nausea and vomiting and pain? Do nurses fail to admit the full extent of patients' problems, perceiving that this would reflect poorly on their nursing practice? One could suggest that none of these questions explain the nurses' responses. A potential explanation could be in the nurses' perceptions of the term 'change in clinical management'. The authors would argue that although the presence of established protocols and interventions for the patient problems of nausea and vomiting and pain exist and imply that 'change' is unnecessary, the WISECARE project may have provided a structure to the assessment and evaluation process which fails to be recognised by nurses as 'change in clinical management'. Consequently, it is also important to evaluate nurses' perceptions of 'change' in more general terms.

The nurses involved in the project perceive that the structured, objective data collection, facilitated by the project, regarding patients' problems of nausea and vomiting, pain, fatigue and oral care has had additional value for the nursing care that they subsequently deliver. Nurses believe this structure fosters the development of a standardised nursing language within not only individual units but also between individual countries participating in the project, leading to an increased sense of affinity to the European nursing community. Generally, this standardised approach to patient assessment has made a positive impact on overall nursing assessments within individual units involved in the project. From a positive stance, this improved assessment practice has been adopted for all patients rather than only patients involved in the project. However, nurses have noted that patients involved in the project are more inclined to discuss their problems freely, which they perceive to be due to the increased length of time spent discussing the patient's problems with them. A slight improvement in general patient education has also been noted, most probably as a result of these enhanced communication practices. As one may hope, nursing objectives are set no differently for patients who are or are not involved in the project while optimistically, there is some suggestion that the planning of nursing care has been improved through participation in the project. In conjunction with this improved planning, the written nursing procedures in each unit are also reported to have improved. In relation to this, it would appear that evaluation of patients' progress has also improved as a result of the project.

To conclude then, from a patient perspective, increased communication and assessment with patients regarding their symptom management is perceived by nurses as the most beneficial change in their clinical management. Regarding the professional perspective, nurses have found sharing information concerning local clinical management of patients' problems beneficial, while benefiting professionally from being involved in collaborative clinical research. Overall, improvements in nursing interventions to ensure enhanced patient outcomes and sharing information between Sites were identified by nurses as the most crucial changes instigated by the project within their clinical management. Continued improvements and changes in clinical management until the end of the project are anticipated by the nurses involved as a result of increased feedback of the project's results. Optimistically, nurses involved in the project believe that commercialisation of the data collection and feedback tool used in the project is a real possibility following completion of the project. This highlights the positive impact that the integration of information technology into their daily clinical practice has had for them.

5   Prospective Expectations of Nurses' Change to Clinical Management

Nurses in the Demonstration Sites were asked to complete an open questionnaire prior to joining the WISECARE project. From this, we were able to evaluate their expectations.

The vast majority of nurses from the Demonstration Sites hope that participation in the WISECARE project will stimulate further clinical research in their area, the primary belief being that once clinical research has been started, there will be enthusiasm for it to persist. There is the suggestion that the focus of the project on quality of nursing care in relation to patient outcomes will encourage participating nurses to continue this type of work in the future. This relates to the perceived benefits of the Demonstration Sites regarding the value of participating in collaborative clinical research.

With regards to changes in clinical management for specific patient problems, over half the nurses perceive that there will be changes to their clinical management of *patients' oral problems* and expect to see changes to their standard protocols and assessment practices. In contrast with the responses from the Demonstration Sites, the majority of nurses in the Demonstration Sites expect changes in *pain management*. They anticipate that existing protocols will be modified alongside patient assessment and hope that this change in management will be continued into the community setting once the patient has been discharged home. More in keeping with the Demonstration Sites, two thirds of nurses from the Demonstration Sites expect changes to the clinical management of *patients' fatigue*, explaining their expectations in relation to the fact that fatigue is still perceived to be less well managed than the other patient problems within the project. Only half of nurses expect changes to the clinical management of *nausea and vomiting*. This can perhaps be explained by the specialities of new Clinical Sites as these include a short stay surgical ward whose nurses do not perceive nausea and vomiting to be a problem. Furthermore, many of the Sites state that they already have established medical and nursing intervention protocols for the management of this particular problem.

Most nurses from the Demonstration Sites expect that involvement in the WISECARE project will lead to increased emphasis regarding patient assessment, enhanced patient communication due to instant feedback facilities, increased discussions regarding symptom management, interesting discussions with other Clinical Sites regarding clinical management of symptoms and increased understanding and involvement in clinical research. Optimistically, those mirror the Validation Sites in that they perceive improvements in nursing interventions for enhanced patient outcomes and the increased sharing of information as the most important changes to clinical management that involvement in the WISECARE project will bring. Other expected changes include increased understanding of patients' symptoms and the ability to illustrate patterns of patients' symptoms to them, again positively identified by the Demonstration Sites. Nurses' expectations regarding their involvement in the project include improving communication within the multidisciplinary team, identification of resources required to ensure optimal care delivery and improved care following discharge.

Thus, to conclude, the expected benefits of participation in the WISECARE project reflect the perceived benefits of those already involved.

6   The Impact of WISECARE on Nursing Care Delivery

Although looking at specific changes in clinical practice is helpful to evaluate change to an extent, it fails to identify changes in philosophy and attitude towards nursing care delivery. As attitudes are hypothetical constructs they cannot be directly observed and their existence is often inferred from behaviours. As a result, change in philosophy and process of care has been better understood by the authors through discussion with clinically based staff involved in the project. Some quotes from these discussions will be used for illustration.

Over the duration of the project, nurses have become increasingly confident in the use of IT to demonstrate the positive impact of their actions and the benefits of using this data constructively to predict patient problems and plan nursing care appropriately to ensure the positive nature of these outcomes. Although the WISECARE project concentrates specifically on four patient problems, the nurses involved in the project have grown to understand that utilising the WISECARE process for other patient problems would provide a structure to their work. This structure would not only have the potential to clarify patients' problems but would also demonstrate the impact of appropriate nursing care and ensure the visibility of their clinical management.

"(the project) has provided the knowledge of how useful IT can be to visualise patients' problems, measure them more effectively and visualise the effectiveness of the nursing interventions." (Scotland)

"We learned to work in a structured way using patients' clinical indicators to plan our care and make decisions." (Belgium)

The sense of belonging and sharing information facilitated — by the collaborative nature of the project that has influenced — changes in care delivery and that has been valued by clinically-based staff. Sharing useful and meaningful information across boundaries has maintained enthusiasm in the project and fostered the development of collegial relationships that nurses hope will endure past the completion of the project.

"I am grateful for the opportunity of sharing information between clinical Sites." (Finland)

"(The project) has provided the impetus for nurses to learn about clinical management from other nurses and stimulated ideas for future projects." (Scotland)

"We (the nurses involved) have just started on our journey towards better patient care." (Belgium)

Such change in relationships can also be seen in the relationship between nurses and patients. Although always unique in its inherent quality, nurse-patient communication has been enhanced through participation in the WISECARE project. Patients' perception of their involvement in the project includes an increased sense of involvement in their care and the individualisation of their care. Such positive feedback reinforces this enhanced communication and so improves care delivery. That the project has encouraged increased communication regarding the little discussed problem of fatigue is, in itself, positive, however such enhanced communication has extended to other areas of concern for patients outwith the confines of the WISECARE project.

"The project has provided patient with a useful tool for documenting some of their problems while at home and a more accurate record for nursing staff to interpret the severity of their symptoms." (Scotland)

"Patients like to be involved, they feel they receive more attention and care." (Finland)

"(As a result of enhanced communication) we have developed new patient admission forms and chemotherapy follow-up forms." (Belgium)

That these expressions of positive changes to patient care delivery are shared by a number of Demonstration Sites highlights the extent of harmonisation that has grown as a result of the WISECARE project. Such harmonisation in nursing care was not evident at the start of the project and has been fostered through enhanced communication, resulting in an increased sense of European partnership in care.

7   The Practice/Management Link for Total Clinical Management

While the above quotes illustrate a change in nurses' clinical practice as a result of the project, change is also evident in their overall clinical management of patient care. Although the WISECARE project has not resulted in a 'direct' change to all aspects of clinical practice for patient problems, participation has provided those nurses involved with an overall philosophy for care. This changed philosophy of care delivery is evident through nurses' explanations of the altered care delivery strategies and structure for all patients. Nurses have become increasingly aware of their importance in clinical management and its subsequent impact on patient outcomes.

"I am now thinking more about patient' feelings and experiences of their care and I try to communicate more with patients about this." (Finland)

"The project has stimulated the importance of nursing staff in thinking of the interventions that are being delivered and the actual patient outcomes." (Scotland)

"The care for the patient group in our ward is changing rapidly.... Care plans will change as a result" (the Netherlands)

"We have developed structure of care: patient => data => information => decision making that has been implemented within the unit." (Belgium)

Furthermore, while participation in the project has fostered the implementation of this philosophy of care to improve the clinical management of all patients, the WISECARE project has led to the development of a structure and a process for the provision of care. In addition, it has provided means of evaluating this care that can be internalised to facilitate appropriate clinical management. Nurses involved in the project have expressed a deepening sense of empowerment and developed a vision for the future as a result of participation. The WISECARE project has provided nurses with an understanding of the positive impact that IT has, and will continue to have, in illustrating and improving their clinical management and so demonstrating the value of this management. Through this collaborative endeavour, these nurses have seen the benefits of autonomy for their future practice and will consequently be enthusiastic for future nursing innovations for improved clinical management and the identification of the unique contribution of nursing to patient outcomes. At a recent meeting, nurses involved in the project expressed concern as the end of the project draws closer, explaining that now they have experienced WISECARE, they cannot revert to pre-WISECARE nursing management.

8   Conclusions

In concluding, participation in the WISECARE project does appear to have resulted in specific changes in clinical practice and these are reflected in the expectations of the new Sites. However, while considering specific changes in clinical practice is helpful in measuring the impact of the WISECARE project on clinical management, more discrete changes in the process and structure of nursing care are evident through discussions with clinically based nursing staff. It is this change in philosophy of care delivery and process for nursing practice that nurses involved in the WISECARE project are able to internalise and so adapt to all aspects of nursing care.

References

[1]   Jootun D & Fitzcharles A. Change without pain. *Managing Clinical Nursing* 1998; **2**: 19-22.
[2]   Lima-Basto M. Challenges of nurses' professional behaviour change process. *Scandinavian Journal of Caring Sciences* 1995; **9**: 113-118.
[3]   Manion J. Managing change: the leadership challenge of the 1990's. *Seminars for Nurse Managers* 1994; **2**: 203-208.
[4]   Muller PA. Change, conflict and coping. *Journal of Post Anaesthesia Nursing* 1992; **7**: 54-55.
[5]   Zukowski B. Managing change…before it manages you! *Medsurg Nursing* 1995; **4**: 325-330.
[6]   Poggenpoel M. Managing change. *Nursing RSA Verpleging* 1992; **7**: 28-31.
[7]   Cartor RA. Breaking down assumptions, managing change. *Hospital and Health Networks* 1993; **68**
[8]   Pryjmachuk S (1996) Pragmatism and change: some implications for nurses, nurse managers and nursing. Journal of Nursing Management **4**: 201-205
[9]   ENB - The English National Board for Nursing, Midwifery and Health Visiting. Managing Change in Nursing Education. Pack One: Preparing for Change. ENB, London, 1987.
[10]   Lewin K. Field Theory in Social Science. Harper and Row, New York, 1951.
[11]   Post N. Working Balance: Energy Management for Personal and Professional Well-Being. Post Enterprises PA, Philadelphia, 1989.
[12]   Salvage J. Introduction. In Salvage J & Heijnen S (ed.). Nursing in Europe. A resource for better health. WHO Regional Publications European Series 1997; **74**: 1-11.
[13]   Hanks GW. Problem areas in pain and symptom management in advanced cancer patients. *European Journal of Cancer* 1995; **31A**: 869-870.
[14]   Harrison A. Assessing patients' pain: identifying reasons for error. *Journal of Advanced Nursing* 1991; **16**: 1018-1025.
[15]   Latham J. Assessment and measurement of pain. *European Journal of Cancer Care* 1994; **3**: 75-78.
[16]   Grossman SA, Sheidler VR, Swedeen K, Mucenski J & Piantadosi S. Correlation of patient and caregiver ratings of cancer pain. *Journal of Pain and Symptom Management* 1991; **6**: 53-57.

Harmonisation of Data Collection

Derek Hoy

1 Introduction

This chapter discusses how harmonisation of data collection was achieved in the
WISECARE project, with emphasis on the technical issues of harmonisation. Reference is
made where appropriate to European standards, whether existing or under development.

2 Summary of WISECARE Data Collection Process

At the time of writing, data has been collected from 20 units in 11 hospitals in 10
European countries, using 6 different languages.

At the start of WISECARE, no Validation Site had a computer-based information
system for nurses to collect the data required. There were constraints of time, money and
contractual agreements that would stop the procurement of a suitable commercial system
for implementation across all the Sites. As a result, a data collection tool was designed,
built and implemented across the Validation Sites (the WiseTool).

Data was collected on paper and re-entered in the system, or directly entered in some
cases. Paper-based collection proved unavoidable because it became clear very quickly
that much of the data collection would be done by patients themselves, often at home.

Data was exported at agreed periods, and sent as an encrypted and compressed file
via email to be processed at one Site into the WISECARE data warehouse.

3 Requirements for Harmonisation

The WISECARE project has set up a network of cancer units which share an information
system which allows them to describe their own care and compare it to others in the
network. This information system collects data, communicates the data to a central point,
aggregates the data in a data warehouse, and supports feedback of a variety of analyses.
Each of these steps requires data flows that are predictable in order to minimise errors or
'noise'. The process of 'harmonisation' ensures that predictability.

WISECARE uses a 'distributed' information system, in the sense that processes are
performed in different places, at different times, and by different people. Achieving an
acceptable degree of harmonisation requires effort in four areas [1, 2]:

- a shared conceptual framework,
- an information model,
- a communication model and
- a terminology model.

Design decisions made the requirements of WISECARE from some of these models a
very simple exercise, for example the communication model is trivial. This was a
deliberate step to make the working of the project more robust and ensure greater success.

However, each model is discussed as future projects using the WISECARE approach may require greater sophistication.

4   Shared Conceptual Framework

To put it very simply, WISECARE can be compared to a large box, into which people put things. These things are combined into more interesting and useful things, which people can then take out. It might be like a large kitchen, where someone puts in eggs, sugar, flour, and receives a nice cake.

When it works, this is a very good system: everyone gets back a bit more than they put in. But it can go wrong: what if someone puts in duck eggs, which give a strange flavour? Or someone expects a pie?

4.1 Agreeing a Common Purpose

The process of human categorisation is complex, but heavily dependent on context of use, particularly the purpose of categorisation [3]. Agreeing the purpose of data collection in WISECARE has been a difficult, but essential, part of achieving harmonisation.

At first, data collection was heavily influenced by the 'purpose' of ensuring comparison of pre- and post-WISECARE interventions in the Validation Sites. In meetings, this came to be seen as a 'research' view of the world. An alternative view was proposed, identified as being more 'clinical', because it was to do with 'real care', and influencing clinical interventions in individual patients ('research', 'clinical', and 'real care' were terms used in the discussions).

There was also a practical element: the full-standardised measures were large and time-consuming to complete for patients and staff. Smaller, focussed measures were quicker and considered more relevant.

This conflict was resolved with much effort by discussion with all the project partners and Validation Sites, and a shift to the 'clinical' view was agreed. This involved using smaller data sets which focused more on a set of clinical issues, agreed by consensus: pain, fatigue, oral health and nausea and vomiting.

There is certainly a trade-off here, between the use of complete, standardised (psychometric) data collection tools and more simple tools which do not have the same demonstrated validity and reliability.

However, a data collection tool may be very well developed and tested, but if its users are not agreed on the purpose of using it, or its value in use, the resulting data is likely to be of poor quality. Early data analysis seemed to confirm this.

The adoption of a 'clinical' purpose for data collection has certainly been seen as a positive change in the course of the project, and has helped to maintain clinical interest until the end. For example, some nurses are printing out graphs of scores to show individual patients how they are progressing.

4.2 Agreeing Conceptual Categories

CEN MOSE [4] uses a triangle to illustrate the difference between three ways of describing a concept:
- By label
- By definition (intension)
- By example, using things which are that kind of object (extension)

When we work with data, we use 'labels', for example text or codes. We might have a definition, and we could give examples. Table 1 gives an imaginary example for 'mucositis'.

Table 1   Example Descriptions for a Conceptual Category

Text label	'mucositis'
Code	324562
Definition	'inflammation of the oral cavity'
Example	'gingivitis', 'inflamed gums' …

To agree conceptual categories, we must ensure that these boxes are harmonised across all system users.

When a concept is added to our system, we give it a unique code. This should carry no information, but be simply an identifier in our system [4]. Meaning can be agreed by using a definition, and/or examples. Definitions are very attractive, but in real life it is impossible to define every concept in a clinical vocabulary, either because precise definitions cannot be agreed or because it is just too much work.

Text labels need not be standardised as long as they are agreed as referring to the same concept (synonyms). They can also be translated into many languages.

In WISECARE, harmonisation was achieved by using pre-existing standardised tools: the Piper Fatigue Scale [5], EORTC Quality of Life Scale [6], and the Oral Assessment Guide [7]. Using these tools gave an instant set of categories for WISECARE, with text labels in English and other languages. It also gave sets of definitions that could be used to ensure an acceptable level of semantic harmonisation.

These concepts were therefore entered into a project lexicon and given unique codes. A separate table gave the term labels for each concept in each WISECARE language.

By using a common set of semantic categories across all users of the system, an important benefit was gained. The nature of the WISECARE assessment tools was such that for any item, only one response was allowed. For example, in the Oral Assessment Guide, in assessing a patient's voice, the user must choose one of 'normal', 'deep or raspy', or 'difficulty talking/painful'. They must make one and only choice, which is a characteristic of a 'disjunctive' classification.

In this situation, the meaning of any one concept is affected by the other sibling concepts. For example, supposing we had to describe a wine as 'red' or 'white', how would we describe a 'vin rosé'? A definition of 'red', which included any wine with red colouring, would make it 'red', but a definition, which was based on characteristics of the wine, might make it 'white'. So, the category 'red' might include red and rosé wines, but in a classification, which included 'red', 'white' and 'rosé' it certainly would not.

When sets of possible values are small, as in the OAG example, this may make it easier for reliable use of the tool, as the user can make a selection based on not just the meaning of one value, but by excluding the other options as less appropriate.

4.3 Problems of Standardised Conceptual Categories

By using standardised assessment tools across all Validation Sites, WISECARE harmonised conceptual categories in a way, which is very common for multi-centre projects. This was even simpler to implement by using one data collection tool (WiseTool).

If Validation Sites had been able to use their own systems (if these systems had existed), then the assessment tools would require to be added to the local data model and controlled vocabulary.

The main problem with this is, if it is necessary to aggregate data across Sites with different information systems, using existing data. In this case, agreement on conceptual categories must be retrospective by mapping between different vocabularies.

This involves greater effort, and may make harmonisation difficult, for example if the local vocabularies were designed for different purposes, such as administration rather than clinical. However, if it can be done, it can open up more sources of data.

4.4 Information Model

When the system purposes and requirements were agreed, an information model was designed, comprising the objects, attributes, and operations required for the system to perform as the 'use cases' described.

At the lowest level, these objects were constrained by the use of the selected assessment tools. Each item is an attribute of a scale, and the tool would define a set of values for that item. For other data items, for example 'treatment profile', a WISECARE value set was constructed by getting all Validation Sites to send their local value sets.

Operations on these objects were decided by the protocols in the standardised tools (all items in the Oral Assessment Guide are added to produce a total score), or by agreeing a WISECARE protocol (all patients must be allocated to one patient group).

The structure of the WISECARE patient record can be compared to the current CEN TC251 direction for EHCR [8] in Table 2.

Table 2 EHCR Components and WISECARE

EHCR Component	WISECARE component
Folder	The WISECARE patient record
Headed section	For example, all the oral assessments. All WISECARE assessments are recorded as part of an assessment-heading-complex, which 'contains' them.
Composition	An assessment, for example an oral assessment. All recorded items in a WISECARE assessment are recorded as part of an assessment complex, which 'contains' them.
Cluster	An assessment item and its recorded value. For example, 'voice' + 'normal', because neither of these data items are meaningful on their own. They must be entered, processed and retrieved together.

As with harmonisation of conceptual categories, WISECARE used a simple (very common) method for harmonising the information model by standardising across the WISECARE information system.

Achieving this harmonisation across Sites using different information systems would require an additional 'mapping' information model, which could be complex and costly to achieve.

CEN TC251 WGII is beginning the work on standards for such requirements with its work on Domain Term Lists[9]. This would also require standardisation in the terminology model to allow mapping from local terms to standardised terms in a standardised domain term list (see also section 6).

5   Communication Model

In this context, we are talking of communication within and between information systems. It can be considered a 'synchronisation of dialogue' between system modules.

In WISECARE this was achieved in a very simple manner, by use of a common system (WiseTool), which exported 'raw' data in an identical format for each Validation Site. All processing of this data was done centrally on importing it into the data warehouse. This allowed communication between the data collection systems and the data warehouse to be kept simple and consistent.

Where data collection from different local systems was required, more effort would be required for harmonisation. Industry standards are evolving that that will help, for example XML. It seems likely that health informatics standardisation effort will focus on content for example, by using XML to define standards for communication of patient records [10].

6   Terminology Model

It was clear from early in the WISECARE project that there would be a very limited terminological model. Previous experience in EU projects has highlighted the need to separate terminology from the 'dialogue model'[11]. In WISECARE, the lexicon contained a flat file of coded concepts with their terms translated into the required languages. These terms were pre-coordinated to a degree that would be very restricting in a good terminology model.

The 'dialogue' layer was modelled using techniques based on the GALEN project: concepts linked by a network (directed acyclic graph) for generic relations, with constraints added by using semantic links.

An example will make this a little easier to understand. Pain data is collected using part of the EORTC Quality of Life scale, which has two pain-related items. The WISECARE lexicon had a concept coded as 2234 with a standard label of *EORTCPain*. The English term for this is: *'Have you had pain in the last 24 hours?'*

In the dialogue model, there is a statement: *EORTCPain IsComponentOf PainSubScale*, which links this concept to others in the pain assessment. There is also a statement *EORTCPain HasValueSet OneTo4ScaleValueSet*. This tells the system to offer the user a scale of 1 to 4 as sensible values for this item.

Also *PainSubScale IsComponentOf WCAssessment*, allows the WiseTool system to build an assessment form by retrieving all the components of *WCAssessment* from the terminology server. *PainSubScale HasHeading PainHeading* links the pain items so they can be retrieved under a common heading.

Almost all of this relates to the dialogue between parts of the system, giving context to help structure the record, and supporting the user interface. It has very little to do with terminology.

The term *'Have you had pain in the last 24 hours?'* is complex. To begin with it could be simplified to *'perception of pain'*, and the other concepts relating to who suffered it (subject of the record), when (previous 24 hours), where (not mentioned in the term), the certainty of the observation (certain?) would be better recorded as additional attributes in the record. In a terminology model *'perception of pain'* might be linked semantically to other types of perception. *'pain'* might have qualifiers of anatomical site and severity.

None of this additional complexity was required for harmonisation of data collection in WISECARE. However, for collection of data from different information systems using different vocabularies some additional effort would be required.

The current CEN approach is to develop 'categorial structures' [4] as agreed international standards (ISO work on terminology standards may use a similar approach). Categorial structures link conceptual categories with a small set of generic semantic links. They form generic templates, which can then be used for development of localised or more specific vocabularies or classifications. They could also be used to map between vocabularies by providing a common underlying framework.

Work is underway to develop a categorial structure for nursing at CEN and ISO levels. Such a categorial structure could then be used to build a terminology model for future projects using the WISECARE approach.

6.1 The International Classification for Nursing Practice (ICNP)

WISECARE gave careful consideration to the role of ICNP as a terminology for the project. ICNP was not used because, as described above, a standard vocabulary was not strictly required, as the choice of standardised assessment tools fulfilled this requirement.

However, it would have been good to test the ICNP for this kind of use, but some other issues prevented this. Over the course of the project, the ICNP was not stable as it moved from alpha to beta versions. The beta version was substantially different as the phenomena axis changed from a mono-hierarchical classification to a multi-axial system. Until 1999, the beta version was described as 'experimental' [12].

The alpha and beta versions did not provide 100% coverage of WISECARE lexicon. Where terms could be expressed using ICNP, they would need to be pre-coordinated from the 8 axes to be usable, so there would be no advantage from its use as an interface terminology. Finally, ICNP has no (permanent) coding system, but uses hierarchical codes as a temporary measure.

Here is still controversy over the future role of ICNP, as a 'user terminology' (front end vocabulary), or 'unifying framework' (back end' reference model). It may prove to be useful for future projects using the WISECARE approach, which requires harmonising data collection over a variety of information systems.

References

NOTE: some of the CEN references are from working or draft documents. This is unfortunate, but these documents are replacing published standards that are now out of date. Given the choice between only referencing out of date published documents, or referencing work-in-progress, the author considers it more useful to the reader to be directed to current thinking on these topics.

[1]   CEN/TC251/prENV 2443. Medical Informatics - Healthcare Information Framework.
[2]   The HIF is now under review in CEN/TC251/SSS-HII Health Informatics - Short Strategic Study-Health Information Infrastructure- Unpublished at time of writing.
[3]   Roth I & Bruce V. Perception and Representation, 2nd ed. Open University Press, Buckingham. 1995.
[4]   CEN/TC251/ENV 12264. Medical Informatics - Categorial structures of systems of concepts - Model for representation of semantics, 1997.
[5]   Piper B, Lindsey A, Dodd M, Ferketich S, Paul S & Wellers. The development of an instrument to measure the subjective dimension of fatigue. In Funk S, Tornquist E, Champagne M, Archer D, Copp L & Weise R (eds). Key Aspects of Comfort: management of pain, fatigue and nausea. Springer Publishing Company, New York, 1989: 199-208.
[6]   Aaronson NK, Ahmedzai S, Bergman B et al. The European Organization for Research and Treatment of Cancer QLQ-C30: a quality-of-life instrument for use in international clinical trials in oncology. *J Natl Cancer Inst.* 1993; **85**: 373-374.
[7]   Eilers J et al. Development, testing and application of the oral assessment guide. *Oncology Nursing Forum* 1988; **15** (3): 325-330.
[8]   CEN/TC251/prENV 13606-1. Health Informatics - Electronic healthcare record communication - part 1 Extended architecture.
[9]   CEN/TC251/prENV 13606-2. Health Informatics - Electronic healthcare record communication - part 2 Domain term list.
[10] CEN/TC251/prENV 13606-4. Health Informatics - Electronic healthcare record communication - part 4 Messages for the exchange of information.

[11] Rector AL, Glowinski AJ, Nowlan WA & Rossi-Mori A. Medical-concept Models and Medical Records: An Approach Based on GALEN and PEN&PAD. *J Am Med Informatics Association* 1995; **2**: 19-35.

[12] Nielsen GH. Telenurse introduction to β-ICNP. Danish Institute for Health and Nursing Research, 1999 (published as part of EU Telenurse ID-ENTITY project).

European Impact Analysis

Jacob Hofdijk

1 Introduction to the WISECARE Project

1.1 Introduction

The goal of WISECARE is to improve the delivery of nursing care by the use of data stored in electronic patient records. The focus is on improving the different dimensions of nursing management, such as the clinical management, the management of resources and the knowledge management (Figure 1).

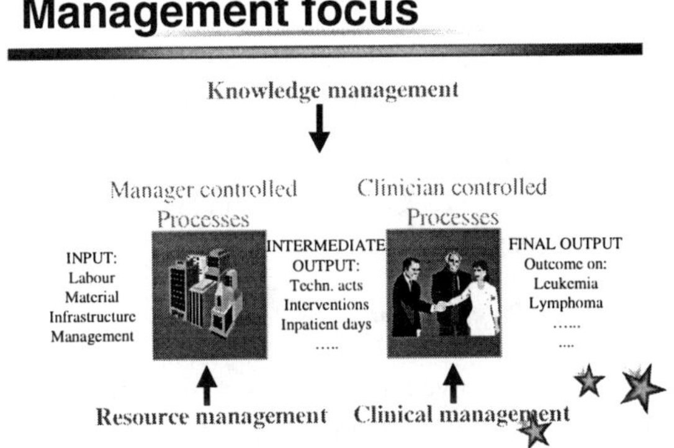

Figure 1   The WISECARE Management Approach

According to Nyberg and Kinnunen [1], Salvage (1997) and other nurse authors have stated that although nurses and midwives comprise the largest single group of health professionals in Europe the impact of nursing care on the total quality of care for the patients has not been evaluated sufficiently. They [1] continue that Turiainen (1999) has shown that there is neither any national database, which would continuously follow up the impact of nursing on patient outcomes. Nor has there been a structured approach to include nursing activities in clinical case mix management systems. Whilst there are attempts to develop nursing classification systems, they are almost never used in any systematic way in Europe. Instead, patients are classified according to medical diagnosis using medical classification systems such as Diagnosis Related Groups (DRGs). Nursing, viewed as supportive to medicine in the DRG system, is not quantified effectively because DRGs are not sensitive enough to quantify or evaluate nursing care [2, 3].

1.2 The Objectives of the Project

The aim of this evaluation paper was to describe the impact of WISECARE on the European market from the perspective of supporting case mix management. To assess the potential of the results of the WISECARE project it is wise to go back to the original objectives [4]:

- To create a workflow information model to systematically exploit clinical nursing data, stored in electronic patient records, for clinical and resource management. The diversity of the patient population, the variability of care, patient outcomes and nursing resources will be quantified using the existing patient classification and coding systems. This information will be made visible using state-of-the-art data presentation techniques. Relations and links between the data will be analysed in a multivariate way, using state-of-the art statistical and analysing tools.
- To establish a network of oncology care centres by using network software (WWW, Workplace servers) in which the clinical practice information will be shared. This will lead to state-of-the art knowledge dissemination and sharing through the network partners.
- The impact of the availability of information on the diversity of the patient population, the variability of care, patient outcomes and nursing resources that have been used and the links between these components, will be evaluated.

The WISECARE project thus seeks to provide a workflow model to monitor nursing activities in relation to the clinical care process, measure the outcomes and evaluate the costs of services to patients. The WISECARE project wanted to use the existing clinical nursing care data for evaluation and development of guidelines and protocols. The WISECARE project aimed to disseminate and share these state-of-the-art international guidelines and protocols and to provide tools to compare actual practice with the benchmarks. The WISECARE project focuses on oncology care as a domain of demonstration, as oncology care covers, by its nature, the complete variety of nursing care in a number of clinical settings.

1.3 The WiseNurses User Requirements

The WiseNurses have been involved in each step of the WISECARE project. An analysis of the user requirements reformulated the focus of the project from the original eight questions that had been raised on the basis of one country evaluation in the original project description [4]:

(1) To what extent is nursing care related to the aim of care (diagnostic, curative, palliative)?

(2) To what extent is the dependency level of the patient different according to the aim of care?

(3) To what extent is treatment influenced by the age of the patient?

(4) To what extent will the organisational structure (number of nursing staff, qualification level, care environment) influence nursing care?

(5) To what extent will the medical diagnoses and the medical treatment influence?

(6) To what extent will the choice of treatment and nursing care influence the quality of life?

(7) To what extent is the quality of life influenced by the continuity of care and emotional support during the caring process?

(8) To what extent will the cost of treatment and the related expected quality of life influence the choice of treatment?

The WiseNurses decided to focus on particular patient groups and problems. The patient groups included adult patients, mostly receiving chemotherapy due to acute lymphoid leukaemia, acute myeloid leukaemia, Non-Hodgkin's lymphoma, breast cancer, lung cancer or osteosarcoma. The WiseNurses originally identified oral health, fatigue, and quality of life as the most specific problems for patients in their care. After a lengthy experiment to utilise measures related to these it was realised that the project would end up with overwhelming data, which would have been difficult to make ready for clinical decision-making. Thus, the project participants decided to focus on more specified patient problems through which the new method of developing nursing care would be easier to test. The refocused areas of clinical concern were decided to be oral health, fatigue, pain, and nausea and vomiting. The focus on patient problems instead of on the use of nursing resources caused a diversion from the original objective.

At the same time, to start the development of a workflow information model to systematically exploit clinical and resource management data, a survey of the WISECARE Validation Sites was undertaken to analyse, how the actual computer-based systems manage these data in the different Validation Sites. The survey revealed that in all the Sites computer-based systems were used for organisational and management purposes but not for clinical nursing management. Therefore the requirements for a clinical nursing information system were studied and a plan to develop tools to meet these requirements was proposed. This plan considered how to meet the broad user requirements by integrating WISECARE tools in existing resources at the Validation Sites [5].

1.4 The WISECARE Data Cycle

Based on these findings, the focus was to create tools to support a complete 'WISECARE data cycle' (Figure 2): data collection, processing for the data warehouse, feedback and communication of the developing knowledge base for the user defined patient groups. The WiseTool helps to collect clinically sensitive personal data across the five cancer nursing Validation Sites. It is a masterpiece of user-friendly data entry, which has been enhanced during the course of the project [5]. The WiseTool focused on the selected patient groups and the assessment of a set of nursing problems selected by the WISECARE community. The data collected at the Validation Sites, and in the last phase of the project, also in the Demonstration Sites, were analysed in Leuven in the WISECARE data warehouse.

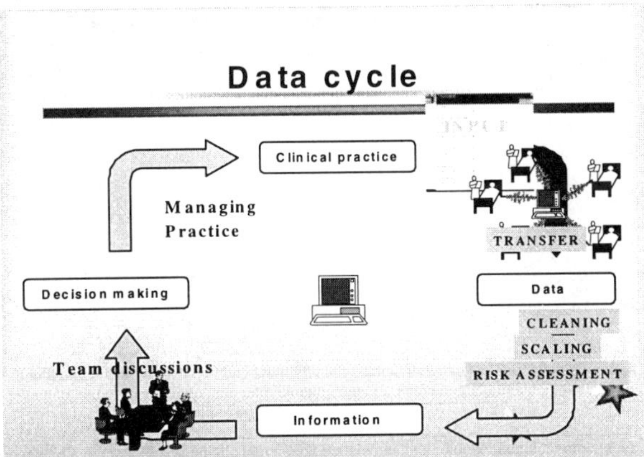

Figure 2   The WISECARE Data and Information Cycle

The aggregated data were analysed to study the diversity of the patient population, the variability of care, patient outcomes and nursing resources [6]. The data-warehouse comprises three central fact tables: *patient descriptors* (based on existing patient records), *clinical activities* and *resources*. There are six associated dimension tables: time, patient, *risk assessment*, staff, unit, *episode*, and clinical vocabulary [7].

The analysis of the data collected during the process created feedback based on each sites' own practice and a comparison with the nursing process at the other Sites. This proved to be a very complex process as there was no agreed nursing care process model as a common basis for comparison. The introduction of 'clinical time' as a reference model created a new challenge in the common understanding of the processes involved. This discussion illustrated the need for the development of a more generic model to link nursing activities to a clinical model. The WiseTool provides a clinical framework introducing the patient group (acute lymphoid leukaemia, acute myeloid leukaemia, Non-Hodgkin's lymphoma, breast cancer, lung cancer or osteosarcoma) and the stage of therapy. Through this approach a logical link to the clinical care process has been established, which provides an interesting basis for a more integrated approach of a clinical information system for both nurses and doctors.

The introduction of measuring instruments, scales, the exchange of protocols and the introduction of an active human interaction network by the Internet and regular user meetings created a new dimension in nursing practice. This process directly supported and promoted the work of bedside nurses by dealing with day-to-day oncology nursing. Assessing the specific health problems of the patients within the hospital and at home enlarged the knowledge of the WiseNurses remarkably.

1.5 Impact on Nursing Resource Management

As the objective of the WISECARE project was to learn about the treatment process across the participating Sites, the process of Global Feedback was an important part of the project. Data collected with the WiseTool were sent to the WISECARE Data Warehouse Centre in Leuven. There the comprehensive process of cleaning the data took place before preparing the feedback information. The data were put into a clinical perspective by relating them to 'clinical time', by modelling the data by patient group and the chosen therapy.

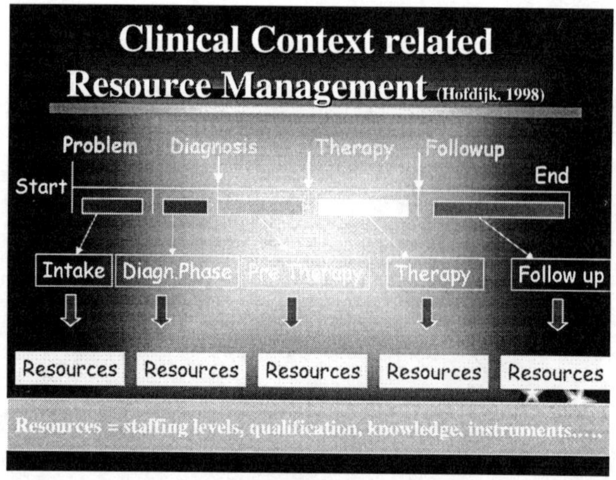

Figure 3   The Clinical Context Model

The modelling of the data was a major contribution to the objective of supporting nursing resource management. It is important to relate the interventions to patient groups for nursing resource management. The concept of clinical time helps to relate nursing events to specific clinical events, like a surgical procedure or the start of a new series of chemotherapy. The process of global feedback has given an important boost to the discussion on these issues. As linking nursing and clinical data is still a rather new concept, the first results emerged from clouds of misunderstanding and passionate discussion. In the last user group meeting, the feedback data were better understood and the appreciation for the information generated increased.

Many more loops of the global feedback cycle have to be made to enhance the model and the information instruments to contribute to the continuous learning process. To support nursing management in all its dimensions it is agreed that the next steps in the process should be focused on collecting data on the nursing treatment of all patients in the department. This has been one of the conclusions of the WISECARE Validation and Demonstration Sites as the departments know they are faced with a diversity of patient groups, each with a great variability of nursing problems, different patient outcomes and nursing resources. In the discussion regarding the modelling of nursing resource use, the episode structure has been used as an example of a method of the modelling (Figure 3). The episode concept has been elaborated in the CHAINE project [8]. Gradually the episode approach is being tested across Europe and in the next stage the linking between the nursing and the clinical care in the episode structure should be further tested and discussed.

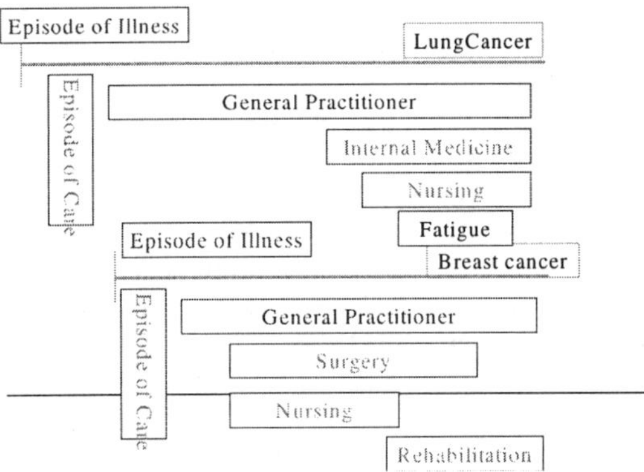

Figure 4   Episode Model linking Care Delivery to a Health Problem

A next step in this process has to be the gradual introduction of an effective concept of nursing interventions. The WISECARE project has contributed to the awareness of recording the assessment of nursing care for patients, the outcome of nursing interventions, but the nursing activities as such were not identified nor recorded. To truly manage the nursing equation of care demand of patients and required nursing capacity, nursing interventions have to be defined. Measuring the health / nursing needs of the patients on a continuous basis is a basic requirement for the ideal nursing management. The identification of nursing activities will be a major step for the further development and use of nursing resource management. Nursing resource management has different dimensions: (1) the management of the resources needed for the actual 'caseload' of a nursing ward, (2) the human resource management of the department taking into account the skills of a team of nurses, (3) the planning process of nursing resources associated with the projected case mix of a clinical department.

The introduction of the Moffitt resource scoring system was a first step, but further development is required. The linkage between the nursing needs of the patient and the available staffing resources is the basis for planning and controlling the resources of a nursing ward.

1.6 The WISECARE Tools

The introduction of the WiseTool supporting the collection and presentation of nursing data was a major breakthrough for the WISECARE project. It encouraged the data collection process, it introduced the benchmarking of sites' practice and supported the knowledge sharing on protocols/guidelines/ interventions. For many WiseNurses it was their first real life experience with information systems and especially through support of those who developed the tool, it built confidence and trust in technology. The WiseTool development has created a natural friend for nursing, which hopefully will be further developed in the coming years.

The electronic patient records of the WISECARE patients have been used not only for interaction purposes and individual patient care, but also for feedback on clinical and resource management. With the cycle of the WiseTool and the WISECARE data warehouse the process of sharing experiences and database with other institutions has lead to the development of a knowledge base of European "practices" in nursing. This allows participants to compare and measure their performances against the practices of other institutions. Many challenges have been identified around the interpretation of the 'knowledge' database and the process of comparing. One of the major results of the process was the strong demand from the Sites to include direct feedback functions in the WiseTool. The introduction of graphics in the tool has shown the way to an easier 'processing' of patient data by nurses.

The process has promoted the shift from individual knowledge to knowledge sharing and thus has promoted better patient care. The first barrier towards the use of an electronic patient record for nursing has been successfully managed. As the WISECARE project was focused on a selected group of patients and a restricted set of nursing problems the results can be the basis for further knowledge and software development. A major achievement from a European perspective was the adoption of the WISECARE project/ process by the European Oncology Nursing Society (EONS).

This will hopefully provide a solid basis for the next steps in the process of knowledge sharing and supporting and broadening the human network of oncology nurses using a Web of WiseNurses. The tools developed and used during the WISECARE project did not produce to marketable products. However the concepts can certainly be used for the next generation of tools supporting nurses. Another issue relevant for the assessment of the European impact analysis has been that the project could not start from a wide selection of clinical information systems among the WISECARE Validation Sites, so no contribution could be given to the use of existing nursing data for case mix analysis. The global feedback cycle with the WISECARE data warehouse has initiated a debate on nursing data, both from a knowledge sharing perspective as from a clinical modelling exercise. So the impact of WISECARE on nursing resource management within clinical case mix systems could not be assessed.

2   The Impact of the WISECARE Tools

The WISECARE approach has made a valuable contribution to documenting the care process and the benchmarking of processes and outcomes. The use of information systems, one of the objectives of a project funded by the fourth framework programme has been archived by the project. Several tools were developed during the WISECARE project supporting the different functions of the learning process. Each of the tools have a wise name, like the WiseTool for data collection, the WiseHoos for the data warehouse, the WiseCompass for the assessment, the WiseWeb for the Internet communication and the WiseMailingList supporting the electronic human network. These tools have supported the WISE community in the WISE learning process.

These tools have helped to prepare the shift from paper documentation and planning systems to an electronic Wise Nursing System. This process has been evaluated by the assessment and evaluation of information technology of the WISECARE approach. The data have been used here to assess the impact of WISECARE. In the following section the assessment is presented for each of the WISECARE tools and a general conclusion is made.

2.1 The WiseTool

To standardise the data collection activities of the WISECARE project a dedicated information system was developed. As the WISECARE project focused on a small group of patients, a standalone approach could be used. The system has been highly appreciated by the WiseNurses, but for a wider use in nursing departments it needs to be 'expanded' for other patient groups and nursing problems.

Analysis found that over half of the nurses thought data collection was meaningful although it added to their daily work.

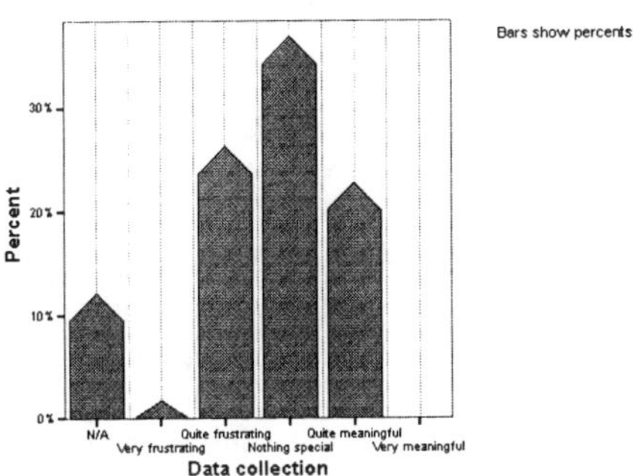

Figure 5 The Assessment of the Data Collection by the WISECARE Sites

Because as over 40% of the nurses indicated that the data collection was frustrating (Figure 5), tools for data collection should be looked after very carefully. Especially as more than half of the WiseNurses have indicated that they think they will not use the WiseTool after the end of the project (Figure 5). When a data collection system as WiseTool is introduced in nursing practice the golden rule should be obeyed of providing *registration should pay in 'cashable added value'*.

So the WiseTool has contributed to the collection of data and been the core tool for nurses to develop an appreciation of the benefits of structured data collection for a better evaluation of the care given. More than one third of the respondents (38%, N = 32) stated that the WiseTool programme would be used in their units after the closure of the WISECARE project. These nurses represented unevenly the different Sites which had participated in the project. Especially some of the nurses from the Validation Site B felt strongly that they would use the instrument also in the future. Surprisingly, three quarters of non-WiseNurses thought that the use of the programme would be likely to continue in their units after the end of the project.

2.2 The WiseWeb

The network of oncology care centres was established by using network software: Wise Web (WWW), the public homepage of which is 'http://wisecare.dn.uoa.gr' and the BSCW (Basic Support for Cooperative Work) server for sharing information between WISECARE members. The networking was also supported by use of an electronic mailing list called WiseMailingList.

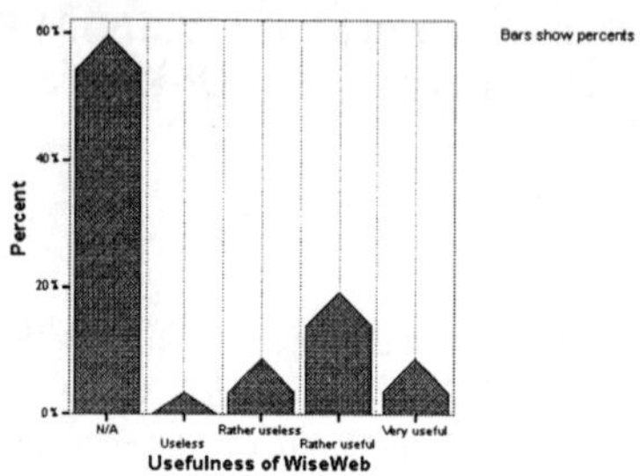

Figure 6   The Assessment of the WiseWeb

For most of the WISECARE Validation Sites the introduction of these services meant a paradigm shift, entering a new world of communication. It took some time before the ease of use was identified, because initiating such services required a change in the IT infrastructure. The appreciation was not overwhelming, but related to the scope of the project, it was positive (Figure 6).

2.3 The WISECARE Feedback

The feedback focus of the WISECARE project was on the global feedback, which was more or less at the end of the WISECARE data / information processing loop. However, during the WISECARE project the need for an instant feedback function in the WiseTool became evident. Direct feedback on data collected on patient care is a basic requirement for success and outcome. The findings about the instant and global feedback as evidence basis [1] suggest that to some degree the WISECARE concept had given the nurses that kind of feedback, which they were able to use in clinical judgement on both individual patients and patient group level. This may have depended on the use of the WiseTool and the WiseFeedback. If the data input to WiseTool had been regular, preferably daily, the nurses were able to receive the instant feedback in graphics of the patient's situation which allowed comparison to the patient's previous data. This finding is supported by the fact that some nurses reported changing their way of evaluating patient's progress. The WiseTool was the WISECARE product that would have helped them to do so, because of the facility of individualised instant feedback. [1]

The appreciation for the feedback function increased towards the end of the project, which illustrates the value of the exercise and raises the return on investment (Figure 7).

2.4 Concluding Remarks

The most important impact of the feedback of the project might be illustrated by the assessment of the importance of evidence based nursing, which is qualified as "rather" to "very" important by over 80% of the nurses (Figure 8). The future will see this investment flourish among the new WISECARE users, through the support the European Oncology Nurses Society.

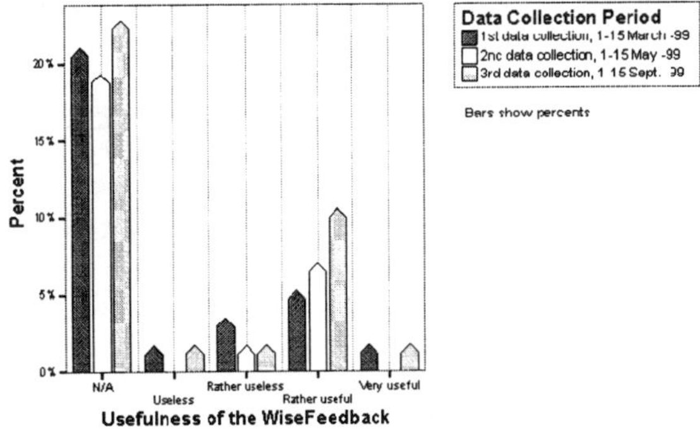

Figure 7   The Growing Appreciation of the WiseFeedback

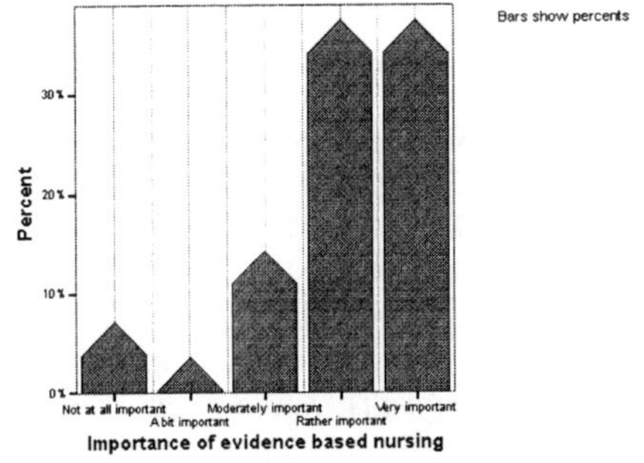

Figure 8   Scoring the Importance of Evidence Based Nursing among the WiseNurses

3   The European Impact

The adoption of the series of WISECARE tools to support the nursing care process in many dimensions is a positive indication of the transition process towards the use of IT. The enthusiasm generated during the WISECARE conferences both in Leuven in June 1999 and in Glasgow in December 1999 is an indicator of a greater market for the approach and the tools. The discovery of clinical context related patient care management has the potential to create a generic model for the support of nursing management with a logical integration in the clinical care process. Although this approach will take quite some time to be accepted and implemented, it seems logical when considering the acceptance of information technology as a basic tool for documentation and communication. The WISECARE project has shown how slowly the process of the adoption of an information technology strategy for nursing takes within a living organisation. But the project has proven that nurses are eager to adopt new technological tools to improve the quality of their work. The focus on a broader implementation of WISECARE should thus be on creating support at a managerial level in hospitals across Europe for the use of ICT for nursing. The development of WISECARE for nursing strategy should be consistent with the increased need for the introduction of an electronic patient record within hospitals and other health care institutions. A balance should be found between a step-by-step approach of the introduction of WISECARE tools supporting nursing care, within a strategic framework at institutional level. Even with the introduction of WISECARE for new Sites focused at the same patient groups and the same nursing problems, it seems essential to embed such an implementation within the ICT strategy of the hospital to ensure a long term perspective and the basis for a step by step approach for a further and broader implementation of the WISE nursing tools.

Based on experience with WISECARE and other CPR related projects the following lessons can be learned:

- Introduction of new tools should be managed in a project with the focus on a sound implementation in a living organisation.
- A project must be user driven and focused at improving the quality of life of the nurses in their process of care delivery.
- Nurses / users should be the promoters of the ICT system.
- The unique selling points will be the improvement of the processes by gaining nursing time and improving the quality of care given to patients.
- A project should be embedded in the ICT strategy of the hospital.
- A project should contribute to the communication on patient care within and across the boundaries of the hospital.
- A system used should be embedded in a network of other clinical systems, which share valuable clinical and administrative data.

These arguments need to be taken into account when defining a market strategy for the WISECARE results. The WISECARE project has created a series of products used for the project: including not only the WiseTool, the WISE net, the WISEcompass and the WISE protocols, but also the WISE approach of supporting nursing care with Information Systems. The latter forms the basis for a wider application of WISE ICT for nursing, which requires a proactive approach and an investment in new WISE based tools.

The products have to be seen as results from a research product, so more or less half products on the way to develop fully applicable tools to support nursing care in practice. So they do not have great commercial value, but are very important steps in the process of operational support for nursing care. During the process the concept of a WISE-Station for nurses has emerged, which integrates both the tools supporting direct nursing care, as functions for nursing resource management, nursing quality assurance, nursing knowledge management, and functions for communication with clinicians, nurse practitioners outside the hospital and patients. The concept of the WISEStation will stimulate the use of health telematics systems in nursing by providing proof of the impact of a better use of information by nurses. The WISECARE project has created a great market potential, which needs an impressive follow up. The commitment of the EONS organisation is a proof of concept, which might lead to the creation of a second life of WISECARE. The integration of the WiseTool concept within the Mirador Clinical Workstation concept of HISCOM might lead to the initiation of the WISE Station in practice.

Another important parameter in the adaptation process will be the change of the funding system of Health Care in Europe. The past twenty years have shown how changes of funding system are drivers for changes within the organisation of health care institutions. External changes lead to major adaptations of the internal systems of the health care organisations. As the costs of health care have risen enormously during the last decade governments have tried to adapt the systems by introducing incentives to control costs. The funding systems have changed from a fee for service orientation towards a more output-oriented system where a price is given for a specific type of treatment. This has raised interest in the process of care, because a better understanding of the care delivered is a good basis for controlling the costs of treatment. The clinical debate starting from clinical knowledge, measuring the actual process of care and the output and based on actual benchmarking of best / known practices will lead to changes in the care process and a more efficient use of resources. This approach can be qualified as consistent with

WISECARE and the basis for an elaboration of the concept in practice. As the hypothesis is that the changes of the funding system are an important parameter in the decision making process, a focus on nursing resource use is needed in the further development of case mix funding systems in Europe. This might be the key for a wider adoption of the WISECARE approach towards a comprehensive and complete nursing record within European health care systems. Time will tell when the policy making process will shift to a higher gear and become the co-driver towards Wise Nursing Management. But the most important fact is that the EONS has decided to continue the WISECARE project, which is the best guarantee for having impact on an European level.

References

[1]   Nyberg T & Kinnunen J. Report on the impact of WISECARE on clinical behaviour of oncology nurses. Deliverable 5.2 in WISECARE project, 1999.

[2]   Halloran E. Nursing workload, medical diagnosis related groups and nursing diagnosis. *Research in Nursing and Health* 1985; 8 (4): 421-433.

[3]   Sermeus W. Variabiliteit van de verpleegkundige verzorging in algemene ziekenhuizen. *Acta Hospitalia* 1992; 4: 5-13.

[4]   Contract 1997 between EU DG XIII and the WISECARE partners.

[5]   Hoy D. Deliverable 3.4 Data Input Programme in WISECARE project, 1998

[6]   Hoy D. Deliverable 3.2 Record layout of the database in WISECARE project, 1997.

[7]   Sermeus W. Annual project review: Workflow Information Systems for European Nursing Care. Belgium: Katholieke Universiteit Leuven, Centre for Health Services Research, 1998.

[8]   Sanderson H. Final Report on the CHAINE project : Episodes for Resource Management in the community, 1999.

Part V

Future

Future Development and Methodological Issues

Luc Delesie

1   From Design to Decision Making

The previous sections on methodological issues, problems and options (chapter 2) enumerated many pitfalls including:

- Good intentions do not lead automatically to a good design and good variables.
- A good design and good variables do not automatically lead to good data.
- Good data do not automatically lead to valuable information.
- Valuable information does not automatically lead to good feedback.
- Good feedback does not automatically lead to better management of the nurses' workflow in the nursing care for cancer patients.

1.1   Good Design and Good Variables

Several variables have been reshaped during the WISECARE project while some others have been added. The time issue proved to be particularly difficult. Incidence oriented, longitudinal designs are of more of interest than prevalence oriented, cross-sectional designs for the management of nursing care. The project had to decide on a cross-sectional design for the resources and only arrived at a workable longitudinal design for the clinical variables after many false starts and months of discussions. It is indeed a burden to stick to a longitudinal design from day to day. The instant feedback motivates to stick the Clinical Sites to the design.

1.1.1   Good Data

The collection of data is still far for the most energy and time consuming part of WISECARE. It is however a necessary, though insufficient, step to arrive at communication on the basis of evidence about the diversity of the patient population, the variability of care, patient outcomes and nursing resources on the aggregate level among nursing units and patient groups.

As a result, much attention should go to the collection of data by way of electronic means. As of now data registration still takes 90% of all time and energy and should be made as attractive, informative, supportive as possible. This implies the clear-cut definition of variables as well as the use of software to render this tedious task easier. WISETOOL version 2 did the job.

The introduction of "instant feedback" was a big step forward. Unfortunately, it is not yet a true feedback as any export or import of data is involved. It does familiarize the nurses with data and data variables, patient classifications, computers, ICT, coding systems, electronic nursing patient records, communication with other nurses beyond the walls of their own nursing unit. This may eventually lead to communication on the diversity of patients and the variability of care from the nursing perspective with other professionals or health care managers such as human resource managers, economic managers, and quality management. This communication may eventually lead to decision-making on the basis of workflow information. It also familiarized the nurses with computer generated graphs and data visualization products. The introduction of the clinical time vector in the instant feedback was a benefit. Unless some automated procedure based on electronic records becomes widely available, the manual data collction will always be subject to a high level of incompleteness. Indeed although all precautions were taken, the data available by December 1999 showed still a lot of missing, incomplete or unreliable data.

1.1.2   Valuable Information

Data analysis is simple: tables, lists, sums and averages are well known and easy to compute. Sensible and meaningful data analysis is somewhat more complicated. The project solved the issue somehow by introducing a clear-cut division between "instant feedback" and "global feedback". Instant feedback does not involve aggregation or benchmarking. Every nurse can see for herself patient scores on daily basis. Instant feedback organises the original data in an accessible and interpretable way: an accessible summary of individual patient parameters and indicators. Global feedback requires aggregation and benchmarking, see above. It is unavoidable that feedback generates more questions than that it gives answers. The nurses are slowly becoming aware of the possibilities as well as the limitations of hard facts on the aggregate level. Any aggregation pushes the individual patient, the individual nurse and his most specific and typifying characteristics to the background in order to stress such abstract and ephemeral aspects as a group of patients or a nursing team. Even the most complete and detailed multivariate database will never be able to cover all aspects of all patients and all detail. The aggregation operations on which feedback information relies have proven to be at least as important as the benchmarking operations that any feedback entails. This is particularly the case in health and health care feedback where the classifications and scales in use remain soft and subjective notwithstanding all attempts to clearly delineate the different categories, gradations or levels. The "official" classifications and scales all aim by way of semantics and syntax to fix the relations between the categories, gradations or levels. However, real life nurses and patients do not always adhere to these rules-of-logic. Subjective estimates, opinions, drifts of opinion and temporary moods result in variety, shifts and some chaos. Unreliable and corrupt data is run of the mill: patients do not always want to state that they feel lousy and very unhappy. State-of-the-art statistical and analysing tools have their space but should be sensibly used. The most advanced database and datamining methods only produce information and do not guarantee knowledge and understanding. Sensible data analysis remains a prerequisite.

1.1.3   Good Feedback

The user is the ultimate criterion for good feedback. Several attempts led to the global feedback presented below. Unfortunately, little experience with feedback could be built up during the project. Consequently, we do not know from the users how good this feedback is or how it can be improved beyond the addition of explanatory tools for example glossaries. The implementation of Information and Communication Technology – ICT in health care is lagging in comparison to other sectors of economic activity: agriculture, service industries such as banking and legal services. This fact meant that hardly any of the participating nurses had ever encountered clinical nursing data on the aggregate level beyond some scientific and professional publications. Few nurses were concretely aware of what feedback could possibly mean for them. Hence, the opinions that circulated were to say the least, divergent. The contact with the first feedback products was a new, maybe even "alien", experience for most of them and raised a lot of questions. We anticipate the actual global feedback to improve on the basis of a larger experience as a consequence of a larger – continuing - database in the future. More refined and more reliable data analysis during the global feedback production will through gauging and calibration in more reliable classifications and scales. The volume of data will result in greater stability of reference, mirror, base distributions among the WISECARE Sites. Trends may start to appear, hopefully in the anticipated direction: better patient outcomes and improved resource management in the participating nursing units.

1.1.4   *Better Management on the Basis of Feedback*

The introduction of feedback about clinical nursing data as a method to improve clinical and resource management has proven to be much more difficult than anticipated. Though everybody approved the objective and was enthusiastic to participate from the start, the road to implementation was much more tiresome. It remains too early to look for signs of better patient care management as a result of participation in the WISECARE project.

2   Clinical Resource Interface

As explained in detail before, the WISECARE project basically investigates clinical characteristics of the WISECARE patients on the one hand and the resource characteristics of the nursing team on the other hand. However, at one point in time it becomes necessary to link the one with the other. Indeed, the main goal of WISECARE is: *"the evaluation of the impact of nursing care in the whole quality care for patients, through a systematic exploitation of data in electronic patient records, the definition of a model for integration of the nursing component in DRG-based systems and a development of a knowledge base of "best practices" in nursing care."* These objectives meant that the impact of nursing care, the nursing component or the nursing resources in view of the patients, their electronic patient records or clinical needs had to be reviewed.

Though the project is almost ready to link up the clinical feedback with the resource feedback in order to develop a knowledge base of "best practices" in nursing care, this step has not yet been taken.

We will discuss the reasons why we are convinced that going through that process is an integral part of the WISECARE project experience and are a lesson for future efforts. The WISECARE patient data variables changed quite a lot during the course of the project. The final variable list was available by May 1998. However, first global feedback was produced in November 1998 and presented the nurses the experimental design of the patient data. Historically nurses are geared towards individual care for individual patients. Best practices, however, demand aggregation of individual data in order to transcend this individual level to arrive at group level. Individual clinical data follow the incidence approach or longitudinal design. Events and markers are recorded along the road in the medical record. This introduces the notion of clinical time.

It took until December 1998 to incorporate the meaning of the clinical time concept into the project. By May 1999, a refined registration procedure was implemented and actual data was being recorded and information becoming available.

Resources deal with the nursing unit as a whole. Every WISECARE nursing unit has some WISECARE patients. Nursing care follows a somewhat different logic than the medical care or pharmaceutical care. Medical and pharmaceutical care overwhelmingly focus on the individual patient. The nursing team's resources involve as well the individual patients and the group of all patients on the unit. Resources are shared among the team members. The nursing team takes responsibility for the group of patients on the unit. Consequently it is useless to evaluate nursing care solely on the level of an individual patient. If the workload is heavy, all patients will receive less care. If the workload happens to be light, then all patients will get more care, e.g. nursing care in the weekend differs strongly from nursing care during the week, nursing care in the morning differs significantly from nursing care in the afternoon due to scheduling deficiencies imposed upon the nursing unit from the outside or just habit. Naturally priorities and minimum thresholds are set but this reality forces us to look at nursing resources from a cross-sectional or prevalence point of view (see Figure 1).

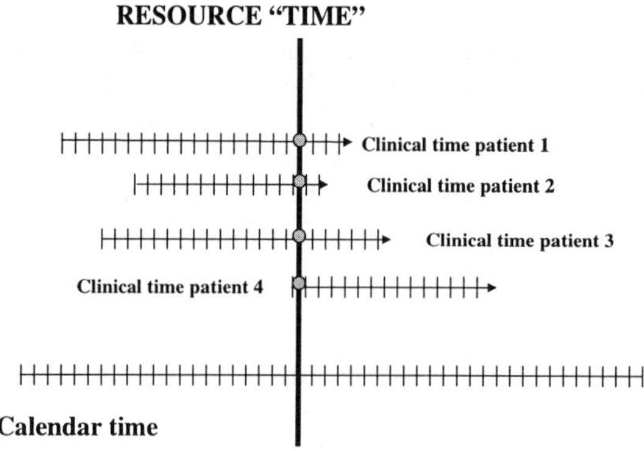

Figure 1   Variation of Nursing Resources during Patient's Hospital Stay

This design takes into account that nursing care varies over the total stay of the patient. There is no such thing as an "average" nursing care for a patient. The design becomes even more complicated as WISECARE patients may only comprise a minority of patients on the nursing unit. Hence the two questions become:

- *What resources go to WISECARE patients and what resources go to NON-WISECARE patients?*
- *How are the WISECARE nursing resources divided among the individual WISECARE patients at their individual clinical times?*

In order to investigate these questions, one has to investigate the association or relationship between the aggregated clinical indicators and the aggregated resource indicators.

By the end of 1999 sufficient data started to become available to allow investigation the relationships between the aggregated clinical indicators and the aggregated resource indicators in a sensible way. It will be most interesting to establish: if WISECARE patients whose assessment indicators show higher care needs are indeed associated with more nursing resources: if nursing resources in every participating nursing unit are allocated over time according to care needs or not. How the different units differ with respect to their allocation performance? Unfortunately, knowledge and understanding of these questions is prerequisite to start the discussion on "best nursing practices" from an operational rather than a theoretical or consensus point of view.

Starting up a WISECARE Oncology User Group

Nora Kearney, Morven Miller

1   Introduction

The development of pan-European nursing research is in its infancy as nurses across the Continent struggle to deal with numerous barriers, which prevent collaborative projects [1]. Issues such as language, distance, culture and lack of resources have hampered nurses' attempts to develop collaborative research programmes across Europe, making the comparison of cancer nursing care problematic. The WISECARE project has given European cancer nurses the opportunity to overcome these problems and develop a network with the aim of harmonising patient care and so improving patient outcomes. In Europe, nurses account for the largest group of health care professionals within cancer care and these is an increasing requirement for them to articulate their contribution to patient outcomes.

2   Collaboration within the WISECARE Project

In developing a framework for the WISECARE project it was clear that a strong clinical focus was required to ensure optimal use of any information system developed. To this end, the European Oncology Nursing Society (EONS) was approached to become key partners in the project. EONS was established in 1984 as a Federation of Oncology Nursing Societies, institutions and agencies involved in cancer care. Currently EONS has a membership of 23 National Oncology Societies, 207 individual members, representing 22,300 nurses in 30 countries. This established network provided the platform for the clinical development of the WISECARE project thereby ensuring the clinical orientation of the project.

From the outset, EONS has been an integral member of the WISECARE team and has taken responsibility for identifying and supporting the nurses in the clinical areas involved in the project. Chapters 1.1, 2.1, 4.2 and 4.4 in this book clearly demonstrate the added value of this clinical orientation and act as an impetus for the establishment of a WISECARE User Group.

3   Clinical Results of WISECARE

The nurses involved within the project have identified the value of the project to their own clinical practice and following the WISECARE conference in Glasgow in December 1999 are keen to both continue with the project and inform others of the benefits of the

WISECARE model of working. There have been many outcomes from the project, which directly impact nursing practice. Nurses are able to compare and measure their patient outcomes against the other Clinical Sites and established benchmarks and from this information, emulate the nursing practice of those sites with the best patient outcomes. Within individual Clinical Sites, individual patient outcomes are being evaluated in conjunction with nursing interventions, facilitating evaluation of specific interventions on specific patient outcomes. This process is also valued by patients who now have a shared language with which to communicate effectively with health care professionals and illustrate their experiences and symptoms. The nurses are also able to communicate and discuss best nursing practice through information technology systems across Europe. Consequently, the project has markedly altered the way in which nurses transfer knowledge and develop nursing practice. There is now evidence to support the belief that not only the project has resulted in a change to nurses' clinical management over the course of the three years, but that patient outcomes for the clinical indictors have also clearly improved.

4   Network

One of the major factors in the success of the WISECARE project has been the establishment of a network of clinically based nurses. Without the enthusiasm of the nurses involved in WISECARE, the project would not have been able to establish such a collaborative network. Having developed in terms of not only the structure of their care provision and the evidence base behind this, they are concerned about a future without WISECARE and the benefits that it has provided for them. Therefore it is intended, by utilising the EONS infrastructure, to maintain some form of interaction between these nurses and if possible, expand the network to other areas of Europe.

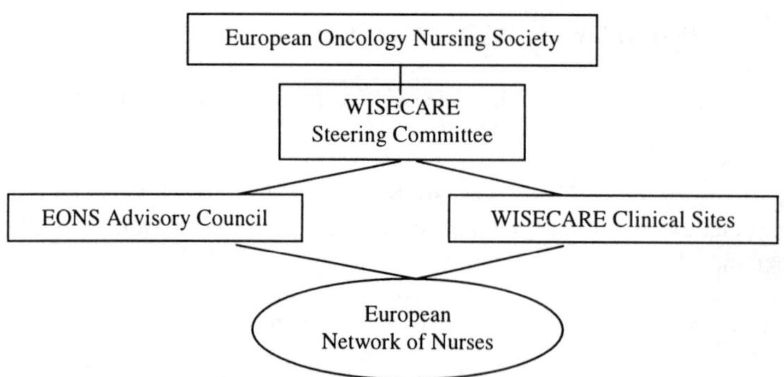

Figure 1   Proposed Structure for the Future for WISECARE

5   EONS WISECARE User Group

It was always the intention to hand over the ownership of the outcomes of WISECARE to EONS who has played a vital role in the development and support of the project over the last three years. EONS would be responsible for the dissemination of the project throughout the European cancer nursing community. In order to achieve this, the Society has considered the most appropriate method for dissemination and proposes the development of a WISECARE Steering Committee to oversee future developments of the project. This Steering Committee will be composed of three members of the Executive

Board of the Society and will collaborate closely with the EONS Advisory Council.

This proposed structure for the future for WISECARE (Figure 1) would facilitate the dissemination of the project's benefit on a pan-Europe basis, utilising the network of cancer nurses already known and established through the European Oncology Nursing Society

6   Outcomes of the WISECARE User Group

Through this proposed new structure, the WISECARE project would continue to provide benefits to oncology nurses across Europe. The collaborative process would continue to be fostered, so overcoming the barriers that have previously prevented this. Knowledge sharing for the development of best nursing care will result in the development of inductive, experience based knowledge, driven by clinical practice and patient requirements. Through such knowledge sharing, patient outcomes will continue to improve. Furthermore, cancer nursing will continue to reap, and extend, the benefits already seen in the project relating to the nursing profession as a while. The philosophy of care delivery the WISECARE has developed will continue as this has been shown to give nurses a deepening sense of empowerment and optimism and a vision for the future. Cancer nurses across Europe will continue to realise the benefits of autonomy in their future practice. Furthermore and perhaps more importantly, continuing the project will facilitate the visualisation of the process of nursing and identifying the unique contribution of nursing to patient outcomes, so proving the value of nursing and securing its place within today's health care system.

References

[1]   Kearney N, Campbell S & Sermeus W. Practising for the future: utilising information technology in cancer nursing practice. *European Journal of Oncology Nursing* 1998; **2** (3): 169-175.

WISECARE
W. Sermeus et al. (Eds.)
IOS Press, 2000

Exploitation Plan

Walter Sermeus, Lieve Goossens, Tonny Gypen, Kenny Willems

A major intention at the start of WISECARE was to hand over the ownership of the outcomes of WISECARE to EONS who has played a vital role in the development and support of the project over the last three years. EONS will be responsible for the dissemination of the project throughout the European cancer nursing community. In order to achieve this, the Society has considered the most appropriate method for dissemination and proposes the development of a WISECARE Steering Committee to oversee future developments of the project.

Ten WISECARE-products have been identified. Eight of them will be internally exploited within the new WISECARE consortium: The Leuven Chemotherapy Risk Assessment Scale (LCRAS), the standardised clinical scales for measuring fatigue, nausea and vomiting, pain, oral problems and nursing intensity, the patient models, the instant and global feedback, the WiseTool-HIS links, the WiseWeb, the WiseHoos and the WiseCompass. Two products will be externally exploited. For the WiseTool a license will be taken in order to incorporated it in any Hospital Information System. Special rights are reserved for EONS and the partners in the project. For the WISECARE network, a trademark on name and logo will be taken. Moving into the world of evidence-based clinical practice, the whole WISECARE project has to breathe a spirit of trust: trust in the reliability and validity of the scales, the design frames, the analysis, the guidelines, the links, the partners in the network, the feedback. A WISECARE Trademark should help to support a high level of trust. Protecting the WISECARE name and logo by a Trademark allows the label to be selectively assigned to highly reliable and valid standardised scales and guidelines. It can be used to help software vendors to build in the WiseTool functionalities in the electronic patient record as 'WISECARE compatible', meaning that the required functionalities are incorporated to load reference scores into instant feedback modules, to generate global feedback reports etc.

Is there a market for WISECARE? The WISECARE project has been designed as a general application system within health care. The demonstration domain is oncological care. The very specific demonstration domain of oncological care has limited impact on the software which has a very flexible and open design. The highest impact is on the WISECARE knowledge server which is very oncology specific given the standardised scales, data collection design and risk appraisal tools. The first aim to launch the project in a production environment will be in oncological care. In a second phase, the project knowledge could be expanded to other health care domains.

Potential benificiaries are patients and their representatives: social insurance companies and governments; professionals represented by health care organisations and professional associations, pharmaceutical companies and ICT-companies.

1   Products and Services

1.1   Description

Evaluating the impact of the WISECARE project on nursing care, it is clear that the opportunity to discuss and compare nursing interventions and consequent patient outcomes using the latest IT facilities on a pan-European basis has been an entirely novel concept for nurses. WISECARE has required a new way of thinking and developing the spirit of evidence-based nursing with a close connection to clinical reality. Use of research findings or utilisation of feedback, received from outside one's own organisation, is not common in nursing care.

Two types of products emerge from the WISECARE-project: the WISECARE Knowledge Server, called Wise^2 and the WISECARE software: the WiseTool and the WiseWeb, WiseHoos and WiseCompass.

1.2   The WISECARE Knowledge Server

The core value of the WISECARE-project is definitively in the Knowledge Server. Davenport & Prusack [2] define knowledge as "a fluid mix of framed experience, values, contextual information and expert insight that provides a framework for evaluating and incorporating new experiences and information." This definition explains that knowledge is not neat or simple but rather exists within people. If information is to become knowledge, we work at this. The transformation happens through such "C" words as:

- Comparison: how does information about this situation compare to that of other situations we have known? Benchmarking activities can support this transformation process.
- Consequences: what implications does the information have for decisions and actions? The focus on outcomes and a systematic evaluation and review of effects and outcomes is supportive
- Context: How does this bit of knowledge relates to others?
- Conversation: what do other people think? Networking is the way to tackle this issue.

The WISECARE Knowledge Server consists of five contributional parts: categorizing patients according to their risk; standardised scales; modelling for understanding relations between problems, interventions and outcomes; instant and global feedback and networking.

1.2.1   Toxicity Level of Chemotherapy Evaluation

The first contributional part of knowledge is done when evaluation of the toxicity level of chemotherapy according to some specific side-effects as pain, fatigue, nausea and vomiting and mucositis. For measuring this level of toxicity, the Leuven Chemotherapy Risk Assessment Scale (LCRAS) has been developed [3]. The scale shows the risk that 36 chemotherapy products can have on 47 side effects. It was developed in 1994 by an interdisciplinary group of Belgian nurses, pharmacists and doctors, in close co-operation with Glaxo Wellcome and the Flemish Oncology and Radiotherapy Society. It was part of the Nurses Cytostatic Compendium, Practical Guide for Nurses. For 36 chemotherapy products, it provides information on about the product, incompatibilities, skin contamination, eye contamination, spilling, extravasation, excretion and frequent side effects.

Added value from the WISECARE project are:
- Sensitivity and specificity in evaluating the LCRAS in predicting the impact of the

chemotherapy product on fatigue, pain, nausea & vomiting, oral problems.
- Adjusting references scores on fatigue, pain, nausea & vomiting, oral problems per LCRAS-risk category risk and per day after administration of chemotherapy. Although, the scores are adjusted by the toxicity level of chemotherapy and clinical time (days after chemotherapy), there still is a high variability from one centre to another centre. The scores can be used to evaluate clinical performance in the management of side effects of chemotherapy.

The LCRAS is still in phase of development. The analysis shows that:
- Not all treatment profiles have been categorised in the LCRAS-frame: 36 out of 185 different treatment profiles. Many treatments use a combination of chemotherapy drugs. The interactions and effects of this on the LCRAS-scoring is not completely known. Some products (because of the main university environment of the Clinical Sites) are experimental in the context of phase III clinical trial, making LCRAS-coding impossible.
- The risks have been classified based on the expertise of the clinicians and the knowledge about the toxicity levels of the chemotherapy drugs. Based on the analysis, some LCRAS-coding are valid. Some of them certainly need review.
- In the LCRAS, risks for side-effects have been associated with chemotherapy regimens. However some symptoms are not associated with treatments but with the underlying pathology.
- The impact of the prescribed dose of a product on the risk profile is still unknown.

Based on the LCRAS, an adjusted risk assessment scale for breast cancer surgery on pain, fatigue, nausea & vomiting and oral care has been developed. Based on empirical evidence, nurses working on the AZ Groningen ward for more than 2 years, created their GBRAS.

WISECARE shows added value in:
- Sensitivity and specificity in evaluating the GBRAS in predicting the impact of the chemotherapy product on fatigue, pain, nausea & vomiting, oral problems.
- Adjusting references scores on fatigue, pain, nausea & vomiting, oral problems per GBRAS-risk category risk and per day after administration of chemotherapy. Although, the scores are adjusted by the toxicity level of chemotherapy and clinical time (days after chemotherapy), there still is a high variability from one centre to another centre. The scores can be used to evaluate clinical performance in the management of side effects of chemotherapy.

1.2.2 Standardised Scales for Measuring Clinical Outcomes

The second contributional part of knowledge provides standardised scales for measuring clinical outcomes for guiding clinical practice. They are useful to guide communication among nurses, from nurse to doctor, from nurse to patient and vice versa. As with all scales, psychometric criteria such as reliability, validity, sensitivity are important. Because of use in daily practice, the use of the scale should be not too time-consuming and be user friendly by nurses as well as by patients or their relatives. Within the WISECARE project, following tools have been selected and evaluated:
- The Oral Assessment Guide (OAG) [4] which is a concise, clinically useful tool comprising of 8 questions, developed through clinical expertise and literature review, to record and communicate oral cavity status and determine changes expected with stomatotoxic treatments. A clinical guide with photographic material was provided by Glaxo Welcome as learning material for teaching patients or relatives how to evaluate the mouth status in a valid and reliable way.

- The Piper Fatigue Scale (PFS) [5] which is composed of 22 numerically-scaled items (0-10) which measure 4 dimensions of subjective fatigue, behavioural/severity, affective/meaning, sensory and cognitive/mood. Both subscales and total fatigue scores can be calculated. The Piper Fatigue Scale was not retained in period 3 of the project. Although very useful in a research environment, it was found to be too time-consuming for patients to complete in a real life clinical environment.
- The European Organisation for Research and Treatment of Cancer Quality of Life Questionnaire (EORTC QLQ-C30) [6] which is a modular approach for evaluating quality of life. It incorporates 9 multi-item scales: 5 functional scales (physical, role, cognitive, emotional and social), 3 symptom scales (fatigue, pain, nausea and vomiting) and a global health and quality of life scale. Several single-item symptom measures are also included. In period 3 of the project, only the 3 symptom scales were retained for further evaluation.

Although many clinical scales are evaluated on their psychometric properties in literature, most of these evaluations are done in controlled research environments. The added value of WISECARE is on the evaluation of these standardised scales in real life environments.

- Providing a standardised patient monitoring design per indicator. In the project, the data collection design has been standardised for 10 days after chemotherapy. This standard way of patient monitoring and data recording will enhance the comparability of data among different Clinical Sites and will enhance the knowledge on the course of side-effects of chemotherapy. These data can be used to evaluate the impact of treatment during the course of chemotherapy.
- Most of the standardised scales are aggregated in a simple Likert-type way of adding up all item scores. The added value of WISECARE is in a more sensitive aggregation of the different item scores improving the psychometric properties of the scale (e.g. sensitivity, validity, reliability).

The work in analysing standardised clinical scales is still in phase of development. The analysis shows that:

- The use of standardised clinical scales for monitoring daily practice is very new to many nurses. This many leads to low reliability figures and a lot of missing values (days as well as items). It is important that the data collection is triggered by the software actively asking for data. Another problem encountered in daily practice is the data input. Currently, the data are collected on paper first (by patient or nurse) before being put into the computer system. Although the input is very user friendly, the effort is double and can lead to many forms waiting for input. There is a need for portable input devices, that can be used as well by nurses and patients (even to take home), and is linked with the automated patient record.
- During the project, several patient monitoring designs were tested. The final one was highly structured and focused on a standardised daily data collection design until 10 days after administration of chemotherapy or surgery. The analysis shows that for some indicators, 10 days is probably too long (e.g. nausea and vomiting). However for other indicators such as fatigue and mucositis, it is much too short. Further analysis should be done to determine the length of patient monitoring for side effects and the optimal frequency of data collection e.g. each day, every other day.
- To keep the project manageable, it focused on a selection of 4 clinical indicators. A library of clinical indicators has been built, according to a selection of patient problems (pathology, treatment or patient characteristic oriented). For each indicator, the patient monitoring design (length and frequency of follow up) can be determined.
- Further development in the psychometric properties of the scale (e.g. sensitivity, validity, reliability) should be performed by more sensible aggregation of item scores. In WISECARE, the Oral Assessment Guide has been processed as an example. For all

other scales in the library, these further developments should be started.

- Developing specifications for electronic patient records. Most of the EPR are developed from a data or thesaurus/lexicon point of view, supporting transactional communication processes. The use of these data for management/research purposes is a result of the availability of the data. There is however no guarantee that, even if all possible data are recorded at 'atomic data level', the data are useful to support the relevant management questions. An example illustrates this remark more concretely: to calculate incidence/prevalence rates, it is not only important knowing the presence of an event but also the absence of an event. Recording the absence of an event requires an active measuring process to distinguish it from missing values. The alternative is that first the information needs of the users are addressed, which leads to a selection of relevant variables, a level of detail, confounding variables and the design of a concrete sampling frame. It is certainly new that the design in which data are collected is part of the specifications of a EPR.

1.2.3   Developing Patient Models [7]

The third contributional part of knowledge is in enhancing the level of understanding of the relations between problems, interventions and outcomes, through the development of patient models. The developed model is coded in a simulation language EpiScript.

The status of the product is in prototyping for general health care problems. The use of this methodology in nursing care, is still in a developmental stage. Further needs are:

- In the WISECARE project, the model generates virtual patients that will undergo chemotherapy ("with-protocol" and "no-protocol"). Measuring intervention strategies could turn this 'virtual' scenarios into real scenarios with real results and output. These kind of simulations needs a lot of data.
- Opening the project in collecting intervention strategies, is very complex but worthwhile. It certainly attracts the interest of pharmaceutical companies who are interested in the effectiveness of treatment protocols in which their drugs are part (instead of just evaluating the efficacy of the drug in the controlled environment of a Randomised Clinical Trial). It opens up the disease management perspective in which pharmaceutical companies are not only addressing their products to clinicians, but are interested in improving the way the drugs are delivered to patients (right dose, right time, right way). The information and instructions that comes along, compliance rates, the final result and patient perspectives. It is complex because of time lag effects in therapy and the high variable nature in which treatments are combined.

1.2.4   Feedback

The fourth contributional part of knowledge is in feedback. Two types of feedback are generated.

The first type of feedback is instant feedback, in which the feedback loop is very short. The recorded data are plotted in a graph. The 'instant feedback' facilitates the demonstration of the impact of nursing interventions on individual patient outcomes, going some way to prove the tangible difference that nursing interventions confer to patient outcomes.

The second level of feedback is 'global' feedback, which requires a much larger feedback loop. Data are send regularly (with an agreed periodicity: e.g. every 6 weeks, every 2 months) to the datawarehouse in which the data from all Clinical Sites are stored. Before transfer, the data are anonymized and encrypted. These data are processed to develop the global feedback. Before producing feedback, data are cleaned and organised.

Developing and selecting the right indicators and the right reports in the right presentations for the first time can take quite some time. Global feedback reports are on paper, use a graphic interface and are made available on the Website. Their main goal is to position each Clinical Site, in relation to all other Clinical Sites in the network, regarding the clinical management of side-effects of chemotherapy and surgery (fatigue, nausea & vomiting, pain, mucositis).

Besides the clinical management global feedback, the WISECARE project provides feedback on nursing resource use for example qualification level and staffing levels. The purpose is similar as for the clinical management feedback: positioning and understanding. The added value of WISECARE is in the standardised reports for oncological nurses, the reference data (average, median, range,....) on fatigue, nausea & vomiting, mucositis, pain, nursing resources.

The global feedback report is in a developmental stage:

- Global feedback become more and more useful when a trend (moving, stable) become visible so that a Clinical Site is able to position itself in a reliable way over time. Three feedback report should be the starting position. More feedback reports will necessary.

- In the actual WISECARE project, the reports are covering a standard time period (1 months, 2 months, 3 months). During the project the content and format of the feedback report was under development and changing. The impact of the global feedback reports on clinical behaviour can not been assessed to date.

- The more advanced level of feedback is realised through integrating instant and global feedback. This can be done by completing the instant feedback score with a reference score (according to the clinical time and risk score for that particular patient). From the global feedback, reference scores can be regularly uploaded into the instant feedback module.

1.2.5 Networking

The fifth contributional part of knowledge is in networking. There is a large agreement in management literature that three types of assets of an organisation can be identified [8]: the financial capital (the numbers, plain resources), the human capital (the knowledge, skills, experiences, attitudes of all people) and the social capital (the accessible networks with specific resources). Burt (1992) shows that real value of a network is not in the number of contacts, but in the quality of the contacts [8]. Well-structured networks archive much higher results than non-structured networks. Benefit-rich networks have (1) contacts established in the places where useful bits of information are likely to be aired, (2) provide a reliable flow of information to and from those places. Networks are most effective when there is a good balance between cohesion and diversity.

An important fact is that EONS has two types of members: individual nurses and national associations of oncological nurses. There is no organisational membership. The WISECARE network consists of organisational membership (mainly hospitals, research institutes,....) in:

- Sharing information on clinical managment and nursing resource management by contributing to the global feedback
- Exchanging clinical guidelines and protocols
- Formal and informal meetings, contacts etc.
- The network is in the prototype phase, is dealing with eleven Clinical Sites across Europe. Further development of the network need consideration for:
- Selection criteria: Some selection criteria were explicit (having access to Internet, being computerised at the nursing ward level). Some selection criteria were more

implicit (being able to speak or understand the English language, a high reputation of performance in clinical oncological care, member of EONS). These selection criteria should be more explicit for creating a high performant network of oncological Sites

- The network should be more organised. A network of ten Clinical Sites can be managed by one co-ordinator (WP2-co-ordinator within the WISECARE-project). Nevertheless, it already became complex when starting up new Clinical Sites: installing software, basic training, providing a helpdesk. Enlarging the network to more Sites, will make co-ordinative work more complex. It is necessary to build a more structured network.

All five elements of knowledge generation (categorizing patients according to their risk; standardised scales; modeling for understanding relations between problems, interventions and outcomes; instant and global feedback; networking) are incorporated in the software tools that have been developed within the project: the WiseTool, WiseWeb, WiseHoos and WiseCompass.

1.3 WISECARE Software Tools

1.3.1   The WiseTool [9]

The WiseTool has to support the activity of clinical networking, from local data collection, to aggregation in the data warehouse, analysis, and finally feedback of new information.

At each Site a tool was required which would support data collection and management, and feedback of new information from the project. Users spoke multiple languages, were not generally experienced in use of the IT and had poor systems support. The tool therefore had to be: very easy to use by nurses at the Sites; require minimal training; easy to install and maintain by non-IT professionals; secure and confidential and support local customisation.

The agreed requirement was for a stand-alone PC-based software tool with minimal duplication with existing local systems. Further, there should only be one integrated tool for data collection and local feedback. The WISETool was developed to meet these requirements.

The WiseTool is in a prototyping stage:

- The functionality of the WiseTool should be plugged into electronic patient records. So far one link between the WiseTool and an electronic patient record system (the HISCOM MIRADOR system) has been linked using Windows Dynamic Data Exchange protocols.
- Because of the various natures of electronic patient records, standards for data transfer (e.g. HL-7) should be specified.

1.3.2   The WiseWeb [10]

The WiseWeb is the communication module within the WISECARE project. The WiseWeb is organised in the WiseWeb and the WiseNet. The WiseWeb is a common Webserver (http://wisecare.dn.uoa.gr) for communicating the project to external visitors.

The WiseNet is a BSCW-server (Basic Support for Cooperative Work). The BSCW enables collaboration over the Internet. BSCW is a 'shared workspace' system which supports document uploads, event notification, group management and much more.

1.3.3   The WiseHoos [9]

The WiseHoos is the relational database of the WISECARE-project. More than 13000 patient assessments have been done during the project lifetime. The data are anonymous to patients, not to Clinical Sites.
Further development in structuring and securing the database is required:
–   Securing the database access by trusted third parties protocols
–   Limitations in the use of the database by internal and external interest groups according to European and national laws

1.3.4   The WiseCompass

The WiseCompass is a technology assessment tools which enables to evaluate the introduction of this new technology on the nursing ward. ComPass is based on the European Foundation of Quality Management (EFQM). The questions have been obtained from various sources. The questions about the management of the Hospital/Department/Ward are adapted from the original (EFQM) tool and were incorporated for Oncological Care Management.

2   Markets and marketing

The core question is if there is any interest in the WISECARE products. What is the market? Who are the primary stakeholders?

2.1 Segmentation

The WISECARE project has been designed as a general application system within health care. The demonstration domain is oncological care. The very specific demonstration domain of oncological care has limited impact on the software (WiseTool and WiseWeb) which have a very flexible and open design. The highest impact is on the WISECARE knowledge server which is very oncological specific given the standardised scales, data collection design and risk appraisal tools. The first focus to launch the project in a production environment will be in oncological care.

It is obvious that cancer poses a major burden on society. One in four deaths can be attributed to cancer and it ranks second on the list of causes of death, after cardiovascular diseases [11]. It has been estimated that in the European Community in 1990, 1,3 million incident cases of all forms of cancer were diagnosed. In men, the major forms of cancer were cancer of the lung (21%), large bowel (13%), prostate (12%), bladder (7%) and stomach (7%). In women, major forms were cancer of the breast (28%), large bowel (15%), lung (6%), uterine corpus (5%) and stomach (5%) [12].

Taking only the impact of ageing into account, it is estimated that the number of cancer patients will have increased by 20% during the 1990s. It should be kept in mind that, with the current state of medical knowledge, on average, 40% of all cancer patients are cured [13]. This average shows wide variations depending on the tumour site and ranges from a relative 5-year survival rate of as high as 93% for testis carcinoma to as low as 4% after pancreatic cancer. The group of cured citizens, however, may face serious problems of social and professional rehabilitation and reintegration after cure and of restoration of physical, mental and social health, which is a problem that is all too often ignored.

Several treatment modalities exist to manage cancer: surgery, radiotherapy, chemotherapy, immunotherapy or a combination of these. Surgical removal of the tumour tissue, usually applied to relatively limited tumours, is at present the most generally successful mode of cancer treatment (60% of all cures). Radiotherapy is given to approximately 50% of all patients and is involved in approximately one-third of the cures. Chemotherapy is increasingly used for haematopoietic malignancies, germinal tumours and paediatric tumours. It is increasingly used in the adjuvant setting. It is estimated that chemotherapy plays a role in approximately 10% of cancer cures. Immunotherapy is promising but still in the infancy stage.

There has been an explosive growth in scientific know-how, resulting in an increasing availability of new drugs, equipment, materials that are expected to be beneficial in the struggle against cancer [14]. Based on the data from the National Cancer Institute, Maryland, USA, it can be calculated that the share of cancer spending in total pharmaceutical research spending has increased from 9% in the late 70s to 15% in the late 80s. Many clinical cancer projects are underway than in most other areas of medicine. Under the Biomedical and Health Research programmes of the EU, cancer research takes up more than 20% of the research funds [15].

In chemotherapy, new and more expensive cytostatic drugs are available. Many of the existing drugs are now used in combination and/or in higher dosages resulting in a higher exposure and levels of toxicity. This increased treatment intensity also requires additional monitoring of patients and necessary supportive therapies to counter the side effects. For these side effects, new drugs have been developed, such as antiemetics against nausea and growth factors to prevent episodes of febrile neutropenia and fever. Jones et al [16] found that the new antiemetics cause an increase in total hospital costs for these patients of 12-34%.

Finally, demands and opportunities not only result in an increase in direct medical care. There is a growing awareness that psychosocial care and rehabilitation should not be neglected either. Cancer patients may suffer from fatigue, leading to difficulties for holding or re-entering a job. Having cancer may lead to a reduction of self-esteem. Adequate prevention of such cancer and successful rehabilitation requires a multidisciplinary approach.

The actual project is at the moment active in 11 Clinical Sites in 9 countries across Europe. All Clinical Sites are university hospitals or Sites with a high reputation in oncological care.

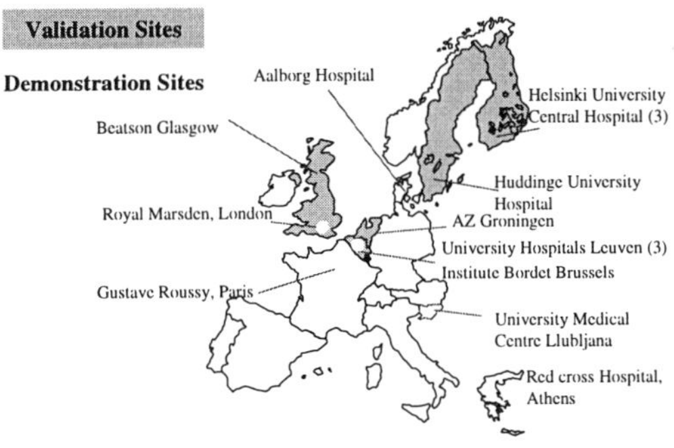

Figure 1   WISECARE Network on December 31, 1999

The systematic Minimum Basic Data Set collection for Belgian hospitals gives some idea about the impact of oncological care on hospital care. Out of 794 AP-DRG codes, 58 codes can be identified as malignancies. In 1995, Belgian general hospitals had 1,64 million admissions, resulting in 13,97 million inpatient days. 102000 patients (6,2%) were admitted for malignancies (28% of them received surgery). This resulted in 888000 inpatient days (27% of which were for surgery). Because of the lack of specificity in the DRG-system for cancer diagnoses, the incidence and prevalence rates could be underestimated. On the other hand, most oncological patients are being treated in ambulatory way or in day-clinics and so are not included in the figures. In 1995, there were 168000 admissions for chemotherapy in Belgian hospitals, 90% (152000) of these were performed in one-day clinics.

This means 102 admissions per 10000 inhabitants; 888 inpatient days for 10000 inhabitants and 168 chemotherapy administrations / 10000 inhabitants.

Extrapolation of the Belgian figures to the EU (375 million inhabitants) results in 3,8 million admissions/year; 33,3 million inpatient days (comparable to a bed capacity of 90000 beds); 6,3 million chemotherapy administrations/year.

The prevalence of side effects that has been described in the WISECARE project (Table 1), gives some estimation of the prevalence of the problem WISECARE is addressing in Europe. More than 70% of oncological patients in hospitals experience fatigue, 2 out of 3 have some oral problems, 50% experience pain and 25% have nausea & vomiting problems.

In interpreting these figures, it is important to notice that the WISECARE consortium is not representative of all oncological patients in hospitals (because it does not include radiation therapy and focused on a limited number of patient groups).

Moreover, some WISECARE patients are at home and not in the hospital context.

Table 1   Overview of the prevalence of patient problems of chemotherapy and general oncological care in the WISECARE-project.

Severity of patient problem	Fatigue	Nausea & Vomiting	Pain	Oral problems
No problem	2329 (27,5%)	3381 (77,7%)	1542 (47%)	655 (30,7%
Mild problems	1262 (14,9%)	707 (16,2%)	1304 (39,8%)	617 (28,9%)
Moderate problems	4333 (51,2%)	180 (4,1%)	343 (10,5%)	266 (12,5%)
Severe problems	537 (6,3%)	81 (1,8%)	87 (2,6%)	596 (27,9%)
TOTAL	8461	4349	3276	2134

Coding scheme:

Severity of side-effect	F	N&V	P	OP
No problem	0	2	2	8
Mild problems	1	3-4	3-4	9-10
Moderate problems	2	5-6	5-6	11-12
Severe problems	3	7-8	7-8	13-24

2.2 Competition:

Knowledge Management in health care is an emerging field (Figure 2). Two types of domains can be identified:

- Evidence-based initiatives focusing on the process of health care delivery: summarizing scientific literature, looking for hard evidence, development of clinical guidelines.

A first goal is creating evidence and the development of guidelines. A good example is the Cochrane-collaboration[1]. The principal output of the Collaboration are the Cochran

---

[1] http://www.cochrane.org/cochrane

Reviews (*The Cochrane Database of Systematic Reviews*). It is the responsibility of over 40 international collaborative review groups which cover most of the important areas of health care. The members of these groups are researchers, health care professionals, consumers, and others who share an interest in generating reliable, up-to-date evidence relevant to the prevention, treatment and rehabilitation of particular health problems or groups of problems.

The second goal is the dissemination of the available information. An example is the National Guideline Clearinghouse[TM] (NGC)[2], a public resource for evidence-based clinical practice guidelines. NGC is sponsored by the Agency for Health care Research and Quality (AHRQ) (formerly the Agency for Health Care Policy and Research [AHCPR]) in partnership with the American Medical Association and the American Association of Health Plans. The National Guidelines Clearinghouse[TM] (NGC) is an Internet Web site intended to make evidence-based clinical practice guidelines and related materials widely available to health care professionals.

- Quality indicator initiatives focusing on the outcomes of patient care: developing indicators, providing benchmarks, ...

In the quality indicator initiatives, two main goals can be identified:

The first goal is to develop and disseminate clinical indicators. A good example is the Centre of Disease Control (CDC)[3]. The CDC has a mission to promote health and quality of life by preventing and controlling disease, injury, and disability. It is realised by setting up surveillance and monitoring systems.

The second goal is to help organisations to benchmark their own results. Examples are the 220 Performance Measurement Systems[4] accredited by the Joint Commission of Health care Organisations in the USA. More-over, many of the systems are focusing on a very specific care problem (e.g. CDC focusing on infection control) or are very general. Many systems lack a very specific focus on specific patient groups (and the interactions between different patient problems) to support clinicians in their daily decision making.

The interaction between guidelines and patient outcomes in a structured way is not supported by most of the systems.

WISECARE has a special niche in this market by focusing for a very specific patient group (e.g. oncological care) on process by disseminating guidelines and outcomes for benchmarking at the same time. The WISECARE project is using existing information, guidelines, scales and indicators as much as possible. However to enhance benchmarking and clinical decision, some limited effort is put on development of scales and indicators

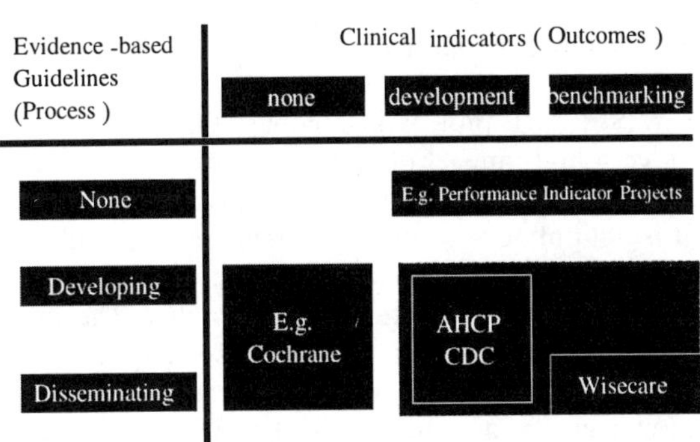

Figure 2   Schematic Representation of Knowledge Management Initiative in Health Care

---

[2] http://www.guideline.gov/
[3] http://www.cdc.gov/aboutcdc.htm
[4] http://www.jcaho.org/perfmeas/perfmeas_frm.html

2.3 Market Strategy

The WISECARE adoption of a series of WISECARE tools to support the nursing care process in many dimensions is a positive indication of the transition process towards the use of IT. The enthusiasm shown during the WISECARE conferences both in Leuven in June 1999 and in Glasgow in December 1999 is an indicator of a greater market for the approach and the tools. The discovery of clinical context related patient care management has the potential to create a generic model for the support of the management of nursing with a logical integration with the clinical care process. Although it can be stated that this approach will take quite some time to be accepted and implemented, it seems the way to go, taking into account the acceptance of information technology as a basic tool for documentation and communication. The WISECARE project has shown how slowly the process of the adoption of an information technology strategy for nursing moves forward within a living organisation. However the project has proven that nurses are eager to adopt new technological tools to improve the quality of their work. The focus on a broader implementation of WISECARE should thus be on creating support at a managerial level in hospitals across Europe for the use of ICT for nursing. The development of a WISECARE nursing strategy should be consistent with the increased need for the introduction of an electronic patient record within hospitals and other health care institutions. A balance should be found between a step-by-step approach of the introduction of WISECARE tools supporting nursing care, within a strategic framework at institutional level. Even with the introduction of WISECARE for new Sites focused at the same patient groups and the same nursing problems, it seems essential to embed such an implementation within the ICT strategy of the hospital. This ensures a long term perspective and the basis for a step by step approach for a further and broader implementation of the WISE nursing tools.

2.3.1 Interest shown by Prospective Customers: Stakeholder Analysis

The stakeholder analysis has two main goals:
- to find out who is interested in WISECARE and
- to find out who is willing to pay for it.

Potential stakeholders are patients and their representatives: social insurance companies and governments; professionals represented by health care organisations and professional associations, pharmaceutical companies and ICT-companies.

2.3.2 Patients and Patient Representatives

The benefit of the WISECARE-project is obvious. Oncological care is not only life threatening but has a very high impact on the quality of life of patients under treatment. The WISECARE approach aimed to reduce the negative impact on the quality of life of patients. The benefit is not only due to improved interventions and better monitoring, but also by an active involvement of patients in the care process. The project shows that patients with cancer can be in therapy for several months. The number of admissions varies from 1 to more than 15. However, despite these frequent episodes of admission, patients are mainly at home. Frequently, they experience many negative side-effects of their treatment, such as pain, fatigue, mucositis. The WISECARE study reveals that the most mucositis problems following chemotherapy are not experienced in the hospital environment, but at home between treatment cycles. Thus, it is vital that patients or their family members are taught how to manage these problems effectively. Professional care is only appropriate when patients or family members require additional assistance. Nurses should concentrate their efforts to improve the self-care abilities of the patient and the family rather than taking over the care in a ritualistic way.

The role of patients goes beyond more active patient involvement. Instead of viewing patients as passive recipients of information or care, patients can be viewed as active participants in their care delivery process. This means that they actively participate in creating the different alternatives for care. A first way is by valuing patient knowledge about their illness. Many patients are very well informed about their illness. High personal concern, a lot of time and a concentrated focus can help a patient to be even more informed about the illness than his or her GP or medical specialist. Doctors may resent patients' extensive knowledge, but instead they should cooperate and use it. A second step is to learn more from patients' experiences. Many patient organisations, mainly for chronic diseases, help patients to gain control over their lives, give psychological support and practical advice. The involvement of professional caregivers, such as medical doctors or nurses, in these organisations has traditionally been very low. In most health care relationships, the direction of information is seen as one-way from professional to "layman". However it is becoming more obvious that these patients are in fact the real experts because of their experience, networks, and living knowledge. The relationship between patients and professionals is increasingly shifting to a dialogue, in which these patient organisations are supporting professional organisations to improve their care, identifying priorities and creating the right environment. A third step is by having the patient as co-author of his or her treatment plan with the patient or family taking an active and responsible role. This can have large impact on the professional organisation. Patients may be invited to develop their own health care teams in whom they have most confidence. It means that the patient is seen as a member of the health care team with equal access to information, briefings etc.

So far no patient organisations are informed about WISECARE. The plan is to do this in future developments. WISECARE can become an accreditional body where patients can get information on which hospitals and other health care organisations actively involve patients in their treatment plan and have an explicit focus on the quality of life.

It is obvious that the WISECARE-service is freely provided to patient in an easily accessible way (on the Internet) and will not require payment. It is different for social insurance companies and government, who want to provide the best service for their members or citizens.

2.3.3   *Professionals and their representatives*

The feedback from Validation & Demonstration Sites shows very clearly that the network is seen as very valuable. Nine out of eleven Clinical Sites want to continue WISECARE networking after finishing the project. There is an agreement among partners and Clinical Sites to continue at least for 6 months, without further development, limited maintenance support, only one global feedback report in April 2000. Even based on these limited conditions, more than 100 new patients have been entered in the WiseHoos database.

Based on this success, the European Oncology nurses Association took the commitment for further support, develop and maintain the WISECARE network.

The problem is funding. Although nurses are very enthusiastic about the WISECARE endeavour, they are not in the position to make financial decisions. Nurse managers, or general managers, should be informed about the WISECARE project. It is not obvious that they would invest in WISECARE:

- When nursing units are part of a European network, the management team would loose an element of control. Guidelines and protocols are derived from the network (evidence-based) and less from in-house rules and regulations. Conflicts between in-house regulations and information from the network are possible.

- The outcomes and resource use are compared through Europe. Exchanging information is very threatening.
- The benchmarking is restricted to oncological care. Only a limited number of nursing units is involved, making it less interesting for general management.
- Incentives to invest in a better quality of care are generally lacking in European health care with most incentives focussing on cost control. For this reason, the nursing resource module should stay an integrative part of the WISECARE feedback.

Professional associations are driven by individual membership. The WISECARE-project takes an organisational perspective. It is not the aim of an individual nurse to subscribe individually to the WISECARE network to enhance his/her individual practice or have benchmarks about his/her patient care etc. Theoretically, it should be feasible but practically, nursing care is highly involved in the organisation.

2.3.4 Pharmaceutical companies

Pharmaceutical companies are highly interested in the WISECARE project, because of two main reasons:

- Traditionally, Pharmaceutical companies and clinicians are having two kinds of relationships. The first one is in testing out the efficacy of a new drug. The pharmaceutical company is involving clinicians to test new drug under very strict conditions (randomised clinical trial). In fact, clinicians are "selling" their knowledge & client network to the pharmaceutical company. When the drug is on the market, the relationship reverse and pharmaceutical companies are selling the drugs to the clinicians. In this last relationship, the weak point is that the selling stops by delivering the drug to the clinician. However, it is known that the clinician-patient delivery process will have a high impact on the final effectiveness of the drug. Sharing patient outcomes with pharmaceutical companies, will give information on effectiveness (real life results) instead of efficacy (results in controlled environments). Clinicians and patients never question their role in the effectiveness of the drug (right dose, right way, right time, interaction with other drugs). When a drug is not doing the job as expected (or promised), the drug is to be blamed. It means that also in the selling part, a two directional relationship between pharmaceutical companies and clinicians is required.
- Secondly, there was a very explicit option in WISECARE to involve pharmaceutical companies in this nurse-patient delivery process: in describing the toxicity levels of chemotherapy, producing leaflets which can be used to explain side-effects to patients, to teach them how to assess their mouth status.

The interest in WISECARE is low for various reasons. The difficulty is the evaluation of effectiveness of a specific drug. However in most cases, therapy is a mixture of various drugs, interventions and treatments. It is not easy to isolate the effect of one drug in the real world environment. Pharmaceutical companies are only interested in the effect of their own drugs. In clinical practice, a mixture of drugs from various companies for a variety of clinical indications is used.

Several interest groups of pharmaceutical companies have been identified:
- Producers of chemotherapy products which should be interested in the side effects that go along with the drug;
- Producers of co-selling drugs against specific side effects (fatigue, pain, mucositis, nausea & vomiting) could be interested.

2.3.5 ICT-companies

WISECARE is focused on telematics in health care. There is high interest in WISECARE from the wide range of ICT-companies:

The main interest comes from ICT-companies in the field of developing hospital or health care information systems. WISECARE can be a module within a hospital information system as part of the electronic patient record. Most of the data stored in patient records are used for individual patient care or for operational communication between individual caregivers, hospital and community etc. So far the introduction of computerised patient records hasn't changed this use very much.

The high potentiality of the electronic patient record is in the exploitation. Beyond individual caregivers and individual use, there are many possible users of clinical data: clinicians, managers, teachers, researchers. They can access patient records for a variety of uses — such as screening for subjects to enroll into clinical trials, determining best practices, and describing health care resource utilization. Manual patient records have been accessed in the past for these uses, but it requires large investment in time and effort to do so. The advent of the computer-based patient record, with its capability of querying large databases, retrieving data on variables being studied, and downloading data into statistical analysis programs, means that if anything, researchers will increase their demands for patient data and information. In other words, the use of this data for further exploitation purposes will be driven by its simple availability. From WISECARE however it becomes more and more obvious that the structure and content of the EPR will not determine its exploitation. It is the need for exploitation that will determine the structure and content. So, for developer of EPR-software it is important that they are involved in project such as WISECARE as soon as possible.

A second group of ICT-companies interested in WISECARE are the EPR-exploitation companies. All kind of applications are offered by these firms: Resource Enterprise Systems, executive information systems, management information systems, data mining, scheduling and planning systems. WISECARE offers an alternative to the various existing systems. They are interested because of the highly involvement of users in the development of the WiseTool. It is obvious that the result is very close to the needs of the users.

Stakeholders	Added value				Willing to pay
	Y/N	Level			
		High	Medium	Low	Comments	

Stakeholders	Y/N	High	Medium	Low	Comments	Willing to pay
Patient	Yes		X		increase quality of care	No
Professionals	Yes		X		increase image increase wages	No
Providers	Yes	X			increase quality of care professionalisation of nursing care increase in patient satisfaction benchmarking	+/-
Insurance firms	Yes		X		more knowledge about care	Yes
Government	Yes		X		quality of care	Yes
Pharma-industry	Yes	X			improve image access to the network feedback on the effect of drugs	Yes
ICT-firms	Yes		X		access to the network	Yes
Educational organisations	Yes		X		access to the network collection of useful data	No

Figure 3   Stakeholder Analysis

A third group of ICT-companies interested in WISECARE are the networking companies. Networking across Europe, setting up knowledge centres, creating virtual organisation by providing a highly performant network environment is a major goal.

The main interest of all ICT-companies is the availability of Clinical Sites across Europe, willing to co-operate. The weak point is that the WISECARE network focuses on one patient group (oncological care). It means practically that linking several health care organisations means that several ICT-systems have to be linked and connected. Within the WISECARE-project, we couldn't solve that problem within time and budget constraints. More over the priority was in building the knowledge base network. However any commercial investment has to deal with this issue. Web-based technologies, well defined specifications and standards should be build to overcome the intersystem-communication problem.

There is definitively interest from the ICT-companies for WISECARE, but so far they don't want to undertake financial investment without a major binding factor (government, pharmaceutical industry).

3   Management and Financial Forecast

A major commitment at the start of WISECARE was the intention to hand over the ownership of the outcomes of WISECARE to EONS who has played a vital role in the development and support of the project over the last three years. EONS would be responsible for the further dissemination of the project throughout the European cancer nursing community.

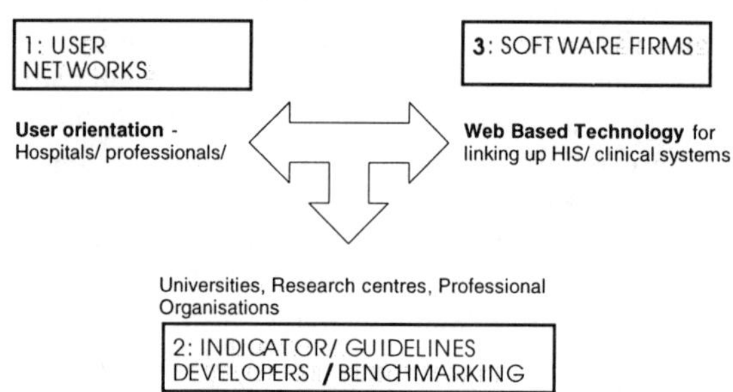

Figure 4   WISECARE Collaboration Model

There are three basic roles in any further project consortium.

3.1 Network Co-ordination

- Management of data and information flow
- Installation & education of new Sites
- Helpdesk
- Listening to Clinical Sites for questions about new functionalities

This role is highly dependent on the number of Sites involved, their geographical location, the different languages involved.

3.2 Knowledge Development (Guidelines, Indicators, Scales, Feedback)

- The functions are highly technical and specialised
- It is the core-business of the network
- Unique combination of specialised professional content and methodology (teamwork)
- Depends on the availability of libraries of scales, indicators, etc.

This role is independent of the number of Sites involved. It depends on the number and quality of indicators that will be provided. Knowledge that is necessary to fulfil these roles: very specialised professional knowledge, statistical knowledge, scientific methods in developing scales.

3.3 IT-development

- The network is IT-supported
- The development of a WiseTool with all functionalities foreseen in knowledge development (data input, feedback, network links, structured guidelines,...)
- The WiseTool should be able to communicate with the local systems (Web-base applications, standards, specifications,...
- Dealing with privacy: passwords, encryptions, data transfer,
- Maintainance and upgrade of systems

This role is independent of the number of Sites involved. It depends on the functional specifications, the different languages, the different platforms the system has to run (95/98/NT, UNIX, Apple,...), network versus stand-alone versions, and the different systems that have to be connected.

Table 2 Cost and Personnel Estimation

Number of Sites	Network co-ordinator	Knowledge development	IT-development	Cost	Real cost per Site
10	1	3	3	442050	44205
20	1	3	3	444050	22203
30	1	3	3	446050	14868
40	1	3	3	448050	11201
50	1	3	3	450050	9001
60	2	3	3	502900	8382
70	2	3	3	504900	7213
80	2	3	3	506900	6336
90	2	3	3	508900	5654
100	2	3	3	510900	5109
200	4	3	4	709300	3547
300	6	3	4	831000	2770
400	8	3	4	952700	2382
500	10	3	5	1151100	2302

* Cost calculations
  Network co-ordinator / Knowledge developer: 50000 Euro/year
  IT-developer: 75000 Euro/year
  Travel budget for network co-ordinator: 20% of the Sites at 1000 Euro/year
  Computer infrastructure (3y depreciation): 850 Euro/year for network co-ordinator; 1700 Euro/year for knowledge developer/IT-specialist
  1 Server infrastructure: back-up server after 50 Sites: 4000 Euro/year

The analysis shows that 50 Clinical Sites are needed with a Site subscription rate of 10000 Euro/year. When the subscription rate is lower to 5000 Euro/year, at least 100 Clinical Sites should be part of the network. Extending the network to 500 Clinical Sites, subscription rates can be go down to 2500 Euro/year.

The cost-benefit analysis shows that this kind of activity still needs to be subsidized. There is no tradition in European hospitals to pay more than 5000 Euro for this kind of information on a yearly base.

References

[1] OECD. The reform of health care systems: a review of 17 OECD countries. *Health Policy Studies*, 1994, **5**.
[2] Davenport T & Prusack L Working knowledge: how organizations manage what they know, Harvard

Business School Press, Boston, 1998.

[3] Dhaenekint C. et al. Nurses Cytostatic Compendium, Practical Guide for nurses, Glaxo Wellcome, 1994.

[4] Eilers J. Bergen A.M., Petersen M.C. Development, testing and application of the oral assessment guide, *Oncology Nursing Forum* **15** (1988):325-330.

[5] Piper BF, Lindsey AM, Dodd MJ, Ferketich S, Paul SM, Weller S. The development of an instrument to measure the subjective dimension of fatigue. In management of Pain, Nausea and Fatigue Funk SG Torniquist EM Champagne MT Copp LA Wiese RA (Eds) Springer Publishing Company: New York, 1993.

[6] Aaronson N, Ahnedzai S, Bergman B, Bullinger M, Cull A, Duez N, Fiiberti A, Fletcher H, Fleischman S, de Haes J, Kaasa S, Klee M, Osoba D, Razari D, Rofe P, Schraube S, Sneeuw K, Sullivan M, Takdea F. The European Organisation for the Research and Treatment of Cancer QLQ-C30: a quality of life instrument for use in clinical trials in oncology. Journal of the National Cancer Institute, 1993 **85**(5): 365-376.

[7] Tansley J. Modeling and Simulation of patients undergoing chemotherapy. WISECARE project, 1999.

[8] [Burt R.S. The social structure of competition in Networks and Organisations: Structure, Form an Action. Harvard Business School, 1992: 57-91.

[9] D. Hoy D. Deliverable 3.2 Record layout of the database in WISECARE project, 1997.

[10] Dounavis P, Karistinou E & Mantas J. WISECARE www-server in WISECARE project, 1998.

[11] Landis (S.), T. Murray, S. Bolden, Ph. Wingo, Cancer Statistics 1999, CA *Cancer Journal for Clinicians*, January/February, **49**(1), 1999, p. 8-31.

[12] Black (RJ), F. Bray, J. Ferlay, DM Perkin, Cancer incidence and mortality in the European Union: cancer registry data and estimates of national incidence for 1990, *European Journal of Cancer*, **33**, 1997, p.1075-1107.

[13] Van der Schueren E, Kesteloot K & Cleemput I. Economic evaluation in cancer care: questions and answers on how to alleviate conflicts between rising needs and expectations and tightening budgets. *European Journal of Cancer* 1999 **0**, 1-24.

[14] Yarbro JW. Changing cancer care in the 1990s and the cost. *Cancer* 1991, **675**, 1718-1727.

[15] Neymark N. A review of economic evaluations in oncology. Working paper. Brussels, EORTC Data center, 1996.

[16] Jones AL, Lee GJ, Bosanquet N. The budgetary impact of HT_3 receptor antagonists in the management of chemotherapy-induced emisis. *European Journal of Cancer*, 1993, **29A**, 51-56.

Appendices

<h1 align="center">Executive Summary</h1>

HC3003 WISECARE

Workflow Information Systems for European Nursing Care

INTRODUCTION

WISECARE is a knowledge sharing project on quality of life indicators for oncological nursing care. The project, focused on fatigue, nausea & vomiting, pain and oral care, was able to network 15 oncological Sites in 10 European countries.

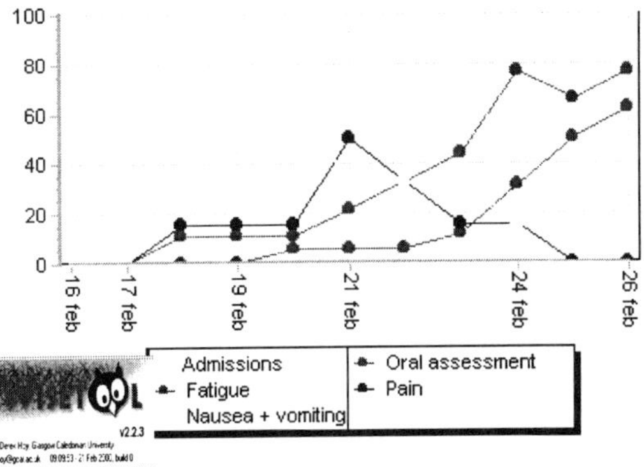

Setting the Scene

Great amounts of data are stored in electronic or manual patient records. They are used for transactional and clinical purposes. They are seldom exploited for management and learning.

Throughout Europe, costs for nursing services take up 40-60% of the health care budget, but the impact that nursing has on the quality of care for Europe's citizens is not evaluated. Given the changes in health care financing that are taking place across Europe, it is imperative that hospitals focus their cost containment and quality development in this area.

Approach

WISECARE focused on the use of existing data for the use of clinical management, resource management and knowledge sharing.

For clinical management purposes, four domain of quality of life were selected: fatigue, pain, nausea and vomiting and oral care. Standardised scales (EORTC-QLQ-30 and Oral Assessment Guide) were used.

These data were collected during ten consecutive days after a clinical event (chemotherapy, surgery). For resource management purposes, the intensity of nursing care (Moffitt patient classification tool), the hours worked and the qualification level of the nursing staff were collected on a random day per week. For knowledge sharing purposes, an internet network was setup to exchange guidelines and protocols.

Results and Achievements

A network of oncological Sites across Europe has been established. In December 1999, fifteen oncological Sites in ten countries participated in the network.

A tool, called WiseTool, was developed to collect the data, to produce first feedback and to structure guidelines. During 18 months, more than 13000 patient assess-ments were made for 280 patients and 590 treatment cycles.

The local feedback graphs were used to discuss symptom control with patients, nurses and physicians.

The data were sent quarterly to the project datawarehouse, called WiseHoos to develop global feedback.

The global feedback served as a benchmark for the oncological Sites.

Secondly, it was possible to monitor trends in clinical outcome and resource use. To enable these comparisons, the indica-tors were adjusted for clinical time and treatment toxicity levels (assessed by the LCRA-Scale).

Main results showed a decrease in the average fatigue score of 44% in the beginning of the project (04/98-12/98) to 33% in period 3 (04/98–09/99), a decrease in the average nausea & vomiting score from 11,8% to 5,6%, a decrease in the average pain score from 23% to 19% and a decrease in mouth problems (OAG) from 22,3% to 18,5%.

For measuring the impact of the project, a WiseCompass Tool, based on EFQM was developed. Main results were an improvement in job satisfaction by the nurses, by being part of a larger network. However, the project imposed more mental demand and effort upon nurses, because of the focus on effectiveness and outcome. The overall evaluation was very challenging.

Conclusions and Plans for the Future

Main plans are the enlargement of the WISECARE Network by the European Oncological nursing Society. More clinical indicators have to be developed. The data collection design, toxicity adjustment profiles have to be updated. A WISECARE knowledge centre (on scales, guidelines and benchmarks) has to be further developed.

Contact Details

Project Name:
WISECARE – Workflow Information Systems for European Nursing Care

Research Area:
Knowledge sharing, Evidence-based Clinical Practice, Clinical Outcome research

Timescale:
01.04.97 - 31.12.99

Budget:
Overall budget: 1.034.950 Euro
European Commission contribution: 938.000 Euro

Keywords:
Clinical indicators, resource management, knowledge sharing

Key Project Participants:

Catholic university Leuven	(BE),
European Oncology Nursing Society	(BE),
University of Glasgow	(GB),
University of Edinburgh	(GB),
Glasgow Caledonian University	(GB),
HISCOM	(NL),
Kuopio University	(FI),
University of Athens	(GR),
Arthur Andersen	(BE),
An Teallach Limited	(GB),
National Health Service Scotland	(GB)

Project Coordinator:
Prof. Walter SERMEUS
Tel:+32 16 336975
Fax:+32 16 336970
E-mail: Walter.sermeus@med.kuleuven.ac.be
Project URL:http://WISECARE.dn.uoa.gr

Glossary

ALL	Acute Lymphoid Leukaemia
AML	Acute Myeloid Leukaemia
ATL	An Teallach Limited
Br Ca	Breast Cancer
C.S.	Clinical Sites
Case Mix	A generic term for Patient Classification Systems, grouping algorithms for clustering patients according to specific variables
Clinical time	Number of days after the start of the treatment episode. Day 0 = Day of start of treatment episode
D.S.	Demonstration Sites
EFQM	European Foundation for Quality Management
EONS	European Oncology Nursing Society
EORTC QLQ-C30	European Organisation for the Research and Treatment of Cancer, Quality of Life Questionnair version C 30
Deliverable	Project report to the European Commission
GBCRAS	Groningen Breast Cancer Risk Assessment Scale
GCU	Glasgow Caledonian University
HISCOM	Hospital Information Systems Company Leiden, the Netherlands
KUL	Katholic University Leuven
LCRAS	Leuven Chemotherapy Risk Assessment Scale
Lu Ca	Lung Cancer
MIRADOR	Clinical Workstation developed by HISCOM
N&V	Nausea & Vomiting
NHL	Non Hodgkin Lymphoma
NHSiS	National Health Service in Scotland
Non-Wise Nurse	A nurse not straight involved in the project but working on one of the units, which participated the project
OAG	Oral Assessment Guide
Ost Sarc	Osteosarcoma
PFS	Piper Fatigue Scale
Risk 0	No risk or risk unknown
Risk 1	Mild risk
Risk 2	Moderate risk
Risk 3	High risk
Scores 0-100	Indicators aggregate responses to individual items into one overall number called the score. This aggregation is always the result of some logical, mathematical or statistical operations on the response data. The EORTC manual suggests summing the item response data that vary from 1 to 4. Hence with 3 items the sum varies from 3 tot 12. This range is standardised into a score 0-100 by way of the formula: 100 x [(sum - minimum sum) / (maximum sum - minimum sum)]
Time period	All WISECARE DATA is collected in the period April 1998- September 1999. This total period is subdivided in 3 time periods for presentation purposes: Time period 1: April 1998 – December 1998 Time period 2: January 1999- April 14, 1999 Time period 3: April 15, 1999 - September 1999
V.S.	Validation Sites
WHO	World Health Organisation
Wise Compass	A technology assessment tool, which was developed to gather follow-up information about the impacts of the project
Wise Feedback	Global feedback about the clinical outcome indicators and resource indicators derived from the shared database. Serves as benchmark for the sites

Wise Nurse	A nurse who has worked closely in the WISECARE project attending the data collection and utilisation of the feedback
Wise Station	A Desktop composed of a series of functions to support the different tasks of a nurse in her / his daily practice, providing access to data, information, programs and functions within and across the institution
Wise Web	Project's home pages, chosen links and under authorisation the BSCW server for sharing information between WISECARE members
WISECARE	An EU funded health telematics project; Workflow Information Systems for European Nursing CARE
WiseMailingList	Networking was also supported by use of an e-mail list; all partners and Wise Nurses were members of the list.
WiseTool	A computer programme, which was developed to collect data, send them regularly to a shared database, give feedback on clinical practice and to contain information about the chosen clinical indicators, it is a mini electronic patient record
WP1	Work Package 1, team responsible for a part of the project.
WP2	Work Package 2, team responsible for a part of the project.
WP3	Work Package 3, team responsible for a part of the project.
WP4	Work Package 4, team responsible for a part of the project.
WP5	Work Package 5, team responsible for a part of the project.
WP6	Work Package 6, team responsible for a part of the project.

List of Annexes

Annex 1 Oral Assessment Guide (Wisecare Form)

Please complete this questionnaire by ticking the box that best represents how your mouth feels or looks today

1. Voice	Normal	☐
	Deep or Raspy	☐
	Difficulty talking/painful	☐
2. Swallow	Normal swallow	☐
	Some pain on swallow	☐
	Unable to swallow	☐
3. Lips	Smooth and pink and moist	☐
	Dry and cracked	☐
	Ulcerated or bleeding	☐
4. Tongue	Pink and moist and papillae present	☐
	Coated or loss of papillae with shinny appearance with or without redness	☐
	Blistered or cracked	☐
5. Saliva	Watery	☐
	Thick or ropy	☐
	Absent	☐

6. Mucous membranes	Pink and moist	☐
	Reddened or coated (increased whiteness) without ulceration	☐
	Ulceration with or Without bleeding	☐
7. Gingiva	Pink and stillped and firm	☐
	Oedematous with or without redness	☐
	Spontaneous bleeding or bleeding with pressure	☐
8. Teeth/dentures	Clean and no debris	☐
	Plaque or debris in localised area (between teeth if present)	☐
	Plaque or debris generalised along gum line or denture bearing area	☐

Thank you for taking the time to complete the whole questionnaire.

Annex 2   Piper Fatigue Scale (Wisecare Form)

Fatigue Assessment Form

Name ________________________

Reference ________________________

Date ________________________

For each of the following questions, circle the number which best describes the fatigue you are experiencing now.
Please make every effort to answer each question to the best of your ability.
Thank you very much.

---

1   How long have you been feeling fatigue? (tick one response only)

minutes

hours

days

weeks

months

other please describe

2   To what degree is the fatigue you are feeling causing you distress?

no distress   great distress

0	1	2	3	4	5	6	7	8	9	10

3   To what degree is the fatigue you are feeling interfering with your ability to complete your work or school activities?

none   a great deal

0	1	2	3	4	5	6	7	8	9	10

4   To what degree is the fatigue you are feeling interfering with your ability to visit or socialise with your friends?

none   a great deal

0	1	2	3	4	5	6	7	8	9	10

5   To what degree is the fatigue you are feeling interfering with your ability to engage in sexual activity?

none   a great deal

0	1	2	3	4	5	6	7	8	9	10

6   Overall, how much is the fatigue which you are experiencing now interfering with your ability to engage in the kind of activities you enjoy doing?

none   a great deal

0	1	2	3	4	5	6	7	8	9	10

7   How would you describe the degree of intensity or severity of the fatigue which you are experiencing now?

mild   severe

0	1	2	3	4	5	6	7	8	9	10

To what degree would you describe the fatigue which you are experiencing now as being:

8   pleasant   unpleasant

0	1	2	3	4	5	6	7	8	9	10

9   agreeable   disagreeable

0	1	2	3	4	5	6	7	8	9	10

10   protective   destructive

0	1	2	3	4	5	6	7	8	9	10

11   positive   negative

0	1	2	3	4	5	6	7	8	9	10

12   normal   abnormal

0	1	2	3	4	5	6	7	8	9	10

To what degree are you now feeling:

13   strong   weak

0	1	2	3	4	5	6	7	8	9	10

14   awake   sleepy

0	1	2	3	4	5	6	7	8	9	10

15   lively   listless

0	1	2	3	4	5	6	7	8	9	10

16   refreshed   tired

0	1	2	3	4	5	6	7	8	9	10

17   energetic   unenergetic

0	1	2	3	4	5	6	7	8	9	10

18   patient   impatient

0	1	2	3	4	5	6	7	8	9	10

19   relaxed   tense

0	1	2	3	4	5	6	7	8	9	10

20   exhilarated   depressed

0	1	2	3	4	5	6	7	8	9	10

21   able to concentrate   unable to concentrate

0	1	2	3	4	5	6	7	8	9	10

22   able to remember   unable to remember

0	1	2	3	4	5	6	7	8	9	10

23   able to think clearly   unable to think clearly

0	1	2	3	4	5	6	7	8	9	10

24   Overall, what do you believe is most directly contributing to or causing your fatigue?

____

____

25   Overall, the best thing you have found to relieve your fatigue is:

26   Is there anything else you would like to add that would describe your fatigue better to us?

27   Are you experiencing any other symptoms right now?
    No   yes

              please describe

Annex 3   Quality Of Life C30 (version 3) Wisecare Form

WISECARE

Quality Of Life
Assessment Form

Name _________________________

Reference _________________________

Date _________________________

We are interested in some things about you and your health. Please answer all of the questions yourself by circling the number that best applies to you. There are no 'right' or 'wrong' answers.
The information that you provide will remain strictly confidential.
Thank you very much.

		no	yes
1	Do you have any trouble doing strenuous activities, like carrying a heavy shopping bag or a suitcase?	□	□
2	Do you have any trouble taking a long walk?	□	□
3	Do you have any trouble taking a short walk outside of the house?	□	□
4	Do you have to stay in bed or a chair for most of the day?	□	□
5	Do you need help with eating, dressing, washing yourself, or using the toilet?	□	□
6	Are you limited in any way in doing either your work or doing household jobs?	□	□
7	Are you completely unable to work at a job or to do household jobs?	□	□

During the past week:

		not at all	a little	quite a bit	very much
8	Were you short of breath?	□	□	□	□
9	Have you had pain?	□	□	□	□
10	Did you need to rest?	□	□	□	□
11	Have you had trouble sleeping?	□	□	□	□
12	Have you felt weak?	□	□	□	□
13	Have you lacked appetite?	□	□	□	□
		not at all	a little	quite a bit	very much
14	Have you felt nauseated?	□	□	□	□
15	Have you vomited?	□	□	□	□
16	Have you been constipated?	□	□	□	□
17	Have you had diarrhoea?	□	□	□	□
18	Were you tired?	□	□	□	□
19	Did pain interfere with your daily activities?	□	□	□	□
20	Have you had difficulty in concentrating on things, like reading a newspaper or watching television?	□	□	□	□
21	Did you feel tense?	□	□	□	□
22	Did you worry?	□	□	□	□
23	Did you feel irritable?	□	□	□	□

24	Did you feel depressed?	☐	☐	☐	☐
25	Have you had difficulty remembering things?	☐	☐	☐	☐
26	Has your physical condition or medical treatment interfered with your family life?	☐	☐	☐	☐
27	Has your physical condition or medical treatment interfered with your social activities?	☐	☐	☐	☐
28	Has your physical condition or medical treatment caused you financial difficulties?	☐	☐	☐	☐

For the following questions please circle the number between 1 and 7 that best applies to you

29   How would you rate your overall physical condition during the past week?

    very poor   excellent

        0   1   2   3   4   5   6   7

30   How would you rate your overall quality of life during the past week?

    very poor   excellent

        0   1   2   3   4   5   6   7

Annex 4 Medical Oncology Acuity Tool (Moffitt)[1]

Date: _________

Instructions:

Start at the top of the tool and check off the first indicator that applies to the patient. It is not necessary to make any other check marks because the first check mark absorbs other care time associated with the indicators.
Each patient should be classified according to his/her current status for the unit's selected time frame.

The admitting nurse on any shift should classify any new admission immediately after orders are received.

Therapeutic indicator/Category	Example	Room Number									
		413	414	415	416	417	418	419	420	421	422
IV. This category of indicators requires an average of 14 hours of care in a 24-hour period or 4.7 hours of care in an 8-hour period.											
Potential for injury (severe) related to											
Chemotherapy infusion requiring nurse at bedside	Arterial chemotherapy										
Immediate post-op (major surgery) < 72°	Total pelvic examination, radical abdominal, head and neck, thoracic										
Acute cord compression											
Anaesthesia/airway clearance	Respiratory distress										
Electrolyte disorders (severe)											
Acute pulmonary oedema requiring diuresis	Congestive heart failure, lower renal function, pulmonary overload										
Seizures/increased intracranial pressure											
Unstable cardiac status/MI or major arrhythmia	Pericardial effusion										
Unstable haematologic status/blast crisis/ disseminated intravascular coagulation	Frequent infusion of blood products > two per shift										
Self-care deficit secondary to age, surgery/ semi-comatose or comatose state	Requiring total daily care; severe dementia, confusion										
Sepsis/uncontrolled fever	Temp > 102°, + blood culture, > four antibiotic drugs or > six IV antibiotics doses daily										
Impaired gas exchange related to unstable respiratory status requiring intensive intervention	Frequent arterial blood gases > 40 % O_2 therapy										
Acute support needs	Grieving situation, new diagnosis, intensive teaching, impending death										

(Continued on next page)

[1] From Lovett RB, Reardon MB, Gordon BK, McMillan S. Validity and reliability of medical and surgical oncology patient acuity tools. *Oncology Nursing Forum* 1994; **21**(10): 1709-1717.

(Continued)

Therapeutic indicator/Category	Example	Room Number									
		413	414	415	416	417	418	419	420	421	422
III. This category of indicators requires an average of 10 hours of care in a 24-hour period or 3.3 hours of care in an 8-hour period.											
Potential for infection related to aplasia	WBC < 1000 and/or granulocytes < 500, antibiotics										
Fluid volume deficit requiring aggressive parenteral therapy	> 3 l fluid/day, chemotherapy induced severe nausea/vomiting, multiple-agent chemotherapy protocol										
Impaired gas exchange related to compromised respiratory status requiring respiratory therapy	Severe shortness of breath, pneumothorax										
Potential for injury related to											
Electrolyte disorder (mild or moderate)	Diabetics requiring ac/hs urines, bloods, sliding scale insulin, frequent lab monitoring/ frequent blood drawing per nurse										
Potential/adverse reaction(s9 requiring intensive monitoring	Phase I drugs, post-chemotherapy regimen, special procedure										
Superior vena cava syndrome	Respiratory support, complete activities of daily living (ADL) support, bed rest										
Impaired physical mobility/severe pain	Complete ADL support, bed rest traction										
Impaired skin integrity/decubitus ulcer/ mucous membranes	Open and draining wounds requiring frequent (> q4h) irrigation or dressing changes										
Altered ADL related to											
Infectious complication requiring strict isolation	Herpes zoster, resistant pathogens										
Knowledge deficit requiring intensive patient/ family education	Discharge teaching, aplasia, chemotherapy teaching, tracheostomy teaching										
Nutritional deficit requiring intensive enteral/ parenteral nutrition	Hyperalimentation, gastrostomy tube feeding										
Potential for haemorrhage	Innominate/carotid artery precautions										
Severe gastrointestinal disturbance(s)	Severe nausea and vomiting unresponsive to standard antiemetic treatment; copious diarrhoea, nasogastric suctions/small bowel obstruction										
Impaired sensory function as evidence by											
Unstable neurologic signs/ disorientation/ emotional disturbance	Neuro checks, delirium, restraints										
Ineffective coping by patient/family	Requiring frequent support interventions										
Self-care deficit secondary to age, surgery semi-comatose or comatose state	Total care uncomplicated										
Impaired haematologic status requiring blood transfusions	Multiple packed cells, volume expanders										

(Continued on next page)

(Continued)

Therapeutic indicator/Category	Example	Room Number									
		413	414	415	416	417	418	419	420	421	422
II. This category of indicators requires an average of 6 hours of care in a 24-hour period or 2 hours of care in an 8-hour period.											
Fluid volume deficit requiring parenteral therapy	Simple IV therapy, > 3l/day, heparin lock, "keep vein open" –fluid rate, single agent or continuous chemotherapy protocols										
Fever, potential for infection	Febrile < 102°, fever of unknown origin, conservative measures, including blood cultures										
Impaired haematologic status requiring blood transfusions	Simple blood component therapy										
Fluid volume deficit requiring aggressive parenteral therapy	> 3l fluid/day, chemotherapy induced severe nausea/vomiting, multiple agent chemotherapy protocol										
Altered protective mechanism or sensory function related to											
Infectious complications requiring enteric isolation	Resistant organisms										
Potential post-op complications	Bronchoscopy, endoscopy, node biopsy, central line or port placement										
Impaired bowel/bladder function related to incontinence	At least one linen change per shift, frequent skin care										
Sensory/neuro deficit (hearing, vision, speech)	Non-native language speaking, profound visual impairment, slightly ataxic gait, mild confusion										
I. This category of indicators requires an average of 4 hours of care in a 24-hour period or 1.3 hours of care in an 8-hour period.		413	414	415	416	417	418	419	420	421	422
Anxiety, mild to moderate	Requiring support/observation										
Altered ADL related to therapy requiring radiation precautions/isolation/self-care	^{131}I, thyroid ablation, iridium implants										
Altered health status related to diagnostic or stating workup											

Annex 5   Surgical Oncology Acuity Tool (Moffitt)[2]

Date: _______

Instructions:

Start at the top of the tool and check off the first indicator that applies to the patient. It is not necessary to make any other check marks because the first check mark absorbs other care time associated with the indicators.

Each patient should be classified according to his/her current status for the unit's selected time frame.

The admitting nurse on any shift should classify any new admission immediately after orders are received.

Therapeutic indicator/Category	Example	313	314	315	316	317	318	319	320	321	322
					Room Number						
IV. This category of indicators requires an average of 14 hours of care in a 24-hour period or 4.7 hours of care in an 8-hour period.											
Potential adverse reaction(s) requiring intensive monitoring	Arterial chemotherapy, vital signs every 15 minutes										
Ineffective airway clearance, actual or potential	Tracheostomy, major head/neck surgery										
Unstable cardiopulmonary status	Congestive heart failure, lower renal function, pulmonary overload, superior vena cava syndrome, potential septic crisis										
Neuro status, alteration in	Seizures, increased intracranial pressure, change in level of consciousness, dementia										
Unstable haematologic status	Frequent infusions of blood products > two per shift, disseminated intravascular coagulation										
Severe self-care deficit secondary to age, surgery, mental status	Requiring total daily care, < 72 ° post-op (major surgery)										
Unstable respiratory status requiring intensive intervention	Frequent arterial blood gases, > 40 % O_2 therapy										
Multiple complex procedures	Multiple dressings/wound irrigation > every four hours										
Infectious complications requiring strict isolation	HIV positive with copious secretions, disseminated herpes zoster										

(Continued on next page)

[2] From Lovett RB, Reardon MB, Gordon BK, McMillan S. Validity and reliability of medical and surgical oncology patient acuity tools. *Oncology Nursing Forum* 1994; **21**(10): 1709-1717.

(Continued)

Therapeutic indicator/Category		Example	Room Number									
			313	314	315	316	317	318	319	320	321	322
III.	**This category of indicators requires an average of 10 hours of care in a 24-hour period or 3.3 hours of care in an 8-hour period.**											
	Infection, actual or potential	WBC < 1000, granulocytes < 500, infected wound requiring irrigation or dressing changes every four hours										
	Fluid volume deficit requiring aggressive parenteral therapy	> 3l fluid/day, multiple antibiotics, multiple agent-chemotherapy protocol										
	Impaired gas exchange related to compromised respiratory status	Chest tube, shortness of breath, incentive spirometry, O_2										
	Impaired physical mobility/moderate self-care deficit	Day 2-4 post-op patient who consistently requires assistance with toileting, ambulation, bathing, feeding etc.										
	Impaired skin integrity	Decubitus ulcer, wounds requiring irrigation or dressing changes every four hours, incontinence										
	Knowledge deficit requiring intensive patient/ family education	Discharge teaching, chemotherapy teaching, tracheostomy or ostomy teaching										
	Sensory deficits (hearing, vision, speech)	Deaf/blind, non-native speaking										
	Alteration in bowel or urinary elimination	Incontinence with > one linen change per shift										
	Coping, ineffective	Patient or family crisis situation										
II.	**This category of indicators requires an average of 6 hours of care in a 24-hour period or 2 hours of care in an 8-hour period.**		313	314	315	316	317	318	319	320	321	322
	Fever, potential for infection	Febrile < 102°, fever of unknown origin, conservative measures, including blood cultures										
	Fluid volume deficit requiring parenteral therapy	Simple IV therapy, > 3l/day, heparin lock, single agent chemotherapy protocol										
	Haematologic status requiring simple blood transfusions	Single blood product										
	Mild self-care deficit	Assistance with some activities of daily living										
	Comfort, alteration in	IV analgesics every two to four hours, pain assessment, patient controlled-analgesia										
	Nutrition, alteration in, less than body requirements	Total parenteral nutrition, tube feeding										
	Neuro status, alteration in	Neuro checks every four hours										
I.	**This category of indicators requires an average of 4 hours of care in a 24-hour period or 1.3 hours of care in an 8-hour period.**		313	314	315	316	317	318	319	320	321	322
	Anxiety, mild to moderate	New diagnosis, requiring support/observations										
	Therapy requiring radiation precautions/minimal care	^{131}I, thyroid ablation, iridium implants (exposure in room < one hour per shift per nurse)										

Annex 6   Wisecare Patient Questionnaire on Pain, Fatigue, Nausea and Vomiting and Oral Care

For completion on ....

Patient I.D. number ....

Please answer all of the questions yourself by circling the number that best applies to you. There are no 'right' or 'wrong' answers. The information that you provide will remain strictly confidential.

	Not at all	A little	Quite a bit	Very much
Have you had pain during the last 24 hours?	1	2	3	4
Did pain interfere with your activities during the last 24 hours?	1	2	3	4
Did you need to rest during the past24 hours?	1	2	3	4
Have you felt weak during the past 24 hours?	1	2	3	4
Were you tired during the past 24 hours?	1	2	3	4
Have you felt nauseated during the past 24 hours?	1	2	3	4
Have you vomited during the past 24 hours?	1	2	3	4

Please move onto the next page now.

Please complete this questionnaire by ticking the box that best represents how your mouth feels or looks today

1. Voice	Normal	☐
	Deep or Raspy	☐
	Difficulty talking/painful	☐
2. Swallow	Normal swallow	☐
	Some pain on swallow	☐
	Unable to swallow	☐
3. Lips	Smooth and pink and moist	☐
	Dry and cracked	☐
	Ulcerated or bleeding	☐
4. Tongue	Pink and moist and papillae present	☐
	Coated or loss of papillae with shinny appearance with or without redness	☐
	Blistered or cracked	☐
5. Saliva	Watery	☐
	Thick or ropy	☐
	Absent	☐

6. Mucous   Pink and moist
membranes ☐

Reddened or coated
(increased whiteness)
without ulceration ☐

Ulceration with or
Without bleeding ☐

7. Gingiva   Pink and stillped and
firm ☐

Oedematous with or
without redness ☐

Spontaneous bleeding
or bleeding with pressure ☐

8. Teeth/dentures Clean and no debris ☐

Plaque or debris in
localised area (between
teeth if present) ☐

Plaque or debris
generalised along gum
line or denture bearing
area ☐

Thank you for taking the time to complete the whole questionnaire.

Annex 7   Nursing Resource Form

DATE ________________

Staffing levels
Please list
Number of qualified staff in your area   ________
Number of Full Time Equivalents   ________
Number of unqualified nurse assistants in your are   ________

Education and experience of nursing staff
Please list the type and level of post-basic cancer nursing education undertaken by each qualified nurse in the area to be involved in the project:

Type of education	*Number of staff*
________________	________________
________________	________________
________________	________________
________________	________________

Please list the number of staff currently undertaking specialist cancer nursing education in the form of:

Type of education   *Number of staff*
Degree/Master's degree in cancer nursing   ________________
Conferences   ________________
Study Days   ________________
Other (Please specify)   ....

Please list the number of years experience in cancer nursing of each qualified nurse in the area to be involved in the project:

Environment of care
Please list:
The nurse/patient ratio in your area   ________________
Number of patients in your area   ________________
Patient dependency in your area   *Grade:*   ________________

Multidisciplinary details:
- Regular multidisciplinary meetings   Yes ________ No ________
- Multidisciplinary documentation   Yes ________ No ________
- Multidisciplinary disease focus groups   Yes ________ No ________

Who is responsible for the management of each of the following aspects of Care
(Please mark the line with an X):

- FATIGUE   Nurse   ________
                         Doctor   ________
                         Psychologist   ________
                         Other *(Please specify)*   ________

- ORAL CARE   Nurse   ________
                         Doctor   ________
                         Other *(Please specify)*   ________

- PAIN   Nurse   ________
                         Doctor   ________
                         Psychologist   ________
                         Other *(Please specify)*   ________

- NAUSEA   Nurse   ________
  + VOMITING   Doctor   ________
                         Psychologist   ________
                         Other *(Please specify)*   ________

Annex 8   Leuven Chemotherapy Risk Assessment Scale (LCRAS)[1]

Chemotherapy Products	Nausea & Vomiting	Oral Care	Pain	Fatigue
Amasacrine	3	3	0	3
Asparaginase	3	0	3	2
Azathiopirine	2	0	0	3
Bleomycine	2	3	0	0
Carboplatine	2	0	0	3
Carmustine	2	0	2	3
Cloormethinehydrochloride	3	0	0	3
Chlorambucil	2	0	0	3
Cisplatine	3	0	0	3
Cyclophosphamide	3	2	0	3
Cytarabine	3	2	2	3
Dacarbazine	3	2	0	3
Dactinomycine	2	3	1	3
Daunarubicine	2	3	0	3
Docetaxel	2	0	0	3
Doxorubicine	2	2	0	3
Epirubicine	3	3	0	3
Estramustine	2	0	0	3
Etoposide	3	2	0	3
Fludarabinephosphaat	2	0	0	3
Fluoro-uracil	3	3	0	3
Gemcitabine hydrocloride	3	0	0	3
Idarubicine	2	2	2	3
Ifosfamide	3	0	0	3
Melphalan	2	0	0	3
Methotrexaat	2	3	0	3
Mitomycine C	3	2	2	3
Mitoxantrone	3	1	0	3
Placitaxel	2	0	0	3
Procarbazine	3	1	0	3
Teniposide	1	0	0	3
Thiopeda	3	0	2	3
Topotecan hydrochloride	2	2	0	3
Vinblastine	2	2	0	3
Vincristine	0	0	3	2
Vindesine	2	0	2	3

[1] Based on Dhaenekint C. et al. Practical Guide for nurses, Verpleegkundig Cytostatica Compendium, Glaxo Wellcome, 1994

Annex 8b   Groningen Breast Cancer Risk Assessment Scale (GBCRAS)[1]

Surgical treatment	Pain	Fatigue	Nausea & Vomiting	Oral Care
Incisional biopsy	2	1	1	1
Incision, drainage abces/fistel	2	2	1	1
Excisional biopsy	2	1	1	1
Breast biopsy after needle localization	2	2	1	1
Excision of fistula	3	2	1	1
Excision of conus	2	1	2	1
Excision of gynaecomasty	1	1	2	1
Excision of tumor	2	2	2	1
Excision of tumor with axillair dissection	3	3	3	1
Mastectomy subcutaneously	3	3	2	1
Modified radical mastectomy	3	3	3	1
Radical mastectomy	3	3	3	1
Mastectomy after breast sparing operation	3	3	3	1
Breast removal	2	2	3	1
Nipple excision	2	1	1	1
Nippel reconstruction	1	1	1	1
Cytology of breast	1	1	1	1
Thoracic wall resection	3	3	3	1
Sentinel node axilla	1	1	1	1
Axillar dissection	3	3	1	1
Skin - reoperation for bleeding postoperatively	1	3	2	1

[2] Based on empirical evidence and Delphi method by AZ Groningen nursing staff

Annex 9   Best Practices Guidelines on Fatigue

1   Assessment

Questions used to assess the patient's level of fatigue and pattern of usual activities should include:
Have you felt fatigued over the past day/week/month? If yes:
- How severe is the feeling of fatigue (scale of 1=not at all - 5=extremely severe)
- What time of day is the fatigue at the lowest? What time of day is the feeling of fatigue most severe? How does the feeling of fatigue relate to your treatment? (How many days post chemotherapy, how many hours after radiotherapy etc?)
- What things have you tired to relieve the fatigue and how well did they work?
Please describe a typical day for you over the past week beginning when you get up in the morning. How does the day you just described differ from your usual day before this illness or before this treatment?
If activities have decreased ask which if the changes were because of fatigue
Which daily activities are most important to you and which ones could be done by someone else?
What activities that you are now doing or stopped doing are things that you really like to do?

2   Interventions

Nursing interventions should be based on patient assessment data. Firstly, it should be determined if the patient has any signs or symptoms of other causes of fatigue such as infection or anaemia. If the most likely cause of fatigue is as a side effect of cancer treatment:
- Utilise data on the severity and pattern of fatigue to guide interventions. If the fatigue is very severe, more adjustment in activity is required than if it is mild. If the fatigue is mild, the patient may decide to maintain the current level of activity but restructure the activities to take advantage of high-energy times.
- Build on what works for the patient. If the patient has identified activities that relieve the fatigue such as exercise, support the intervention rather than trying to substitute it with something else. Discourage the repeated use of interventions that are not effective as they may be contributing to the fatigue.
- When the patient can not identify anything that works, suggest decreasing activities and increasing rest. Focus on identifying important activities with the patient. If the patient is interested in exercise, screen for contraindications and follow the necessary precautions before commencing exercise.
- For those patients receiving treatment, provide reassurance and education that the fatigue is a common side effect of the treatment and that this will gradually improve once the treatment is completed. For those patients whose fatigue is an indication of advanced cancer, planning with the patient and the caregiver regarding the most important activities to ensure they are incorporated into the daily routine, may help to maintain quality of life.

2.1   Education should also include energy conservation techniques that cold be utilised by the patient, such as:

2.1.1 Activities of daily living

- Sit down to bathe and dry off
- Use shower or bath organiser to avoid reaching and leaning
- Install bath handles
- Use extension handles on sponges and brushes
- Use an elevated toilet seat
- Organise time to avoid rushing
- Lay out clothes and toiletries before washing and dressing
- Minimise leaning over to put on clothes and shoes
- Modify home environment to maximise efficient use of energy
- Wear comfortable clothes and low-heeled shoes

2.1.2 Housekeeping

- Schedule household tasks throughout the week
- Do housework sitting down when possible
- Delegate housework, shopping, laundry and child care when possible

2.1.3 Shopping

- Organise the shopping list by isle
- Use a shopping trolley for support
- Shop at less busy times
- Request assistance for returning to the car

2.1.4 Meal preparation

- Use convenience foods/easy to prepare foods
- Use smaller cooking utensils as they are easier to use
- Arrange the preparation environment for easy access to frequently used items
- Prepare meals sitting down
- Soak dishes instead of scrubbing them and allow them to air dry
- Prepare double potions and save half

2.1.5 Child care

- Plan activities to allow for sitting down (e.g. drawing, playing, reading, computer games)
- Teach children to climb onto chairs or laps to avoid lifting

2.1.6 Workplace

- Plan workload to take advantage of peak energy times
- Arrange work environment for easy access to frequently used equipment and supplies

2.1.7 Leisure

- Do activities with a companion
- Select activities that match energy level
- Balance activity and rest (don't get overtired)

Based on information from Donovan E. (1995) 'Energy conservation' In Fatigue initiative through research and education (FIRE) course. Educational programmes sponsored by Oncology Nursing Society and Ortho Biotech Inc.

3   Evaluation of interventions

This should be done on a regular basis, taking the patient's disease status and treatment into consideration. Evaluation should follow the pattern of the original assessment, lead onto further interventions and be cyclical.

Annex 10 Best Practices Guidelines on Pain

These guidelines follow a multimodal approach to pain and will address the nursing care involved in: assessment of patients' pain, interventions for pain management, evaluation of pain management and patient education regarding pain management. These aspects of nursing care have been addressed separately for the purpose of these guidelines however, in clinical practice they continuously overlap.

1   Assessment of patients' pain

Assessment of patients pain should be conducted using a measurement instrument previously shown to be both reliable and valid in the particular patient population in question. The choice of assessment tool should take into consideration the multidimensional nature of pain and the importance of assessing the impact of nursing interventions on the pain. For example, a pain assessment could be carried out using the Pain Assessment Tool in combination with a Pain Flow Sheet.

It is crucial that in assessing pain the nurse should address the:

3.1   Onset

- How long the pain has been present indicates whether it is acute or chronic
- Implications for treatment plan
- Allows for the assessment of any behavioural or physical responses
- Consider the patient's perception of when the pain began (makes the patient believe that you are genuinely interested in their problem, useful insight into what the patient felt caused the pain and which pain he is talking about)

3.2   Anatomical position of the pain

- Be aware that this can change or extend to avoid presumptions about the pain
- Ongoing anatomical assessment may show that there is a different pain in a different place that requires different treatment
- Assists in the decision regarding whether a pain is primary or referred

3.3   Description of the pain

- Influenced by factors such as racial origin, regional variation, age, mental ability and social class
- Allow the patient to describe the pain in his own words as this gives insight into type of pain, pattern/nature of pain and intensity

3.4   Activities of daily living

Factors that may exacerbate or bring on the pain provide valuable information regarding the nature of the pain and include:
- Time that the pain occurs
- Activities/movement
- Food/drink
- Stress/anxiety
- Family dynamics
- Social isolation/social crowding
- Work situation
- Housing

Previous treatment
- May influence the choice of future treatments
- Assess how the patient felt about previous treatments
- Previous side effects from treatment?
- Dosages and length of time other treatments taken
- Overview of other medical treatments and conditions as they may affect the subsequent choice of treatment

Whether or not a pain assessment tool is utilised in gathering this information, it is essential that the information obtained during this assessment is stored in a useful manner. For example, a measure of pain intensity and pain relief should be recorded on the bedside vital sign chart or similar record that facilitates regular review by the healthcare team. The intensity of pain/discomfort should be assessed and documented on admission, following any known pain producing procedure, with each new report of pain, and routinely at regular intervals. The degree of pain relief can then be determined after each pain management intervention, once sufficient time has elapsed to allow treatment to reach peak effect

4   Interventions for pain management

The first interventions for pain interventions must be to establish the patient's beliefs regarding the principles of analgesia and the importance of assessment and open communication. Understanding the patient's opinion of the potential side effects of analgesia is also important. Thus, it is important to:
- Discuss patient's and family's fears regarding the concerns about addiction, tolerance and physical dependence.
- Develop a plan of care with the patient and the caregiver for how to manage the side effects of the analgesia. Provide the patient with written instructions of how to manage these side effects.
- Discuss with patients the deleterious effects of unrelieved cancer pain and the fact that they do not need to be in pain.

After establishing the patient's beliefs regarding analgesia and their wishes about pain control, these should be considered alongside the pain assessment. A multidisciplinary team approach to pain interventions can then be initiated, incorporating both pharmacological and non-pharmacological interventions according to the patient's wishes. These interventions should be continuously evaluated and manipulated to achieve positive patient outcomes and should include the following aspects:
- The prescription of analgesia should follow the guideleines set by the WHO (1990) of the analgesic ladder
- The analgesia prescribed for a patient should consider patients' pain location, type, instensity, other conditions and wishes
- The timing of the administration of analgesia should occur exactly according to the prescription
- Analgesia efficacy should be evaluauted regularly utilising the same assessment scale
- Patients should be given advice and information regarding the benefits of non-pharmacological interventions for pain management and contact numbers for accessing this service

5   Evaluation of pain management

In an effort to evaluate the outcome of pain interventions a pain medication flow sheet could be utilised as suggested by Haviley et al (1992).

Date/time	Medication/ Comfort measures	Assessment Quality of pain	Intensity rating (0-5)	Sedation rating (1-5)	BM	Resp

Intensity rating:
0 = none
1 = mild
2 = moderate
3 = severe
4 = incapacitating
5 = overwhelming

Sedation rating:
1 = awake
2 = drowsy
3 = mostly sleeping
4 = only awake when aroused
5 = unarousable

6   Patient education regarding pain management

Education should include both the patient and family and should be an ongoing process throughout the pain experience.
The education of patients and families about cancer pain management should include
- Causes of pain
- Anticipated effect of therapy on pain
- What to report regarding their pain
- Medication information
- Side-effects of medications and their management
- Expected effects of analgesics e.g. initial drowsiness
- Self-care measures
- Contraindicated treatments or activities
- Information to restructure attitudes about addiction, medications etc.
- Plan for follow-up and contact for emergencies
- Patient's responsibilities for the pain management plan
- Role of the multidisciplinary team regarding pain management

Teach patients and their family caregivers how to use a pain assessment tool. Go beyond teaching them how to record pain intensity ratings in their pain diary. Teach them how to evaluate the pain intensity scores on a daily basis to determine if their pain medication is providing adequate relief.

Teach patients to document the negative consequences of unrelieved pain on their ability to perform activities of daily living, engage in social activities and perform work related activities.

Teach patients how to communicate with their health care providers about unrelieved pain. Teach patients to provide health care providers with data about their pain intensity scores and to understand the deleterious effects of unrelieved pain on the patient's mood and quality of life.

Provide educational information and self-care skills that will restore hope that pain can be relieved (e.g. alternative therapies, all options have not been exhausted)

Elicit patient's and significant other's beliefs and fears regarding pain medication

Teach patient to take their pain medication on a regular basis and the reason why this approach is more effective than an 'as required' approach.

Teach patients and significant others about the concept of dependence, tolerance, withdrawal and addiction in an effort to allay fears

Instruct patient and significant others regarding how to seek help and use resources to assist in implementing a pain management plan

Encourage patients to use a pain diary or other tools to assess their pain to identify factors that may contribute to pain and interventions to alleviate pain

Refer patients to experts for assistance with unrelieved pain

Evaluate the effect of education on those experiencing cancer pain

Refer patients and significant others to self-help groups for education and support

Develop structured educational programmes

Establish procedures to assess patient education following discharge

Participate in public education activities regarding cancer pain

Annex 11 Best Practices Guidelines on Oral Care

1   Assessment

Effective care begins before therapy begins with assessment and prophylactic treatment in conjunction with dental hygiene consultation being the ideal (Madeya 1996, Nieweg 1992).

Patients' mouths should be assessed prior to treatment using a standardised assessment tool such as the Oral Assessment Guide developed by Eilers et al (1988). See below.

Category	Tools for assessment	Methods of measurement	1	2	3
Voice	Auditory	Converse with patient	Normal	Deeper or raspy	Difficulty talking or painful
Swallow	Observation	Ask patient to swallow. Test gag reflex by placing blade on back of tongue and press	Normal swallow	Some pain on swallow	Unable to swallow
Lips	Visual/ Palpatory	Observe and feel tissue	Smooth, pink and moist	Dry or cracked	Ulcerated or bleeding
Tongue	Visual/ Palpatory	Feel and observe the appearance of tissue	Pink and moist and papillae present	Coated or loss of papillae with a shiny appearance with or without redness	Blistered or cracked
Saliva	Tongue blade	Insert blade into mouth, touching the centre of the tongue and floor of the mouth	Watery	Thick or ropy	Absent
Mucous membranes	Visual	Observe appearance of tissue	Pink and moist	Reddened or coated (increased whiteness) without ulcerations	Ulcerations with or without bleeding
Gingiva	Tongue blade + visual	Gently press tissue with tip of blade	Pink and stippled and firm	Oedematous with or without redness	Spontaneous bleeding or bleeding with pressure
Teeth or dentures	Visual	Observe appearance of teeth or denture bearing area	Clean and no debris	Plaque or debris in localised areas (between teeth if present)	Plaque or debris generalised along gum line or denture bearing area

7   Interventions

7.1   Mechanical cleaning

The most effective methods for mechanical cleansing of the mouth are a soft small toothbrush rotated through 45 degrees and unwaxed dental floss (Daeffler 1981, Nieweg 1992, Moore 1995). Brushing should not be performed by thrombocytopaenic patients (platelets<50,000) (Armstrong 1994).

7.2   Mouthwashes

Results concerning optimal mouthwashes remain inconclusive. Chlorhexidine (a broad-spectrum antimicrobial agent that suppresses oral microflora) was found to prevent dental plaque formation, reduce gingival inflammation and decrease the incidence of oral mucositis in patients treated with high dose chemotherapy (Ferretti et al 1990). Conversely, Dodd et al (1996) compared two mouthwashes – chlorhexidine and sterile water- in a placebo-controlled trial and found that chlorhexidine had no significant effect in preventing mucositis in the out-patient chemotherapy setting. Further evaluation is consequently required.

7.3   Lubricants

Artificial saliva is helpful in maintaining comfort if used sparingly but does not have the antibacterial properties of saliva (Holmes 1991). Lubricants used to moisturise lips vary and include aloe vera and lanolin lip lubricant and lanolin petroleum-based lip lubricant to name but a few (Kenny 1990). Additionally, there are a number of commercial products available.

7.4   Frequency of oral care

Increasing the frequency of oral care with the worsening of oral status has been shown to have a positive effect on oral health (Armstrong 1994). Interventions should be performed 2-6 hourly or the benefits of previous care will be lost (Armstrong 1994). Oral care should also be given throughout the night if mouth complications exist (Sweeney and Bagg 1995).

7.5   Patient education

While no 'gold standard' oral protocol exists, the benefits of a systematic oral hygiene teaching programme have been illustrated (Larson et al 1998). The programme requires patients to inspect their mouths, checking for listed signs and symptoms of complications, followed by instructions on brushing, flossing and rinsing with a mouthwash.

7.6   Pain management

The appropriate management of oral pain is essential. Assessment of this pain should be performed utilising a standardised assessment tool such as the visual analogue scale or a graphic rating scale. Pharmacological interventions may range from oral interventions to subcutaneous opiod administration. Pain should be assessed on a regular basis and recorded in an appropriate multidisciplinary record.

7.7   Nutritional advice

Patients both at risk of oral problems and suffering from oral problems should be advised to avoid eating hot and cold foods and also heavily spiced foodstuffs. Smoking and alcoholic beverages should also be avoided.

The education programme described by Larson et al (1998) was:
For non-denture wearers:
- Brush your teeth for 90 seconds twice a day, after breakfast and before going to bed.
- Floss your teeth once a day.
- Rinse your mouth with water for 30 seconds, twice a day, after brushing and flossing your teeth. Swish thoroughly and spit out. DO NOT SWALLOW. Do not use any other mouthwash.
- Inspect your mouth, including your lips and tongue, using a torch, every morning after brushing and rinsing. *Call your nurse* as soon as possible if you have any mouth problems.
- *Avoid* smoking, alcoholic beverages and spicy foods

For denture wearers:
- Remove your denture/partial plate before beginning your mouth care
- Brush your teeth for 90 seconds twice a day, after breakfast and before going to bed.
- Floss your teeth once a day.
- Rinse your mouth with water for 30 seconds, twice a day, after brushing and flossing your teeth. Swish thoroughly and spit out. DO NOT SWALLOW. Do not use any other mouthwash.
- Inspect your mouth, including your lips and tongue, using a torch, every morning after brushing and rinsing. *Call your nurse* as soon as possible if you have any mouth problems.
- *Avoid* smoking, alcoholic beverages and spicy foods
- Wear your dentures or partial plate as little as possible
- Remove your dentures and partial plate at night for soaking
- Clean and brush your dentures or partial plate before soaking
- Soak dentures or partial plate without metal parts in a weak bleach solution (1/2 teaspoon in a cup of tap water). For dentures or partial plate with metal parts, omit bleach and soak in a regular soaking solution. Rinse thoroughly before wearing.

8 Evaluation

Evaluation of care should again be performed using an assessment guide such as that developed by Eilers et al (1988) illustrated earlier.

Annex 12 Best Practices Guidelines on Nausea and Vomiting

1 Assessment

1.1 Baseline assessment using standardised nursing admission documentation prior to treatment, taking into consideration factors including

- Previous emetic history
- History of alcohol abuse
- History of motion sickness
- Emetic history during any previous pregnancy
- Age
- Expectation of treatment
- Nutritional patterns
- Home environments
- Stress response

1.2 Establish patterns of emesis following previous treatment using a standardised assessment scale e.g. NVR-2. Patterns of nausea and vomiting that should be evaluated include:

- Acute nausea/vomiting
- Delayed nausea/vomiting
- Anticipatory nausea/vomiting

1.3 Determine the impact of emesis on patient's life and quality of life through discussing factors such as:

- Social activities
- Employment implications
- Financial implications
- Family role

2 Plan care

Through open communication, set mutually agreeable goals with patient incorporating factors such as:
- Acceptable level of nausea/vomiting
- Tolerable side effects of anti-emetics
- Potential for utilising non-pharmacological interventions

3 Ensure effective communication are utilised to ensure positive patient outcomes. Such communication should involve

- The patient
- The family
- The clinicians
- The community care staff
- The other health care professionals e.g. dietician, psychologist, pharmacist

4   Interventions

4.1 Pharmacological interventions

- Administer anti-emetics as per an established, hospital, research-based protocol
- Educate patient regarding the administration of his anti-emetics at home, anticipated side-effects, how to monitor the effectiveness of the drugs and when to seek assistance
- Highlight the benefits of the patient keeping a note of nausea and vomiting symptoms and antiemetics taken regarding their impact on daily living, nutrition, hydration and quality of life to facilitate assessing drug efficacy before the next cycle of treatment. For example, suggest the patient keeps a log or diary
- Act as patient advocate with regards to recommendation of anti-emetic changes for the patient
- Manage the side effects of anti-emetics effectively and efficiently and document these to ensure appropriate treatment on subsequent treatment cycles
- Monitor the effectiveness of anti-emetics. This should include:
  Ensuring sufficient anti-emetics are administered prior to chemotherapy
  Ensuring a quick response to situations where anti-emetics are not effective
  Ensure anti-emetics are administered on a regular basis rather than 'as required'
  Continue to evaluate the effectiveness of antiemetics throughout treatment using an appropriate assessment tool such as VAS or NVR-2
  Ensure adequate antiemetic cover is in place for delayed emesis once the patient has been discharged

4.2 Non-pharmacological interventions

4.2.1 Dietary adjustments

- Types of food – educate the patient to avoid heavily spiced foods and extremes of temperatures
- Frequency of meals – advise the patient to eat small frequent meals
- Size of servings – educate the patient regarding the advantages of eating small meals rather than large meals
- Avoiding favourite foods when symptoms are increasing – suggest to the patient that avoiding favourite foods while feeling nauseated prevents the development of an association between favourite foods and nausea and vomiting

4.2.2 Environmental adjustments

- Advise the patient to avoid smells of cooking/food within the house
- Educate the patient to avoid smoky atmospheres and strong perfumes

4.2.3 Relaxation and behavioural interventions

- Distraction such as the television, conversation, games
- Guided imagery
- Meditation
- Passive or active relaxation
- Systematic desensitisation
- Acupuncture/acupressure

5   Evaluation

5.1   *Evaluate the effectiveness of the treatment plan*

- Establish the patient's pattern and severity of nausea and vomiting following treatment through the use of patient diary, assessment tool such as the NVR-2, VAS or ordinal scale
- Evaluate effectiveness of anti-emetic regime including the type of antiemetic, patient satisfaction with the outcome and patient compliance with the antiemetic treatment
- In-depth evaluation of the period post-treatment using both established assessment tools and open-ended questions
- With the patient's permission, assess the perspectives of family members
- Report findings to relevant personnel and ensure they are taken into consideration when planning and prescribing future treatment

Reassure the patient that every effort will be made to adjust antiemetic treatment to achieve both optimal and acceptable

Annex 13 EORTC QLQ-C30 Scale

Within the WISECARE project the option was taken to use the EORTC Quality of Life Questionnaire C-30. In the beginning of the project the entire questionnaire was used. Along the project a change in data collection was made and 3 subscales of the EORTC Quality of Life Questionnaire C-30 were retained. This scoring Manual is used to produce all feedback on the indicators fatigue, nausea and vomiting and pain. Also for some data analysis on the results of the Oral Asessment Guide (OAG) the rules of this manual are followed.

The following section gives the scoring procedures for EORTC Quality of Life Questionnaire C-30 as used in WISECARE. This manual is owned by the EORTC[1].

1   The EORTC QLQ-C30

1.1   Introduction

The EORTC quality of life questionnaire (QLQ) is an integrated system for assessing the health-related quality of life (QoL) of cancer patients participating in international clinical trials. The core questionnaire, the QLQ-C30, is the product of more than a decade of collaborative research. Following its general release in 1993, the QLQ-C30 has been used in a wide range of cancer clinical trials, by a large number of research groups; it has additionally been used in various other, non-trial studies.

This manual contains scoring procedures for the QLQ-C30 versions 1.0, (+3), 2.0 and 3.0; it also contains summary information about supplementary modules.

All publications relating to the QLQ should use the scoring procedures described in this manual. This manual will be updated at regular intervals, to reflect future changes to the QLQ and to incorporate new supplementary modules.

2   Background

2.1   EORTC

The European Organization for Research and Treatment of Cancer (EORTC) was founded in 1962, as an international non-profit organization. The aims of the EORTC are to conduct, develop, co-ordinate and stimulate cancer research in Europe by multidisciplinary groups of oncologists and basic scientists. Research is accomplished mainly through the execution of large, prospective, randomized, multicentre, cancer clinical trials.

The EORTC Central Office Data Center, created in 1974, is concerned with all aspects of phase II and phase III cancer clinical trials, from their design to the publication of the final results. Since its inception, over 80,000 patients have been entered in trials handled by the EORTC Data Center.

In 1980, the EORTC created the Quality of Life Study Group, which in 1986 initiated a research programme to develop an integrated, modular approach for evaluating the QoL of patients participating in cancer clinical trials.

---

[1] All rights reserved. No part of this manual covered by copyrights hereon may be reproduced or transmitted in any form or by any means without prior permission of the copyright holder.
The EORTC QLQ-C30 (in all versions), and the modules which supplement it, are copyrighted and may not be used without prior written consent of the EORTC Data Center.
Requests for permission to use the EORTC QLQ-C30 and the modules, or to reproduce or quote materials contained in this manual, should be addressed to:
Quality of Life Unit, EORTC Data Center, Avenue E Mounier 83 - B11, 1200 Brussels, BELGIUM, Tel: +32 2 774 1611, Fax: +32 2 779 4568

2.2. *EORTC QLQ-C30 version 3.0*

Version 3.0 of the QLQ-C30 differs from version 2.0 in that it has four-point scales for the first five items (QLQ-C30(V3).. These are coded with the same response categories as item 6 to 28, namely "Not at all", "A little", "Quite a bit" and "Very much." To allow for these categories, question 4 has been re-worded as "Do you have to stay in a bed or a chair during the day?"

Version 3.0 is currently the standard version of the QLQ-C30, and should be used for all new studies unless investigators wish to maintain compatibility with previous studies, which used an earlier version of the QLQ-C30.

3.   Scoring procedures

3.1. *General principles of scoring*

The QLQ-C30 is composed of both multi-item scales and single item measures. These include five functional scales, three symptom scales, a global health status / QoL scale, and six single items. Each of the multi-item scales includes a different set of items - no item occurs in more than one scale.

All of the scales and single-item measures range in score from 0 to 100. A high scale score represents a higher response level. Thus a

- *high score for a functional scale* represents a *high / healthy level of functioning*,
- *high score for the global health status / QoL* represents a *high QoL*,
- but a *high score for a symptom scale / item* represents a *high level of symptomatology / problems*.
  The principle for scoring these scales is the same in all cases:
- Estimate the average of the items that contribute to the scale; this is the *raw score.*
- *Use a linear transformation to standardise the raw score, so that scores range from 0 to 100; a higher score represents a higher ("better") level of functioning, or a higher ("worse") level of symptoms.*

3.2. *Technical Summary*

In practical terms, if items $I_1, I_2, ... I_n$ are included in a scale, the procedure is as follows:

Raw score

Calculate the raw score

$$RS = \left(I_1 + I_2 + ... + I_n\right)/n$$

Linear transformation

Apply the linear transformation to 0-100 to obtain the score S.

Functional scales: $\quad S = \left\{1 - \dfrac{(RS - 1)}{range}\right\} \times 100$

Symptom scales / items: $\quad S = \left\{(RS - 1)/range\right\} \times 100$

Global health status / QoL: $\quad S = \left\{(RS - 1)/range\right\} \times 100$

Range is the difference between the maximum possible value of *RS* and the minimum possible value. The QLQ-C30 has been designed so that all items in any scale take the same range of values. Therefore, the range of *RS* equals the range of the item values. Most items are scored 1 to 4, giving *range* = 3. The exceptions are the items contributing to the global health status / QoL, which are 7-point questions with *range* = 6, and the initial yes/no items on the earlier versions of the QLQ-C30 which have *range* = 1.

4.   Scoring the EORTC QLQ-C30 version 3.0

Scoring the QLQ-C30 version 3.0

	Scale	Number of items	Item range*	*Version 3.0* Item numbers	Function scales
1.1.1.1.1.1.1.1 *Global health status / QoL*					
Global health status/QoL (revised)[†]	QL2	2	6	29, 30	
1.1.1.1.1.1.1.2 *Functional scales*					
Physical functioning (revised)[†]	PF2	5	3	1 to 5	F
Role functioning (revised)[†]	RF2	2	3	6, 7	F
Emotional functioning	EF	4	3	21 to 24	F
Cognitive functioning	CF	2	3	20, 25	F
Social functioning	SF	2	3	26, 27	F
1.1.1.1.1.1.1.3 *Symptom scales / items*					
Fatigue	FA	3	3	10, 12, 18	
Nausea and vomiting	NV	2	3	14, 15	
Pain	PA	2	3	9, 19	
Dyspnoea	DY	1	3	8	
Insomnia	SL	1	3	11	
Appetite loss	AP	1	3	13	
Constipation	CO	1	3	16	
Diarrhoea	DI	1	3	17	
Financial difficulties	FI	1	3	28	

* *Item range* is the difference between the possible maximum and the minimum response to individual itemsmost items take values from 1 to 4, giving *range* = 3.

† (revised) scales are those that have been changed since version 1.0, and their short names are indicated in this manual by a suffix "2" – for example, PF2.

For all scales, the *RawScore, RS*, is the mean of the component items:

$$RS = RawScore = (I_1 + I_2 + ... + I_n)/n$$

Then for *Functional scales*:

$$Score = \left\{1 - \frac{(RS-1)}{range}\right\} \times 100$$

and for *Symptom scales / items and Global health status / QoL*

Examples:

     Emotional Functioning
$$RawScore = (Q_{21} + Q_{22} + Q_{23} + Q_{24})/4$$
$$EF\ Score = \{1 - (RawScore - 1)/3\} \times 100$$

     Fatigue
$$RawScore = (Q_{10} + Q_{12} + Q_{18})/3$$
$$FA\ Score = \{(RawScore - 1)/3\} \times 100$$

$$Score = \{(RS - 1)/range\} \times 100$$

Glossary

Core questionnaire: the QLQ-C30 is a "core questionnaire" which incorporates a range of physical, emotional and social health issues relevant to a broad spectrum of cancer patients; the core questionnaire should be used, unmodified, in all QLQ assessments.

Items: the individual questions on the QLQ-C30 are called items, and are described as Q_1, Q_2, Q_3, etc., where the suffix corresponds to the question-number on the QLQ questionnaire.

Module: the core questionnaire may be supplemented by diagnosis-specific and/or treatment-specific questionnaire modules. Modules should be used unmodified and in conjunction with the core questionnaire.

Raw score: the score formed by averaging the items that are included in a particular function or symptom scale.

Scales: the QLQ comprises distinct scales, each of which represents a different aspect of QoL.

Scale score: the raw score transformed to a standardised 0 - 100 final "scale score".

List of WISECARE Members and Partners

Wisecare Partners Team

Mrs. Jane **Bryan-Jones** AT Consulting Cnoc nan Cruach by Catlodge, Laggan Bridge UK - Newtonmore PH20 1BT (Scotland) Tel.: +44 152 854 4312 Fax +44 152 854 4360 jane.BryanJones@btinternet.com	Mr. Tonny **Gypen,** Partner Arthur Andersen Healthcare Practice Business Consulting Group Montagne du Parc 4 B-1000 Brussels (Belgium) Tel.: +32 2 545 35 75 home: +32 15 516 406 Fax: +32 2 545 35 99 tonny.gypen@be.arthurandersen.com
Prof. Ir. Luc **Delesie** Centre of Health Services Research & Nursing, KULeuven Department of Public Health, Faculty of Medicine Kapucijnenvoer 35/4 B-3000 Leuven (Belgium) Tel.: +32 16 336 972 Fax: +32 16 336 970 Luc.delesie@med.kuleuven.ac.be	Mr. Stelios **Halkiotis**, BSc, MSc, PhD candidate. University of Athens, Faculty of Nursing Laboratory of Health Informatics 2a Igimonos, Athens GR – 11527, Greece Tel.: +30 1 778 14 60 Fax: +30 1 777 98 34 Stelios@ dn.uoa.gr
Dr. Jaap **De Vries** Oncological Surgeon Academic Hospital Groningen – Dept. Surgery Hanzeplein 1 9700 RB Groningen (Netherlands) Tel.: +31 50 361 23 17 Fax: +31 50 361 48 73 E-mail: j.de.vries@chir.azg.nl	Mr. Jacob **Hofdijk**, MSc Baan Healthcare Solutions Schipholweg 97 NL-2316 XA Leiden (Netherlands) Fax: +31 71 521 98 56 Mobile: +31 6 549 72 808 Jhofdijk@hiscom.nl
Mr. Peter **Dounavis** BSc in Nursing, MSc in Health Informatics, PhD candidate. University of Athens, Faculty of Nursing Laboratory of Health Informatics 2a Igimonos, Athens GR - 11527, Greece Tel.: +30 1 778 14 60 Fax: +30 1 777 98 34 petros@dn.uoa.gr	Mr. Derek **Hoy**, RGN MSc Research Fellow Glasgow Caledonian University Home address for mail: 68 Brunstane Road Edinburgh EH15 2QR (UK) Tel.: +44 (0) 131 669 7508 Fax: +44 (0) 131 657 3638 d.hoy@gcal.ac.uk
Dr. Marianna **Diomidis,** MD in Medicine, MSc, PhD University of Athens, Faculty of Nursing Laboratory of Health Informatics 2a Igimonos, Athens GR - 11527, Greece Tel.: +30-1-7779834 Fax : +30-1-7781829 mdiomidi@dn.uoa.gr	Dr. Alan **Hyslop** IT Strategy Manager, NHS in Scotland Management Executive St.-Andrew's House UK - Edinburgh EH1 3DG (Scotland) Tel.: +44 131 244 23 66 Fax: +44 131 244 34 70 Ahyslop@cix.co.uk
Mrs. Lieve **Goossens**, RN, MSc Centre of Health Services Research & Nursing, KULeuven Department of Public Health, Faculty of Medicine Kapucijnenvoer 35/4 B-3000 Leuven (Belgium) Tel.: +32 16 33 69 91 Fax: +32 16 33 69 70 E-mail: lieve.goossens@uz.kuleuven.ac.be	Mrs. Emily **Karistinou**, BSc ,MSc University of Athens, Faculty of Nursing Laboratory of Health Informatics 2a Igimonos, Athens GR - 11527, Greece Tel.: +30 1 778 14 60 Fax: +30 1 777 98 34 emily@dn.uoa.gr

Mrs. Nora **Kearney** RGN, MSc Nursing and Midwifery School University of Glasgow 68 Oakfield Avenue Glasgow G12 8LS (Scotland) Tel.: +44 141 330 5915 Fax. +44 141 330 3539 Mobile: +44 411 16 90 15 NK16D@clinmed.gla.ac.uk	Prof. Walter **Sermeus**, RN, PhD Centre of Health Services Research & Nursing, KULeuven Department of Public Health, Faculty of Medicine Kapucijnenvoer 35/4 B-3000 Leuven (Belgium) Tel.: +32 16 33 69 91 Fax: +32 16 33 69 72 walter.sermeus@med.kuleuven.ac.be
Prof. Juha **Kinnunen,** RGN, MSc, PhD Department for Health Policy and Management University of Kuopio Harjulantie 1B / PO Box 1627 F - 70211 Kuopio, Finland Tel.: +358 17 162 616 Fax: +358 17 162 999 Juha.Kinnunen@uku.fi	Mr. Martin **Steegh,** MSc Software Engineer, HISCOM BV Central Development and Support Group HIS Schipholweg 97 NL-2316 XA Leiden (Netherlands) Tel.: +31 71 525 68 91 Fax: +31 71 521 98 56 Mobile: +31 655 34 21 43 msteegh@hiscom.nl
Ms. Gillian **Knowles** Department of Nursing Studies University of Edinburgh - Adam Ferguson Building 40 George Square UK - Edinburgh EH8 9LL (Scotland)	Ms. Anne **Tanghe**, RN, PhD Centre of Health Services Research & Nursing, KULeuven Department of Public Health, Faculty of Medicine Kapucijnenvoer 35/4 B-3000 Leuven (Belgium) Tel.: +32 16 33 69 91 Fax: +32 16 33 69 72 mahjoub.a@planet.tn
Prof. John **Mantas** BSc, MSc, PhD, Ass. Dean (Fac. of Nurs. of the Univ. of Athens) University of Athens, Faculty of Nursing Laboratory of Health Informatics 2a Igimonos, Athens GR - 11527, Greece Tel.: +30-1-7779834 Fax : +30-1-7781829 jmantas@dn.uoa.gr	Dr. Jeff **Tansley**, Consultant AT Consulting Cnoc nan Cruach by Catlodge, Laggan Bridge UK - Newtonmore PH20 1BT (Scotland) Tel.: +44 152 854 4312 Fax +44 152 854 4360 jeff.Tansley@btinternet.com
Ms. Morven **Miller**, RN, MSc Nursing and Midwifery School University of Glasgow 68 Oakfield Avenue Glasgow G12 8LS (Scotland) Tel.: +44 141 330 5915 Fax. +44 141 330 3539 mm118p@clinmed.gla.ac.uk	Kris **Vanhaecht**, RN, MSc Centre of Health Services Research & Nursing, KULeuven Department of Public Health, Faculty of Medicine Kapucijnenvoer 35/4 B-3000 Leuven (Belgium) Tel.: +32 16 33 69 71 Fax: +32 16 33 69 70 kris.vanhaecht@med.kuleuven.ac.be
Ms. Tiina **Nyberg,** RGN, CNS, RNE, MSc candidate Academic advisor Department of Health Policy and Management University of Kuopio MSc St. in Health Management Retkeilijantie 7B 16 70200 Kuopio (Finland) Tel.: +358 17 162 685 Fax: +358 17 162 999 Tiina.Nyberg@uku.fi	Mr. Kenny **Willems** Senior Consulent, Arthur Andersen Healthcare Business Consulting Montagne du Parc 4 B-1000 Brussels (Belgium) Tel.: +32 2 545 35 29 Fax: +32 2 545 35 99 kenny.willems@be.arthurandersen.com

WISECARE Validation Sites

Ms. Tiina **Aalto** RN Nurse, Pulmonary ward 82 Helsinki and Uusimaa Hospital Distric, HUCH P.O. Box 340 FIN - 00029 HYKS Tiina.Aalto@hus.fi	Tiina **Kärjä-Lahdensuu** Research nurse, division of haemathology PL340 (P.O.Box 340) 00029 HYKS (Finland)
Ms. Pirkko **Bellaoui** RN Deputy head nurse, Pulmonary ward 82 Helsinki and Uusimaa Hospital Distric, HUCH P.O. Box 340 FIN - 00029 HYKS Pirkko.Bellaoui@hus.fi	Ms. Pirjo **Korhonen-Kivinen** RN, MSc Head nurse, Pulmonary ward 82 Helsinki and Uusimaa Hospital Distric, HUCH P.O. Box 340 FIN - 00029 HYKS Pirjo.Korhonen-Kivinen@hus.fi
Phyllis **Campbell**, Clincal Services Manager Western Infirmary Beatson Oncology Centre Dumbarton Road Glasgow, Scotland G11 6NT (Scotland) p.campbell@nhut.org.uk	Mr. Joacim **Larsen**, RN, PhD-student Department of Nursing, Karolinska Institutet P.O. Box 286 S-171 77 Stockholm, Sweden joacim.larsen@omv.ki.se
Fiona **Ferguson,** Staff Nurse Western Infirmary Beatson Oncology Centre Dumbarton Road Glasgow, Scotland G11 6NT (Scotland) p.campbell@nhut.org.uk	Mr. Xavier **Lefever**, RN, MSc student UZ Gasthuisberg,E 632 Herestraat 49 B-3000 Leuven (Belgium) Xavierlefever@hotmail.com
Ms. Helena **Frimansson** Nurse Heamathology Dept. Huddinge University Hospital S-141 86 Huddinge (Sweden) Helenafrimansson@hotmail.com	Mrs. Helena **Librand**, RN Heamathology Dept., M72 Huddinge University Hospital S-14186 Huddinge (Sweden)
Mr. Jop **Helleman**, RN Nurse Oncology Surgery/Plastic Surgery – B3VA Academic Hospital Groningen Hanzeplein 1 9700 RB Groningen (Netherlands) J.Helleman@chir.azg.nl	Ms. Marika **Liimatainen** RN Head nurse, Cancer Centre, Chemotherapy OPD Helsinki and Uusimaa Hospital Distric, HUCH P.O. Box 180 FIN - 00029 HYKS Marika.Liimatainen@hus.fi
Ms. Anne **Henttinen** RN Nurse, Cancer Centre, Chemotherapy OPD Helsinki and Uusimaa Hospital Distric, HUCH P.O. Box 180 FIN - 00029 HYKS Anne.Henttinen@hus.fi	Ms. Karin **Långstedt** RN, RNA Director of nursing, Department of Internal Medicine Helsinki and Uusimaa Hospital Distric, HUCH P.O. Box 340 FIN - 00029 HYKS Karin.Langstedt@hus.fi
Mr. Rommy **Hoekstra**, Headnurse Nurse Oncology Surgery/Plastic Surgery – B3VA Academic Hospital Groningen Hanzeplein 1 9700 RB Groningen (Netherlands) R.I.Hoekstra@chir.azg.nl	Ms. Ann **McLinton,** Ward Manager Western Infirmary Beatson Oncology Centre Dumbarton Road Glasgow, Scotland G11 6NT p.campbell@nhut.org.uk
Ms. Marja-Leena **Hyvärinen** RN Nurse, Haematological ward 141 Helsinki and Uusimaa Hospital Distric, HUCH P.O. Box 340 FIN - 00029 HYKS Marja-Leena.M.Hyvarinen@hus.fi	Ms. Tamara **Patchev**, RN Nurse Heamathology Dept., M72 Huddinge University Hospital S-14186 Huddinge (Sweden) tamarapatchev@hotmail.com

Ms. Marita **Kaltea** MSc, RN Director of Nursing, , Cancer Centre Helsinki and Uusimaa Hospital Distric, HUCH P.O. Box 180 FIN - 00029 HYKS Marita.Kaltea@hus.fi	Mr. Gert **Peeters,** RN, MSc Head Nurse E 632 UZ Gasthuisberg Herestraat 49 B-3000 Leuven (Belgium) Gert.Peeters@uz.kuleuven.ac.be
Mr. Simo **Pietilä** BSc (Econ) Chief Information Officer Helsinki and Uusimaa Hospital District P.O. Box 440 FIN-00029 HYKS Finland Simo.Pietila@hus.fi	Mr. Lars **Strömberg** The Nursing R&D Unit Huddinge University Hospital S – 141 86 Huddinge Sweden Lars.stromberg@nurssres.hs.sll.se
Ms. Mirjami **Pyykkö** RN Head nurse, Haematological ward 11 Helsinki and Uusimaa Hospital Distric, HUCH P.O. Box 340 FIN - 00029 HYKS Mirjami.Pyykko@hus.fi	Ms. Marja **Tammisto,** Director of nursing HUCH, Department of Internal Medicine, P.O. Box 340 FIN - 00029 HYKS
Ms. Sinikka **Ripatti** RN, Diploma in business information technology Senior information systems specialist, Centre for IT Helsinki and Uusimaa Hospital Distric, HUCH P.O. Box 440 FIN - 00029 HYKS Sinikka.Ripatti@hus.fi	Saara **Vaalas** Helsinki University Central Hospital Haartmaninkatu 4 00290 Helsinki, Finland Saara.Vaalas@huch.fi
Ms. Ann **Roelants**, RN UZ Gasthuisberg, E632 Herestraat 49 B-3000 Leuven (Belgium) aroelants@hotmail.com	Mr. Lars **Wiström**, Head Nurse Head Nurse Heamathology Unit M72-74 Huddinge University Hospital S-141 86 Huddinge (Sweden) Lars.wistrom@hematol.hs.sll.se
Mrs. Catherine **Servaes**, RN UZ Gasthuisberg,E 632 Herestraat 49 B-3000 Leuven (Belgium) nocturne@hotmail.com	Ria **Ziengs**, RN Nurse Oncology Surgery/Plastic Surgery – B3VA Academic Hospital Groningen Hanzeplein 1 9700 RB Groningen (Netherlands) H.Ziengs@chir.azg.nl
Mrs.Karin **Smith**, Staff Nurse Western Infirmary Beatson Oncology Centre Dumbarton Road Glasgow, G11 6NT Scotland p.campbell@nhut.org.uk	

WISECARE Demonstration Sites

Mrs. Geraldine **Baron- Merle**, Infirmière en charge du projet, Service Ardennes, IGR DSSI, Institut Gustave Roussy, 39,Rue Camille Desmoulins, 94805 Villejuif, France cleclerc@igr.fr	Mr. Per **Kloster**, RN, MPM Nursing Manager, The Medical Department Aalborg Hopsital P.O. Box 365 9100 Aalborg pk@aas.nja.dk
Mrs. Marjana **Bozjak**, RN Head Nurse University Medical Centre Division of Internal Medicine Department of Haematology Zaloska 7, 1525 Ljubljana, Slovenia marjana.bozjak@kclj.si	Mrs.Ifigenia **Kostagiorggi**, SRN, Specialist in Pathological Nursing Hellenic Red Cross Hospital 1 Athanasaki 11526 Athens, Greece gikagrnurse@yahoo.com
Mrs. Elisabeth **Charalambidou** Ph.D,Nursing Adm. of Hellenic Red Cross Hospital,Member of the Board of the National Nurses Association&of the Oncology Nursing Section 1,Erytrou Staurou str.,Athens 11526, Greece gikagrnurse@yahoo.com	MrsClaudine **Leclerq**, Surveillant, Service Ardennes,IGR DSSI, Institut Gustave Roussy, 39,Rue Camille Desmoulins, 94805 Villejuif, France cleclerc@igr.fr
Mrs. Alenka **Dobrovoljc**, RN University Medical Centre Division of Internal Medicine Department of Haematology Zaloska 7, 1525 Ljubljana, Slovenia alenka.dobrovoljc@kclj.si	Mrs. Maria **Malama** SRN,Section of Education Hellenic Red Cross Hospital Ieremioy Pacriarthoy 11471 Athens, Greece gikagrnurse@yahoo.com
Mr. Jan **Foubert** Jules Bordet Institute Rue Heger-Bordet 1 1000 Bruxelles FoubertJan@bordet.be	Mrs. Jytta **Moelgaard**, RN The Medical Department Aalborg Hopsital P.O. Box 365 9100 Aalborg U27833@aas.nja.dk
Mrs. Mary **Gika**, Grad. of Theology&Nursing, SRN,Ph.D Hellenic Red Cross Hospital Ieremioy Pacriarthoy 11471 Athens, Greece gikagrnurse@yahoo.com	Mr. Nikos **Efstathiou** SRN,MSc,Ph.D Canditate Hellenic Red Cross Hospital Ieremioy Pacriarthoy 11471 Athens, Greece gikagrnurse@yahoo.com
Mr. Patrick **Crombez**, RN, MSc Aseptic and BMT Unit Jules Bordet Institute Rue Heger-Bordet 1 1000 Bruxelles FoubertJan@bordet.be	Mrs. Darja **Ovijac**, RN, B. Sc Assistant Teacher University of Ljubljana University college of health care Poljanska c. 26 a, 1000 Ljubljana, Slovenia darja.ovijac@vsz.uni-lj.si
Mrs.Jane **Gledhill**, DSSI, Institut Gustave Roussy, 39,Rue Camille Desmoulins, 94805 Villejuif, France gledhill@igr.fr	Mrs. Theodora **Pappa**, SRN,Specialist in Oncology Nursing,Member of the Board of the Oncology Nursing Section,Hospital St.Anargyroi gikagrnurse@yahoo.com

Mrs. Ellen **Riis**, RN Staff Nurse, The Medical Department Aalborg Hopsital P.O. Box 365 9100 Aalborg U27491@aas.nja.dk	Mrs. Vesna **Prijatelj**, RN, B.Sc., M.Sc. Health Care Information System Manager University Medical Centre Information Centre Zaloška 2, 1525 Ljubljana, Slovenia vesna.prijatelj@mf.uni-lj.si
Irena **Skoda**, RN Head Nurse Assistant University Medical Centre Division of Internal Medicine Department of Haematology Zaloska 7, 1525 Ljubljana, Slovenia irena.skoda@kclj.si	Mr. Marc **Vrebos**, RN, MSc Clinical Nurse Specialist Hematology UZ Gasthuisberg Herestraat 49 B-3000 Leuven (Belgium) marc.vrebos@uz.kuleuven.ac.be
Vlasta **Slabe**, RN University Medical Centre Division of Internal Medicine Department of Haematology Zaloska 7, 1525 Ljubljana, Slovenia vlasta.slabe@mf.uni-lj.si	

WISECARE Peer Reviewers

Heine H. Hansen ESMO The Finsen Center, 5072 Blegdamsvej 9 DK-2100 Copenhagen Denmark mbjsekfc@rh.dk
Prof. E. Halloran, PhD, RN School of Nursing University of North Carolina at Chapel Hill CB 7540, Carrington Hall Chapel Hill, NC 27599-7460 USA ehallora@email.unc.edu
Prof. Julita Sansoni, RN, PhD Appointed Professor Dirigenti Assistenza (Nursing Area) Istituto d'Igiene Universita "La Sapienza" Roma ITALY sansoni@axrma.uniroma1.it

Author Index